RECOVERY

FROM

LYME DISEASE

*The Integrative Medicine Guide to
Diagnosing and Treating Tick-Borne Illness*

DANIEL A. KINDERLEHRER, MD

Foreword by Joseph J. Burrascano Jr., MD

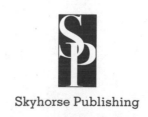

Skyhorse Publishing

Skyhorse Publishing books may be purchased in bulk at special discounts for sales promotion, corporate gifts, fund-raising, or educational purposes. Special editions can also be created to specifications. For details, contact the Special Sales Department, Skyhorse Publishing, 307 West 36th Street, 11th Floor, New York, NY 10018 or info@skyhorsepublishing.com.

Skyhorse® and Skyhorse Publishing® are registered trademarks of Skyhorse Publishing, Inc.®, a Delaware corporation.

Visit our website at www.skyhorsepublishing.com.

10 9 8 7 6 5 4 3 2 1

Library of Congress Cataloging-in-Publication Data

Names: Kinderlehrer, Daniel A., author.
Title: Recovery from lyme disease: the integrative medicine guide to
    diagnosing and treating tick-borne illness / Daniel A. Kinderlehrer, MD;
    foreword by Joseph J. Burrascano Jr., MD.
Description: New York, NY: Skyhorse Publishing, [2021] | Includes
    bibliographical references and index. | Identifiers: LCCN 2020051706 (print) |
LCCN 2020051707 (ebook) | ISBN
    9781510762053 (hardcover) | ISBN 9781510762060 (ebook)
Subjects: LCSH: Lyme disease. | Lyme disease—Alternative treatment. |
    Integrative medicine.
Classification: LCC RC155.5 .K56 2021 (print) | LCC RC155.5 (ebook) | DDC
    616.9/246—dc23
LC record available at https://lccn.loc.gov/2020051706
LC ebook record available at https://lccn.loc.gov/2020051707

Cover design by Daniel Brount
Cover illustrations from Getty images

Hardcover ISBN: 978-1-5107-6205-3
Paperback ISBN: 978-1-5107-7317-2
Ebook ISBN: 978-1-5107-6206-0

Printed in the United States of America

For Jane Kinderlehrer,
who continues to inspire
my life and my work

And for Kay Lyons,
who saved my life—
my deepest gratitude

Contents

SECTION FOUR: WHAT ELSE?

SECTION FIVE: LAST THOUGHTS

Foreword

by Joseph J. Burrascano Jr., MD

D r. Kinderlehrer is not only wise and gifted as a doctor, but he has also experienced Lyme in a most personal way. In addition to having seen thousands of patients with various iterations of tick-borne diseases, he himself had Lyme disease and suffered through the all-too-common path of delayed, inaccurate, and incomplete diagnoses and inadequate and incomplete treatments. When a doctor is also a Lyme patient, he or she immediately becomes better at caring for others with Lyme. The best Lyme doctors are the ones who have experienced it themselves, because there are no medical textbooks or courses in medical school that paint a complete and honest picture of these illnesses or offer useful, accurate advice on treatment. In fact, this is the very problem that has prompted Dr. Kinderlehrer to write this book.

Lyme and the associated tick-borne infections present the doctor and patient alike with one of the most complex group of diseases imaginable. Typically, there are multiple triggers, multiple infections, and multiple imbalances all affecting pretty much the entire body—a real nightmare. All of these issues need to be properly addressed for patients to recover.

Today's world of five-minute office visits does not address complex, multifaceted illnesses. The usual scenario is one problem, one diagnostic test, and one treatment (or no treatment) based on the result of that one test. Unfortunately, far too many Lyme patients go undiagnosed or misdiagnosed, or are offered limited treatments that are doomed to failure. The fact that Lyme is the most prevalent and most rapidly growing vector-borne infectious illness in this and many countries only makes this entire crisis more acute.

In the real world of Lyme, diagnosis is based upon taking a detailed history, review of past records, a careful and thorough physical exam, and not one but a series of direct and indirect tests to look for evidence of infections, and then further tests to help define the scope and extent of the problems. In this book, Dr. Kinderlehrer provides guidelines that will facilitate a deeper understanding of how to evaluate and treat this complex illness. As Dr. Kinderlehrer explains, it is not only important to treat the underlying infections, but also the "terrain."

I recall the early days of Lyme. I began treating patients back in the 1980s, a time when we had basically no idea which diagnostic tests were best, which medications were most effective and at what doses, nor how long to treat. And as we finally developed insight into how to approach patients infected with *Borrelia burgdorferi*, the bacterium that causes Lyme, then a "new" co-infecting germ would be discovered—*Babesia, Bartonella,* new *Rickettsias*—and the process was repeated again and again. At the same time, it became clear that treating the infections was not enough. We had to investigate and remedy the downstream effects of these infections.

A detailed and thoughtful road map is sorely needed. And it is in this context that I am so pleased that we have this book by Dr. Kinderlehrer. I wish I'd had a book like this back in the day to guide me! It covers just about everything—the infections, diagnostic tests, treatments, and yes, the all-important terrain. It gives the reader an in-depth, but easily understandable, guide through the many subtleties of tick-borne illnesses. I am impressed with the knowledge presented and grateful for this information, which has helped so many people recover from chronic illness.

To anyone touched by tick-borne diseases, be they a patient, a caregiver, loved one, or health practitioner, this book is a must-read. It will serve as a continuing reference as it gets read and reread to assimilate all it has to offer. I congratulate Dr. Kinderlehrer and thank him for this most impressive work.

Preface

It is not your responsibility to finish the work of perfecting the world,
but you are not free to desist from it either.
—Rabbi Tarfon, Pirke Avot, Sayings of our Fathers, 2:21

Lyme disease is perhaps the most controversial issue in Western medicine today, but regardless, everyone agrees it is a growing epidemic. Over the past thirteen years the number of reported cases has doubled.[1] In 2017, there were 42,430 new cases of Lyme disease reported to the Centers for Disease Control and Prevention (CDC),[2] and the CDC estimates that Lyme is underreported by a factor of ten to one.[3] However, the more than 400,000 new cases of Lyme disease reported in 2017 is likely far lower than the actual numbers because the criteria the CDC uses for surveillance are extremely narrow.

The CDC states that their criteria for reporting should not be used to make the diagnosis in the doctor's office.[4] When clinical criteria are used instead to make the diagnosis, it is estimated that there are more than 1,000,000 new cases of Lyme disease annually.[5,6] While the Northeast, the Northwest, and the Great Lakes states are particularly notable as places where Lyme is endemic, it has been reported in all fifty states. An editorial in *The New England Journal of Medicine* on August 23, 2018, refers to Lyme and other tick-borne diseases as "a growing threat."[7]

Long-term studies have demonstrated that anywhere from 10 percent to 53 percent of patients diagnosed with acute Lyme disease* develop chronic symptoms, meaning there are literally hundreds of thousands of people every year who become chronically ill after being treated for Lyme disease.[8,9,10] The Infectious Diseases Society of America (IDSA) characterizes these chronically ill people as suffering from post-treatment Lyme disease syndrome (PTLDS). In other words, they are deemed cured from Lyme, and instead are suffering some unknown chronic ailment.

---

* In medical parlance, acute means recent, and chronic refers to long-term.

There are also a large number of individuals suffering from chronic infection with the Lyme disease pathogen, *Borrelia burgdorferi*, a.k.a. *Bb*, who were *never* diagnosed with an acute infection at all. Instead, they are typically misdiagnosed as having chronic fatigue syndrome, fibromyalgia, an autoimmune condition, or a neuropsychiatric disorder, particularly anxiety and depression. Children are often labeled with oppositional defiance disorder, attention deficit disorder, learning disabilities, eating disorders, autism spectrum disorders, or even bipolar disease.

We do not know how many people suffer from chronic infection with the Lyme spirochete.[†] The term "chronic Lyme disease" does not even have an official case definition. The IDSA continues to maintain that there is no evidence that infection with *Bb* persists after a treatment of ten days to three weeks of antibiotics, despite there being a multitude of scientific reports that have documented persistent infection, even after aggressive intravenous antibiotics.[‡] I refer to these people as suffering from *Lyme disease complex*, because there are invariably more issues than simply persistent infection with the Lyme bacteria.

I did not start out specializing in infectious disease. When I finished medical school and residency in Internal Medicine in 1979, I opened a practice called "Nutrition and Preventive Medicine." My mother, Jane Kinderlehrer, deserves a lot of the credit for this decision. She had been food editor of *Prevention Magazine* for twenty-five years, and raised me on wheat germ, dark green lettuce, and no sweets. In the 1950s and '60s, she was considered a health-food nut. (I longed for iceberg lettuce and Wonder Bread.) And later, the values she instilled in me regarding nutrition and prevention were not what I learned as a resident in Internal Medicine. My mother was ahead of her time, and decades later her views are now considered mainstream.

When I started my nutritionally oriented practice, I thought I would see individuals who were interested in treating common maladies like high blood pressure with diet and nutrients instead of relying on drugs. But instead I saw people who had fallen through the cracks. They had consulted with a multitude of physicians but had not experienced relief from their chronic symptoms. Labeled with diagnoses such as migraine headaches, irritable bowel syndrome, chronic fatigue syndrome, and fibromyalgia, they wanted to see someone who thought outside the box—someone who could tell them why they felt ill, and to help them heal rather than treat their symptoms.

Back then, there were only a handful of us practicing Holistic Medicine. Over time our designation changed: Alternative Medicine, Complementary and

---

†   The active form of the Lyme bacterium is a spirochete, a helical microorganism.

‡   Chapter 3 gives a detailed description of research studies that document the persistence of infection after antimicrobial treatment.

Alternative Medicine, and more recently, Integrative Medicine and Functional Medicine. Regardless of the label, we were able to help a lot of patients who had been suffering for a long time, particularly by dealing with food sensitivities, digestive issues, and nutritional supplementation. Unfortunately, there were many patients that were falling through the cracks there as well. When we became aware of Lyme disease, with its propensity to cause so many symptoms, it seemed we had found the answer. And when we began treating this infection, many patients who had been chronically ill improved dramatically.

But there were always outliers—those Lyme patients who continued to suffer—so we kept searching for more answers. We applied principles we had learned from practicing integrative medicine. These people also had chronic issues like hormone imbalances, parasites, and food sensitivities. And we also became aware of co-infections, infections other than Lyme that are also transmitted by the deer tick. We were able to help even more people, but every time we thought we had found a solution to the problem, there were still people who didn't fully recover.

We continued to expand our universe. We became aware of viral activation, detoxification issues, mold toxins, small intestinal bacterial overgrowth, and more recently, mast cell activation disorder. The universe keeps expanding and we continue to find new answers to benefit some of the outliers whom we could not previously help. We are getting better all the time, but I guarantee there will always be unanswered questions and problems we cannot explain. And we will continue to expand our universe.

Those of us who have medical practices devoted to treating people with chronic tick-borne infections, Lyme literate MDs (LLMDs), have long waiting lists of patients. It is imperative that we train more practitioners to fill this need. In that spirit, I created the Lyme Fundamentals course at the International Lyme and Associated Diseases Society (ILADS), which introduces practitioners to the principles of diagnosis and treating these infections. It is offered every year and has been well received. I am also actively engaged in training practitioners in my office. And finally, I am writing this book to help patients seeking more answers, as well as physicians who can benefit from my experience.

While this book cannot contain every piece of clinical and research information on tick-borne infections, it will address the most common issues that impact people with these issues. Currently, over 90 percent of my patients, most of whom have been ill for years or even decades, get 80 to 100 percent better. And as we learn more, our abilities to help more patients will continue to expand.

In the old days of treating Lyme disease complex, most of us treating this illness were individuals who had personal experiences with these infections—either we or a close family member became ill, and the mainstream infectious disease physicians did not have answers. The following section is what happened to me.

Introduction

When you're going through hell, keep going.
—Unknown

Sometimes there is a moment in a person's life that, although seemingly insignificant at the time, heralds a drastic and unalterable change in everything that follows. For me, it was August 15, 1996. The "insignificant event" was, I thought, a virus. I had a fever and chills. The fever was high, 104 degrees, and the chills made my teeth chatter and the bed shake. My body ached so much I felt like a discarded New England Patriots tackling dummy.

But I had no other symptoms commonly associated with the flu, no cough or respiratory congestion, and influenza does not occur in the summer. I didn't have the upset stomach or diarrhea typical of a stomach bug, either. I never saw an insect bite, and I didn't notice a rash. For two days I was so sick I stopped worrying I would die, and started fearing that I would live. On the third day, it was all just a memory.

It seemed quite strange, but since I was able to resume full activity, including several three-mile runs, I didn't think much of it—until one week later, when it hit again. Once more, the fever, chills, and muscle aches lasted two days and then went away. Still pretty strange, I thought, but since I felt well after this relapse I chose to ignore it. Denial works well when you feel okay. But when the symptoms recurred for the third time a week later, the denial stopped working and I began to worry. This time I went to see a physician friend of mine. Upon examination, he palpated an enlarged spleen. He ordered some blood tests, and the laboratory reported a positive antibody test to Lyme. The diagnosis came as a relief. The cause of my problems was a simple bacterial infection. Two weeks of antibiotics would clear it, and then I could resume my normal life.

Was I in for a surprise.

I tolerated the antibiotics without difficulty, and the fever and chills did not return. But instead of feeling better, I felt worse. The next symptom that hit me, and hit me hard, was insomnia. One night I woke up at 4:00 a.m., and couldn't fall back to sleep. The next night I woke up at 3:00 a.m., the next at 2:00 a.m., and then 1:00 a.m., unable to go back to sleep. This went on for weeks. I only slept a few hours a night. I was exhausted. But even worse, I became consumed with anxiety.

I would lie awake through the dark hours of the night riddled with fear. Initially the apprehension focused on my sleeplessness, anticipating the difficulty of getting through the day in my worn-out state. Gradually the anxiety generalized into a constant dread that something terrible was about to happen—impending doom. It wasn't rational. It wasn't something I could control with reason. It was just always there. It felt like a black cloud was enveloping me, cutting me off from any future; it was pure existential terror. It was so intense that some nights, as I lay awake with insomnia, I shook so violently that I added disrupting the San Andreas fault to my list of fears—and I was living in Boston!

Although I'm a physician, I had little experience with Lyme. So I mustered what energy I could—I phoned a Lyme specialist in Boston at the Tufts-New England Medical Center, my alma mater, who was considered a world expert in Lyme disease and asked for advice. He listened courteously to my story as I described my history of symptoms and lab tests, but what he told me came as a shock.

"You don't have Lyme," he concluded.

I was confused. "Well, then, what do I have?"

"Something else," he replied.

"But what about the lab tests?" I asked. "Using the Western blot technique, the assay demonstrated the presence of antibodies highly specific for Lyme. I even repeated the tests one month later, and they confirmed the initial results. Isn't this the CDC criteria for the diagnosis of Lyme?"

"The laboratory must have been wrong," he informed me.

"Why do you think I don't have Lyme?" I responded.

"Because if you had Lyme, you'd be better by now."

I thanked him for his time, hung up the phone, and tried to make sense out of what I had just heard. I considered this doctor's logic: if the cure didn't work, I didn't have the disease. I had had an acute illness with fever, chills, and muscle aches. I had blood tests that confirmed a diagnosis of Lyme. I lived in an area endemic for Lyme. I had seen deer ticks on our dog. I continued to feel terrible, but I didn't have Lyme because I wasn't better. I was getting my first taste of the controversies surrounding Lyme disease.

Next I consulted with a friend and colleague, a physician in upstate New York who treats a lot of people with Lyme. When I told him what the Lyme expert had said he replied, "Welcome to the Lyme wars." He informed me that there are two different Lyme camps: those who maintain that Lyme is hard to get and easy to treat, and those who believe Lyme is easy to get and hard to treat. The so-called

Lyme expert was a strong proponent to the former. Given my personal experience, I now subscribed to the latter.

What is clear now is that while the Lyme expert was categorically wrong when he denied I had Lyme, he was correct that I did indeed have "something else." The something else was a co-infection, specifically *Babesia*. However, this bug was under the radar in 1996. If I were taking my history now, I would immediately suspect this infection.

I have shared my story here because there are millions of people today suffering as I did: people who are losing their cognitive function, are severely depressed, anxious and irritable, in chronic pain, and tired beyond exhaustion; people who are losing their jobs, are disabled, are going bankrupt, and whose families are breaking up; people who are contemplating suicide—and sometimes following through. The toll in medical costs and lost income is huge. The toll in human suffering is beyond calculation.

The bad news I learned on my journey is that there is no single treatment regimen that will cure any chronic illness—no magic pill, no simple injection. Healing from chronic illness requires a multipronged and multidimensional approach. Each person is different, and treatment protocols need to be individualized. It requires assembling the pieces of a puzzle, with each person presenting his or her own clues. There is no single recipe for success.

While Lyme has been the worst thing that has ever happened to me, it has also been the best. This experience has been profoundly humbling. There were times I felt so poorly that the only way I could get through the day was to tell myself that tomorrow I could commit suicide. But Lyme has also blessed me with deep compassion and empathy for others who are suffering. Lyme has stirred in me a passionate commitment to help others who are challenged with this illness. Lyme has filled me with hope that each and every patient coming through my office door will get well. I can't think of anything more rewarding or more gratifying than helping people restore their well-being.

My medical practice is now limited to treating people with tick-borne infections. And despite living in Colorado, where the state Department of Health continues to deny that one can acquire Lyme disease, I have a long waiting list that keeps growing. There is a huge need out there for more Lyme literate practitioners, and I hope this book will help both physicians and patients better address this tremendous demand.

Section One

ANATOMY LESSONS

How do we become ill? Chronic illness cannot be reduced to just one thing going wrong. It is a confluence of interacting issues that devolve into disease. Chapter 1, "Anatomy of an Illness," describes the multiple factors that align and precipitate the disease state.

Likewise, epidemics don't just happen. They are the changing circumstances in the environment and simultaneous alterations in human susceptibility. Chapter 2, "Anatomy of an Epidemic," describes the convergence of issues that have precipitated the epidemic of Lyme disease.

There still remains enormous controversy regarding the persistence of infection with *Borrelia burgdorferi*, a.k.a. *Bb,* after a short course of antibiotics. This present state of affairs is known as the Lyme Wars. Despite the conflict between the Infectious Diseases Society of America and those of us who recognize and treat this infection, there is compelling research documenting persistent infection following treatment. Chapter 3, "Anatomy of the Lyme Wars," provides an overview of the scientific evidence as well as the multiple factors that explain the resistance of this microbe to respond to a short course of antibiotics.

Chapter 1

Anatomy of an Illness

W hy do some people become so ill? A brief history of medicine lays the groundwork of our present understanding of chronic illness.

In 1667, Antoine van Leeuwenhoek, the inventer of the microscope, identified living microbes, but these microscopic organisms were considered harmless. Nearly two hundred years later, the American physician and poet Oliver Wendell Holmes studied the pattern of childbed fever in a Boston hospital and concluded that the disease was spread from one patient to another by physicians. He was angrily denounced and his observations were largely ignored, even when Dr. I. P. Semmelweiss, a Hungarian physician, recorded that the death rate from childbed fever had reached 50 percent when patients were treated by medical students who also participated in autopsies and examined patients. By comparison, less than 3 percent of patients on wards attended by midwives died from childbed fever.[1]

THE GERM THEORY

In 1875, Louis Pasteur proved Semmelweiss right when he isolated bacteria from the blood of women who had died of childbed fever. This was a decade after Semmelweiss entered an insane asylum—driven crazy by his inability to convince his colleagues to wash their hands before examining their patients. Ironically, he himself succumbed to sepsis. Despite ongoing resistance to the concepts of microbiology, surgeons began employing antiseptic techniques with great success. For the first time in history, nascent microbiologists studying the scourges of the late nineteenth century—tuberculosis, malaria, leprosy, cholera, and plague—identified the actual causes of disease.

Or did they?

IT'S NOT JUST THE GERM

An alternate theory holds that the cause of disease is not simply the presence of the germ, but also the susceptibility of the host. Tuberculosis (TB) is a perfect example. The incidence of this illness rose dramatically with the migration of peasants into cities in the sixteenth century. Robert Koch succeeded in isolating the tubercle bacillus, and injected the microbes into guinea pigs that subsequently died of TB. He thereby identified the source of the illness as well as defining and satisfying Koch's postulates, the criteria Koch established to determine a causal relationship between a microbe and a disease.

However, almost all Europeans at the time harbored tubercle bacilli. In many it was walled-off behind a barricade of white cells (granulomas), while in others the bacteria made their way outside these conclaves and into the air sacs of the lungs, resulting in the chronic cough and debilitation then known as consumption. In other words, not everyone exposed to TB gets sick. The condition of the individual appeared to be key.

Despite the apparent breakthrough of a scientific explanation for disease, particularly for epidemics, some physicians maintained that the condition of the host was paramount. Antoine Bechamp, a French physician and medical researcher, was famous for maintaining that germs only became active when a patient's health was compromised.

Louis Pasteur, the father of microbiology, agreed that the condition of the individual, not just the germ, was critical to patient outcome. He brought two caged chickens, both infected with the deadly anthrax bacteria, to a meeting of the French Academy in 1878. He had injected both birds with the anthrax bacteria, but had exposed one bird to cold temperatures while housing the other in a warm pen. The first bird was quite dead, while the other was alive and clucking. Then he uttered his famous pronouncement to the astonished audience, "You see, a microbe is nothing; *le terrain* is everything!"

Le terrain may not be everything, but it is a big deal. It is clear that when a cold virus or influenza infection gets passed around a house or a classroom, some people get sick and others don't. More particularly, after exposure to *Borrelia burgdorferi* (*Bb*), the bacteria implicated in Lyme disease, some people respond quickly to a short course of doxycycline while others become increasingly debilitated. Thus, while the discovery of bacterial triggers for disease is perhaps the foremost scientific advancement in modern medicine, it does not tell the whole story. We need a more comprehensive model, one that includes both "the seed and the soil."

THE ARC OF ILLNESS

Leo Galland, in his excellent book *The Four Pillars of Healing*, describes the anatomy of an illness based on a constellation of factors that include antecedents,

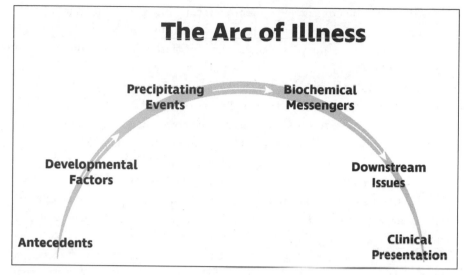

Figure 1–1

developmental factors, precipitating events (also called triggers), and mediators Galland refers to this model as "The Patient Centered Diagnosis." I refer to it as "The Arc of Illness," and it is depicted in Figure 1–1.

Per Galland, antecedents are factors people are born with, such as genetics, epigenetics (modification in the activation of certain genes based on the condition of the parent), and congenital (acquired in the womb) conditions. Antecedent issues are then influenced by developmental factors, such as age, nutritional status, toxin and drug exposure, lifestyle, physical conditioning, traumatic events, and so on. In other words, the developmental issues influencing antecedent factors determine a person's susceptibility to becoming ill.

A history of childhood trauma is a major risk factor for physical illness. Vincent Felitti, Robert Anda, and their colleagues authored a study entitled "Relationship of Childhood Abuse and Household Dysfunction to Many of the Leading Causes of Death in Adults. The Adverse Childhood Experiences (ACE) Study."[2] The inquiry asked 17,000 people to complete a questionnaire asking them to describe their personal histories in various categories of adverse childhood experiences. These included physical and sexual abuse, emotional neglect, parental divorce, and family members who suffered from mental illness, suicide, homicide, alcoholism, or drug problems. The researchers assigned one point for each category of trauma the patients had experienced to get their ACE score.

The authors then compared the ACE scores with the subjects' medical histories. The association of negative childhood experiences with adult outcomes was stunning. There was a linear correlation between the ACE score and the severity of outcome, from addictive behavior to chronic illness. It is not surprising that victims of dysfunctional childhoods suffered more from mental illness; an individual with an ACE score of four or higher is twelve times more likely to attempt suicide. But ACE scores also showed a strong correlation with physical illness: persons with an ACE score of four or higher were twice as likely to have cancer, twice as likely to have heart disease, and four times as likely to suffer from chronic obstructive lung disease. The authors concluded that there is "a strong graded relationship between the breadth of exposure to abuse or household dysfunction during childhood and multiple risk factors for several of the leading causes of death in adults."

The next step on the arc is the precipitating event, commonly referred to as a trigger. This is the factor typically identified as the cause of an illness, whether infection, trauma, toxic exposure, allergic reaction, or stress. The precipitating event acts on a predisposed individual. This in turn results in the release of bio-chemical mediators that generate the signs and symptoms we call an illness. These mediators include hormones (e.g. adrenaline and cortisol), neurotransmitters (e.g. serotonin and norepinenphrine), prostanoids (prostaglandins and leukotrienes that mediate inflammation), cytokines (messenger molecules of the immune system), and so on. Biochemical mediators in turn have downstream impacts, particularly when antecedents and developmental factors are factored in.

Returning to the question of the individual who fails to respond to initial Lyme disease treatment: Rather than infection being eradicated, persistent infection causes cycles of inflammation and contributes to immune incompetence, allergies, and autoimmunity. Nervous system inflammation can cause mood disorders, cog-nitive dysfunction, neuropathy, and dysautonomia. Chronic stress asks the adrenal glands to compensate for the metabolic demands of illness, which over time can lead to lack of adrenal reserve or adrenal insufficiency.

In medical school, physicians are taught to seek the single common denomina-tor that explains a patient's multiple symptoms. While this reductionist approach often works well for diagnosing the vast majority of acute illnesses, it falls short with chronic illness, which typically encompasses multiple issues. Physical injury can have a heightened impact if it is accompanied by the memory of a previous trauma, or if an individual is sleep-deprived due to emotional stress. In similar fashion, an encounter with a specific microbe can lead to varied outcomes depend-ing on whether the individual lives in a moldy house, is exposed to formaldehyde from recently installed carpeting, or suffers from a congenital immune deficiency. Add in antecedents, such as the ubiquitous presence of heavy metals, with their impact on the nervous, immune, and endocrine systems, or the impact of adverse childhood experiences, and one can see how the impact of a microbial infection will vary from one person to the next.

This has been borne out in practice, where patients with severe mold exposure do not become ill with mycotoxin-related illness until they become infected with

Bb; patients who contract Lyme but are asymptomatic until coming down with a viral infection; and patients who are infected with *Bb* and remain asymptomatic until going through a divorce or losing a parent.

WHAT HAPPENS AFTER WE BECOME ILL?

Lyme disease complex is the result of multiple factors acting on many different levels. Healing is not only physical; it is also important to assess each patient's beliefs about illness and their impact on self-worth and self-esteem. And it is essential to determine what support is available to assist patients who are weakened, cognitively impaired, in chronic pain, and depressed. (See Appendix A for a diagram of the anatomy of Lyme Disease Complex.)

The term post-traumatic stress disorder (PTSD) conjures images of veterans of war or survivors of rape and childhood abuse. However, PTSD can also result when a person who is chronically ill, such as with Lyme disease complex, comes face to face with the ignorance and arrogance of the medical profession. Myriad patients with multi-systemic and debilitating symptoms have gone from doctor to doctor seeking answers to their chronic symptoms, only to receive vague labels such as chronic fatigue syndrome or fibromyalgia that don't identify causation. Many are told they are somaticizing, "this is a psychiatric problem," and experience the condescending disdain of physicians who don't have answers but won't admit that to themselves or their patients. Instead of a diagnosis, the patient receives a label. Multiple such encounters often lead to helplessness, hopelessness, and PTSD—which in itself contributes to illness and inhibits recovery.

Consider the common societal feelings and belief systems regarding illness: familial and cultural attitudes absorbed on unconscious levels; individual responses to pain or fear; and issues of self-esteem and productivity that rear their head when a person is not well. Who among us doesn't feel deficient when no longer capable of functioning at full capacity—or functioning at all? Compound this with the anxiety and depression that result from chronic pain, lack of sleep, the inability to engage in active lives, or the fear of going bankrupt due to unpaid bills.

Many of the psychological symptoms result from the neuropsychiatric impact of "bugs in the brain." It is challenging indeed to heal when an infection with *Bb*, *Babesia*, or *Bartonella* results in severe depression, anxiety, panic attacks, irritability, unaccountable rage, and diminished cognitive and executive function. There may not be a lab test for measuring hopelessness, but I know what it feels like, and it does not lead to healing.

Healing begins when patients are given the space to tell their stories, to be heard and believed. Healing occurs when patients are received with compassion, experiences are validated, and questions are answered openly and honestly—including the occasional "I don't know." Healing transpires when patients know they can trust their physicians, when they feel supported and no longer isolated. Healing occurs when patients have reason to hope.

Chapter 2

Anatomy of an Epidemic

L yme disease has only been recognized by medical authorities in the United States for a little more than five decades, but it is far from new; there is evidence that Lyme has been around for a long time. In 1991 the ice-encased corpse of a five-thousand-year-old "Ice Man" was discovered high in the Alps. Scientists established that at the time this forty-year-old man died from head trauma, he was not particularly healthy—he had arthritis, gallstones, vascular disease, parasites, and an arrowhead in his shoulder. He also had foreign DNA in his body that, upon investigation, turned out to be from Lyme bacteria.[1]

THE FIRST REPORTS OF LYME DISEASE

In 1764, the Reverend Dr. John Walker described what is perhaps the first modern account of Lyme disease. He reported seeing patients with limb pains while visiting an island off the coast of Scotland (Jura Island, a.k.a. Deer Island); he also described the tick vector he speculated was responsible for the disease: a "worm . . . with a reddish colour and a compressed shape with a row of feet on each side . . . that penetrates the skin."[2]

In 1909, the Swedish dermatologist Arvid Afzelius described an expanding, ring-like rash on a patient, which he named erythema chronicum migrans (currently referred to simply as erythema migrans). Afzelius speculated the rash had come from the bite of an *Ixodes* tick.*[3] Throughout the 1900s, European physicians reported several cases of tick bites associated with an erythema migrans rash, arthritis, and neurological disorders, particularly meningitis and radiculitis. By the 1950s, European physicians had established that penicillin effectively treated these outbreaks.

---

*   Deer ticks are now technically referred to as blacklegged ticks. There are two main varieties in the United States: *Ixodes scapularis* is predominantly on the East Coast, and *Ixodes pacificus* in the West.

There is evidence that ticks infected with *Bb* have also been present in North America for thousands of years.[4] Researchers examining mice collected in 1894 at the Harvard Museum of Comparative Zoology isolated DNA of the Lyme spirochete in these rodents.[5] There were also likely cases of Lyme in the United States during the past century, reported under different names such as Montauk Knee and Bannworth Syndrome. The first official case of Lyme disease reported in the United States was in 1970, when Rudolph Scrimenti, a dermatologist in Wisconsin, recognized an erythema migrans rash from a description in the European literature, and successfully treated the patient with penicillin.[6]

It took the perseverance of mothers to get the CDC interested in investigating the outbreak of "Juvenile Rheumatoid Arthritis" in youngsters in Lyme, Connecticut. Polly Murphy, author of *The Widening Circle: A Lyme Disease Pioneer Tells Her Story,*[7] was instrumental in getting the CDC to investigate the mysterious ailments plaguing her family and members of her community. The researchers published their findings in 1977 and credited themselves with the discovery of Lyme disease.[8] Since then, Lyme disease has grown from breakouts in a few communities such as Lyme, Connecticut, and Ipswich, Massachusetts, to a fast-growing and full-blown nationwide epidemic. Lyme disease has now been reported in all fifty of the United States, and its numbers are growing.

So, what happened? One answer may lie with changes to our landscape.

FACTORS LEADING TO THE LYME EPIDEMIC

Surprisingly, there are a lot more trees in the United States today than a century ago. The number of trees on the eastern seaboard has doubled in the last seventy years.[9] While in the early 1900s people lived either in cities or on family farms where the land was cleared, over the past century cities expanded into tree-lined suburbs, and small family farms in the Midwest were gobbled up by the mega-farm industries. Factor in the efforts of environmentalists to preserve and maintain forested areas, and the multitude of trees makes sense. Simultaneously, the number of Americans now living in the suburbs has reached 53 percent of the population, where they are in much closer contact with nature and its natural inhabitants than in previous decades.[10]

Here's another surprising fact: in 1930 the population of white-tailed deer in the United States was estimated to be about 300,000. By 2014 this number had grown to 30 million, a hundredfold increase in less than one hundred years.[11] There are many explanations for the explosion of the deer population, but the most credible is the elimination of natural predators like wolves, coyotes, grizzlies, and cougars. As a result, many people who live in the suburbs and small communities regularly see herds of deer wandering down the streets or munching on the vegetables in their gardens. If they have pets that romp outdoors, these animals can essentially collect ticks and bring them home.

Simultaneous to the changes described, people began to have more contact with other tick-carrying wildlife such as rabbits, raccoons, chipmunks, squirrels, opossums, and especially white-footed mice. These once-exclusively rural dwellers became suburban, and often urban, inhabitants. Meanwhile, the tick population began to flourish.

It makes sense that with more host animals available, more ticks will be around to feed on them; but climate change may also account for this uptick. In her book *Lyme: The First Epidemic of Climate Change,*[12] investigative journalist Mary Beth Pfeiffer provides strong evidence that global warming also plays a role. The change in weather patterns now allows tick populations to thrive in places where they previously could not. And how do they get there? Ticks attach to birds as well as mammals, which then carry them to places once considered too cold for them to survive. Indeed, ornithologists such as John Scott, PhD, have linked the pattern of bird migration in the northern hemisphere to that of new endemic regions of Lyme disease.[13]

It appears to be the perfect recipe for an epidemic: a demographic migration to suburbs, closer proximity to the expanding animal world, and a drastic change in ecology that promotes an exploding tick population. But do these recent factors really account for the exponential increase in cases of Lyme? Recall that the *Borrelia burgdorferi* spirochete[†] has been around for millennia, and there have been documented cases of what is now called Lyme disease over the past few centuries. Humans have been living with *Bb* for a long time. Why is it making so many people so ill right now? It may well be that the tipping point in the Lyme epidemic is that *we* have changed.[‡]

THE TIPPING POINT

In 2000, Malcolm Gladwell published his first book, *The Tipping Point: How Little Things Can Make a Big Difference.* Gladwell describes how ideas, products, and behaviors reach a critical mass and become a social epidemic. Gladwell outlines the combination of factors that lead to a tipping point and catapult into a full-blown epidemic. The tipping point is what Gladwell terms "The Stickiness Factor,"[14] the underlying condition that allows the combination of other factors to have an epidemic impact.

So what could be the stickiness factor for Lyme? It might, in fact, have its roots in both diet and environment. Our diets have undergone a radical transformation

---

†   In its active form, *Bb* is a spirochete, which is a helical shaped bacteria. The germ that causes syphilis, *Treponema pallidum*, is also a spirochete.

‡   In her book *Bitten* (New York, NY: Harper Wave, 2019), Kris Newby describes attempts by the US army in conjunction with scientists including Willy Burgdorfer at the Rocky Mountain Laboratories to weaponize and disseminate ticks. The full story is still not known.

from a century ago. The depletion of minerals in the soil, the refinement of grains into white flour, the huge increase in sugar intake, and the addition of preservatives and other additives have all contributed to this transformation. People are increasingly overfed but undernourished, and the effects of this are far reaching. One small example of this change is zinc deficiency.

In 1983, researchers fed pregnant rats a zinc-deficient diet and observed the development of immune suppression, which was expected. Offspring of these rats were fed a normal diet, but the immune deficits persisted. In fact, the next two generations of rats who were fed normal diets replete with zinc were still immuno-suppressed.[15] In other words, a deficiency of one mineral in a single generation negatively impacted the next three generations even when that mineral was replaced in subsequent offspring.

This phenomenon can be explained using a new framework called epigenetics: the study of changes in organisms caused by modification of gene expression rather than changes to the genes themselves. While it takes millennia of natural selection to change the genes themselves, specific proteins can turn genes on and off, and alter gene expression in a single generation. Epigenetics explains how a change in expression of genes can be passed from one generation to the next without actually changing the DNA. The zinc deficiency described above is but one example of epigenetics at work; there are thousands of issues that impact epigenetics and therefore influence subsequent generations.

Nutrient deficiencies can have significant impact. Zinc deficiency has been correlated with attention deficit hyperactivity disorder (ADHD). Deficiency of omega-3 fatty acids has been associated with behavioral disorders in children, and with depression in adults.[16] Maternal undernutrition and maternal obesity during pregnancy have been associated with an increase in cardiovascular disease and other metabolic disturbances in children.[17] *Significantly, nutritional deficiencies can activate epigenetic changes that result in neurological issues from mood and behavioral disorders to cognitive dysfunction,*[18] *and these problems are passed on to subsequent generations.*

Beyond diet is the impact of chemical exposures. Our entire population has been exposed to hundreds of thousands of chemicals that are new to human existence over the past century. Pesticides, insecticides, herbicides, and other chemicals all have the potential to modify epigenetic activity.[19] Countless agents now ubiquitous in daily life, from air pollution to air fresheners and fabric softeners, may negatively impact overall health.[20,21]

But it is not only diet, nutrition, and exposure to toxic chemicals that have changed in the past century. Another factor that has undergone radical transformation is the social milieu. The social sphere, which used to revolve around communities, devolved to extended families, then to nuclear families, then single-parent families, and now tragically, at times, to homeless families.§ People can no longer go next door to be held by Grandma, or move in with aunts and uncles when the going gets rough; in essence, safe shelter has disappeared. This lack of safety is compounded for childhood trauma survivors, who often develop epigenetic abnormalities and thus pass the trauma on to their offspring.[22]

Other social factors also have an enormous impact on health and well-being. Social isolation is a major risk factor for depression.[23] The chronic stresses of poverty, racism, homophobia, and misogyny act on our biochemical pathways impacting immune, hormonal, and neurological function.[24] The long-term release of the "stress hormone" cortisol and of proteins called cytokines (which regulate the body's immune system response) can cause even more damage. These biochemical messengers, in turn, can result in epigenetic changes that are passed on to future generations.[25] In sum, chronic stress plus lack of community support is bad for you, your children, and your grandchildren.

A host of medical problems are increasingly prevalent—autism, obesity, type 2 diabetes mellitus, ADHD, PTSD, autoimmune illnesses, some types of cancer, asthma, food sensitivities, mood and behavioral disorders, heart disease, chronic fatigue syndrome, and fibromyalgia—and have been attributed to the cumulative impact of unhealthy diets, toxin exposure, stressful socioeconomics, trauma, and abuse. Lyme disease is another epidemic that can be added to this list. The evolution of the Lyme epidemic has occurred within a perfect storm: the demographic migration to the suburbs; the surge in deer and tick population; and our increased susceptibility to illness.

HOW CAN WE RESPOND?

At first glance this may feel like a doomsday scenario with no way out, but there is also cause for hope. In the case of the zinc-deficient rats, researchers found that the negative impact on immune competence decreased with successive generations when zinc was replaced in their diets. In a similar vein, there are many things people can do to proactively address this issue, making a difference not only in their own health and well-being but also for their children.

The first step starts with changes in diet, by drastically reducing sugar consumption while increasing intake of fresh fruits and vegetables. Next is addressing our home environments by eliminating air fresheners, scented candles, and fabric softeners. Health improves when people go outside and get some fresh air,

---

§   Many of us don't recall that homelessness was rare and mostly limited to alcoholics and drug addicts until the 1980s, when the Reagan administration stopped subsidizing payments to states for low-income housing and started closing the large mental health hospitals. That is also when there was an acceleration in the transformation of family configurations from extended to nuclear.

exercise regularly, tear themselves away from electronic devices, and get together with friends and family.

But that is not enough. The macro-environment poses as much, and perhaps an even greater threat, to human health and that of subsequent generations. A collective effort is needed to make life on this planet more sustainable for human existence. There have been times when global cooperation has made a huge impact. The last known case of smallpox was in 1977 following a global immunization campaign by the World Health Organization. A decade later, the world came together to sign the Montreal Protocol, a pact that effectively banned all ozone depleting substances, including chlorofluorocarbons.** The Food and Drug Administration and the World Health Organization have both recommended the elimination of trans fats, and New York City took it even further by banning these heart-disease-causing chemicals in 2007. Most recently, 195 nations signed onto the 2015 Paris climate agreement, with the recognition that climate change is a threat to every country and every citizen on this planet.††

When Darwin wrote *On the Origin of Species*, he described two lines of evolution. On an individual level, survival depends on the passing of genes from one generation to the next. This can translate to being incredibly selfish: the best way to ensure individual success is to hoard food or stay at the back of the battlefield. However, Darwin also described group evolution, or survival of the tribe. In this scenario, altruism and the ability of individuals to sublimate their selfish needs enhance the likelihood of clan survival. Think of the brave warriors leading the charge: if the clan survives, so do its members and their progeny.

Now more than ever, all of us need to individually assume responsibility for the fate of mankind and our planet. It is clear that it is not enough for us to sit back passively while politicians make decisions that impact our well-being and that of future generations. It is imperative that our voices be heard, and that we insist on clean air, clean water, clean food, and a habitable planet.

To paraphrase Mahatma Gandhi, we have the capacity to affect the change we want to see. And we would do well to follow the guidance of Rabbi Hillel: "If I am not for myself, who is for me? But if I am only for my own self, what am I? And if not now, when?"‡‡

** Sadly, scientists have recently detected a rise in CFC emissions, and it appears to be coming from China. https://www.cnn.com/2019/05/22/health/china-cfc-pollution-environment-intl-scn/index.html (Accessed June 7, 2019)

†† The impact of the Trump administration's withdrawal from this treaty may not be a catastrophe. Over three hundred cities in the United States as well as thousands of agencies and corporations are working to decrease our addiction to fossil fuels and our carbon footprint.

‡‡ Pirkei Avot, Sayings of Our Fathers 1:14

Chapter 3

Anatomy of the Lyme Wars

The Infection Disease Society of America (IDSA) recognizes that Lyme disease has reached epidemic proportions in the United States. However, they also claim that Lyme disease is easily diagnosed and successfully treated with ten days to three weeks of antibiotics. According to the IDSA, any symptoms that remain after treatment are "something else," and they refer to persisting illness as post-treatment Lyme disease syndrome (PTLDS).

Many practitioners see things differently, particularly those faced with patients who, far from appearing cured, return with mounting problems. These "Lyme literate" doctors (LLMDs) refute the IDSA claim, asserting that a Lyme diagnosis is easily missed, can result in debilitating chronic illness despite short-term antibiotic treatment, is frequently complicated by the presence of co-infections (simultaneous tick-borne infections by multiple pathogenic species), and often requiring long-term treatment. This chapter will explore these divergent claims.

WHAT IS THE EVIDENCE FOR PTLDS?

For decades the IDSA has maintained that any symptoms following treatment of acute Lyme disease were simply the normal fatigue, aches, and pains of daily living. It is now well accepted that at least 10 to 20 percent of patients treated for acute Lyme disease remain seriously symptomatic—particularly fatigue, sleep disturbances, musculoskeletal pains, and depression.[1,2] It is likely that the number of patients who continue to feel ill following antibiotic treatment for acute Lyme disease is much higher.

In 1994, Dr. Nancy Shadick and her colleagues reported on thirty-eight patients in Massachusetts who had been diagnosed with acute Lyme disease. Thirteen of these patients (33 percent) remained significantly symptomatic for an average of 6.4 years after treatment. The most common complaints were joint pains, cognitive dysfunction, and neuropathic symptoms.[3]

Also in 1994, Dr. E. S. Asch and his colleagues reported that 114 out of 215 patients (53 percent) previously diagnosed and treated for acute Lyme disease continued to complain of fatigue, joint pains, and cardiac and/or neurological symptoms after treatment for an average of 3.2 years.[4] Both this study and the Shadick study documented that the longer patients went between the onset of infection and the initiation of treatment, the greater the chance for persistent symptoms.

In 2013, Dr. S. Hook and colleagues reported that 42 percent of Lyme disease patients remained ill six months after treatment, and 12 percent were ill for more than three years.[5] The next year Lorraine Johnson and colleagues published the results of an online survey regarding Lyme disease and the continuation of symptoms.[6] Of 5,357 people who responded, 3,090 met the criteria for chronic Lyme disease as defined by the persistence of symptoms for at least six months after being treated with antibiotics for Lyme disease. The results of this study are summarized in the accompanying tables below. The worst symptoms were fatigue, sleep disorders, pain syndromes, cognitive impairment, and depression, with 75 percent of responders describing their symptoms as severe or very severe. A shocking 72 percent rated their health status as fair or poor—a worse rating than patients with congestive heart failure—and 43 percent had to stop working altogether.

Numerous other studies have documented ongoing or recurrent illness after treatment with antibiotics. These include studies that demonstrated objective neurological abnormalities in patients with PTLDS. Dr. P. Novak and colleagues described small fiber neuropathy with autonomic and sensory dysfunction and abnormal cerebral blood flow.[7] Dr. J. Coughlin and colleagues documented abnormal immune activation in the brains of patients diagnosed with PTLDS.[8]

While it is evident that a significant number of patients treated for acute Lyme disease progress to chronic illness, the cause of the ongoing symptoms is still disputed. In 2017, Dr. A. W. Rebman and colleagues at Johns Hopkins acknowledged that PTLDS is a real phenomenon, but stated that, "the spectrum of symptoms and their impact on quality of life remain largely unexplored . . . [and] the pathophysiology [i.e. the cause] is unknown."[9]

The official guidelines of the IDSA state that "To date there are no convincing published data that repeated or prolonged courses of either oral or IV antimicrobial therapy are effective for such patients. The consensus of the Infectious Diseases Society of America expert-panel members is that there is insufficient evidence to regard 'chronic Lyme disease' as a separate diagnostic entity."[10]

There is clearly a huge disconnect between LLMDs, who ascribe ongoing symptoms to persistent infection, and the IDSA. Although the fact that many patients who acquire Lyme disease progress to chronic and sometimes debilitating illness is now accepted by the medical community, there is widespread disagreement as to whether people who were previously treated for Lyme disease are still infected.

Symptom Severity

75% of chronic Lyme patients experience severe or very severe symptoms. 63% describe two or more symptoms as severe or very severe.

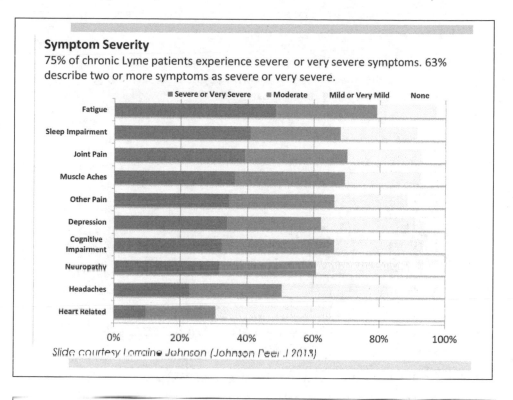

Slide courtesy Lorraine Johnson (Johnson Peer J 2013)

Quality of Life

Chronic Lyme patients suffer worse quality of life compared to most other chronic diseases. 72% report their health status as fair or poor.

- Gen. Pop. — 16%
- Asthma — 31%
- Depression — 32%
- Multiple sclerosis — 37%
- Diabetes — 46%
- Fibromyalgia — 59%
- Congestive heart failure — 62%
- Chronic Lyme disease — 72%

Slide courtesy Lorraine Johnson (Johnson Peer J 2013)

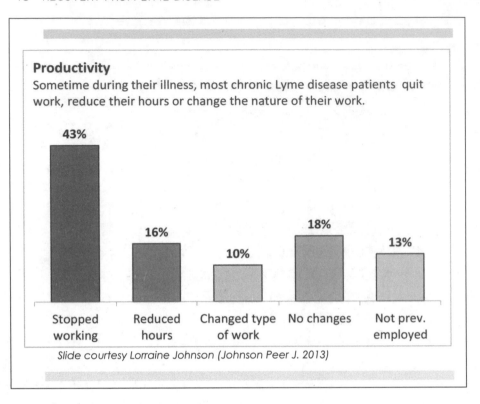

Productivity
Sometime during their illness, most chronic Lyme disease patients quit work, reduce their hours or change the nature of their work.

| 43% | 16% | 10% | 18% | 13% |
| Stopped working | Reduced hours | Changed type of work | No changes | Not prev. employed |

Slide courtesy Lorraine Johnson (Johnson Peer J. 2013)

WHAT IS THE EVIDENCE FOR THE IDSA'S CONCLUSION?

The IDSA bases its conclusion of insufficient evidence for persistent infection on four retreatment trials where an additional course of antibiotics did not demonstrate appreciable improvement of patient symptoms. Two of these trials were performed by the same research team, and are referred to collectively as the Klempner study.[11] The first Klempner trial treated seventy-one patients who were seropositive (i.e. had positive antibodies to *Bb*) and had chronic symptoms after previous treatment for Lyme disease. The second Klempner trial was comprised of fifty-one patients with the same history who were seronegative. Patients in both studies were treated with one gram of IV ceftriaxone daily for one month followed by oral doxycycline 100 mg twice daily for two months. The researchers assessed outcome using the SF-36 questionnaire, a patient-reported survey that measures both mental and physical health, and found no change in clinical symptoms after the two months of treatment.

Dr. Brian Fallon and colleagues conducted a different study consisting of thirty-seven patients who had previously been treated for Lyme disease, were still symptomatic, and had persistent IgG positivity on Western blot (a commonly used lab method for detecting past exposure to a pathogen). Patients were treated with two grams of IV ceftriaxone daily for ten weeks, and reported significant improve-ment in fatigue, pain, cognition, and physical functioning at twelve weeks from the start of the study. However, at twenty-four weeks, fatigue and cognitive issues relapsed, although pain and physical functioning maintained their improvement. [12]

Finally, Dr. L. B. Krupp and colleagues conducted a study of fifty-five patients with ongoing symptoms following treatment for Lyme disease. All were adminis-tered IV ceftriaxone for one month; after four weeks patients reported significant improvement in fatigue but not in cognition.[13]

Do these four studies support the IDSA conclusions? While on the surface this might appear so, the logic doesn't bear up to careful scrutiny. The Klempner studies have so many flaws that some claim they were designed to fail. First, the antibiotic doses and the duration of treatment are considered insufficient by many; LLMDs typically recommend twice those doses and for a longer duration. Furthermore, it turns out that 30 percent of patients had already failed IV antibiotic treatment for at least thirty days (a median of seventy-one days in the seropositive group and fifty-four days in the seronegative group), meaning there was significant selection bias to include subjects who had already failed to respond to retreatment. In addi-tion, statisticians point out that the SF-36 symptom-based questionnaire used to assess outcomes requires a much larger sample size to detect statistically significant differences in results. And finally, while many with Lyme disease are concurrently infected with other tick-borne infections, there was no testing or treatment for co-infections.[14,15]

Then there is the Fallon study. The IDSA cites it as not providing evidence for benefit of retreatment in patients who continue to have symptoms following treat-ment for Lyme disease. However, Fallon documented significant improvement when patients were assessed twelve weeks after completing a retreatment regimen. The IDSA has highlighted the fact that improvement was not fully sustained at twenty-four weeks (when patients had been off treatment for fourteen weeks) and thereby concluded that additional treatment is ineffective. The alternative inter-pretation is that patients would do even better with longer durations of treatment. While this study also did not consider the existence of co-infections, the positive response to treatment provides evidence for persistent infection.

Similar conclusions can be drawn from the Krupp study. Again, the IDSA claims that this study proves that retreatment with antibiotics is ineffective, when in fact the clinical improvement in fatigue after one month of treatment offers solid evidence of persistent infection and the effectiveness of the treatment.

Dr. Allison DeLong and colleagues performed a biostatistical review of these four trials and concluded that ceftriaxone treatment produced clinically meaning-ful improvements in fatigue and cognitive functioning, and that patients with seri-ous baseline pain and poor physical functioning after conventional Lyme disease treatment are likely to experience significant and sustained improvement from more prolonged retreatment.[16]

The bottom line is that the results of these four retreatment trials do not support the IDSA position that "There is no convincing biologic evidence for the existence of symptomatic chronic *B. burgdorferi* infection among patients after receipt of recommended treatment regimens for Lyme disease."[17] But that's it. These four retreatment trials are the sum total basis for the IDSA's claim that there is no evidence that chronic Lyme disease exists.

In fairness to the IDSA, published research findings are often refuted by subsequent evidence. John P. A. Ioannidis authored a paper in 2005 entitled "Why Most Published Research Findings Are False."[18] He states that "There is increasing concern that in modern research, false findings may be the majority or even the vast majority of published research claims."* Simply put, the IDSA bases its understanding on what can be measured with a high probability in a laboratory, and the multifactorial nature of Lyme disease complex does not lend itself to easy evaluation. LLMDs base their understanding on their experience as clinicians. In the scientific world, this experience is considered anecdotal, since it does not conform to a prospective placebo controlled double-blind crossover study with a single variable. But those controlled studies turn out not to be reproducible. The experience of LLMDs treating a seriously ill, complicated cohort of patients flies in the face of the narrow conclusions maintained by the IDSA, which do not hold up to scientific scrutiny. *The fact is, there are no studies that prove that three weeks of antibiotics cures all cases of Lyme disease.*

WHAT DO EXPERTS SAY ABOUT THE QUALITY OF IDSA GUIDELINES?

Dr. A. R. Khan and colleagues reviewed all the guidelines issued or endorsed by the IDSA from March 1994 to June 2009. They determined that "The IDSA guideline recommendations are primarily based on low-quality evidence derived from nonrandomized studies or from expert opinion."[19] Drs. D. H. Lee and O. Vielemeyer analyzed forty-one IDSA guidelines released from January 1994 to May 2010. They concluded that "More than half of the current recommendations of the IDSA are based on level III evidence [expert opinion] only. Until more data from well-designed

---

*   Ionnadis cites Colhoun HM, McKeigue PM, Davey Smith G (2003) "Problems of reporting genetic associations with complex outcomes." *Lancet* 361: 865–872; Ioannidis JP (2003) "Genetic associations: False or true?" *Trends Mol Med* 9: 135–138; and Ioannidis JPA (2005) "Microarrays and molecular research: Noise discovery?" *Lancet* 365: 454–455. The P value has been applied to scientific studies to determine statistical significance. It is now considered obsolete.

controlled clinical trials become available, physicians should remain cautious when using current guidelines as the sole source guiding patient care decisions."[20]

In 2013, Jeanne Lenzer and colleagues published their concerns regarding the integrity of practice guidelines. They stated that "widespread financial conflicts of interest among the authors and sponsors of clinical practice guidelines have turned many guidelines into marketing tools of industry. Financial conflicts are pervasive, under-reported, influential in marketing, and uncurbed over time." They concluded that "Biased guidelines can cause grave harm to patients, while creating a dilemma for doctors who may face professional or legal consequences when they choose not to follow guidelines they distrust. Such guidelines fail to place patients' needs foremost, and instead protect livelihoods and preserve ideologies."[21]

While the IDSA claims that their guidelines are not mandatory protocols, the reality is that they have become the standard of care for medical societies, government agencies, and insurance companies. IDSA member physicians also testify against physicians whose practices do not comply with the IDSA guidelines. In 2006, then attorney general of Connecticut Richard Blumenthal brought an antitrust lawsuit against the IDSA on the basis that the guidelines limited patient access to treatment options. Blumenthal also found significant conflicts of interest among guideline panel members. Under the terms of the lawsuit agreement, the IDSA agreed to review their guidelines. Several physicians with divergent viewpoints applied to be seated on the review panel, but they were rejected. Thus, it was to no one's surprise when the revised guidelines, published in 2006, were no better than the original ones. Notably, they continued to restrict treatment options for patients with Lyme disease.

Johnson and Stricker published an outstanding article detailing the flaws in the development of the IDSA guidelines.[22] Their key issues are summarized in the table on the next page.

As more and more research comes to light, the evidence is mounting that the IDSA Lyme guidelines are flawed both in their development and in their recommendations.

Weakness or Flaw	IDSA Guidelines
Conflict of interest[23]	Key panel members had financial interests related to Lyme disease patents, diagnostic tests, pharmaceutical (vaccines) interests, and insurance consulting fees.[24] Citation by panel members of their own research was high (40 percent).
Overreliance on expert opinion[25]	38 of the 71 recommendations in the guidelines depend on the weakest Level III evidence, namely "expert opinion."[26]
Artificial unanimity of recommendations[27]	The panel excluded competing viewpoints voiced by community physicians and members of its rival, ILADS.[28]
Specialty society self-publication[29]	The guidelines were published in an IDSA journal and were not submitted to normal peer review that would include divergent viewpoints. Letters to the editor critical of the guidelines were not published.
Failure to acknowledge legitimate controversy[30]	The controversy over Lyme disease was well known, but physicians with divergent viewpoints were excluded from participation on the panel and the guidelines failed to mention that other treatment approaches exist.[31]
Limitations on the exercise of clinical judgment and failure to provide treatment options[32]	The guidelines impose severe restrictions on the exercise of clinical judgment and fail to provide treatment options despite a weak evidence base.
Academic researchers setting medical protocols	The IDSA panel consisted almost exclusively of academic researchers.[33]

Table 3–1: Problems with IDSA Lyme Disease Guidelines. Johnson L, Stricker RB (2010)

WHAT IS THE EVIDENCE OF PERSISTENT INFECTION AFTER TREATMENT FOR LYME DISEASE?

In 1996, Dr. M. E. Bayer and colleagues reported on ninety-seven patients presenting with symptoms of Lyme disease complex—all had had documented blacklegged tick bites followed by EM rashes, and most had been treated for extended periods of time with antibiotics. Seventy-two (74.2 percent) had PCR positivity in their urine, meaning the antibiotics failed to eradicate the bacteria.[34] (PCR is a technique designed to detect small amounts of DNA in a laboratory sample.)

In 1999, Dr. J. Oksi and colleagues treated 165 patients with Lyme disease, of which thirty patients continued to be symptomatic. Of the original 165 patients, 136 were retested and fourteen of those were PCR positive for Lyme: "We conclude that the treatment of Lyme borreliosis with appropriate antibiotics for even more than three months may not always eradicate the spirochete."[35]

Both Drs. Fallon and DeLong published lengthy reviews of the four retreatment studies cited by the IDSA and concluded that IV antibiotics in these patients can be effective, which in itself is a priori evidence of persistent infection.[36,37]

There are several smaller examples of antibiotic failure after short-term treatment that provide evidence for persistence of infection. The most compelling are those that directly identify bacteria via culture or PCR detection. M. B. Chancellor and colleagues describe seven patients with neurologic and urologic issues associated with Lyme disease. All were treated with IV ceftriaxone, but four of the seven relapsed and were re-treated with IV ceftriaxone. One patient who continued to have symptoms had *Bb* present in a bladder biopsy.[38] M. J. Middelveen and colleagues studied twelve patients with Lyme disease symptoms who had been treated or were being treated with antibiotics. Cultures of blood, urogenital secretions, or skin demonstrated *Bb* in all twelve patients; the control group all had negative cultures for *Bb*.[39] A. C. Steere and colleagues reported that six out of twelve patients treated for Lyme arthritis continued to have spirochetes in their joints.[40]

There are multiple case reports of people who were treated aggressively for Lyme disease but continued to have evidence of persistent infection. For example, a twenty-four-year-old woman developed an EM rash after camping in Pennsylvania, then developed arthritis years later, and lab tests confirmed Lyme disease. She was treated with recurrent courses of antibiotics: two courses of IV penicillin, three courses of IV ceftriaxone, one course of IM penicillin, and thirteen months of doxycycline, as well as arthroscopic synovectomy. She always felt better during treatment but would relapse when the antibiotics were discontinued, and repeat evaluation of the synovial fluid remained positive for Lyme spirochetes by silver stain and PCR analysis.[41]

Multiple animal studies have demonstrated persistent infection in animals despite aggressive treatment with antibiotics. These include mice, rats, hamsters, guinea pigs, gerbils, dogs, and nonhuman primates, including baboons and rhesus macaques.[42] Monica Embers and colleagues infected rhesus macaque monkeys with *Bb*, and twenty-seven weeks later treated them with antibiotics analogous to the Klempner trial—IV ceftriaxone followed by oral doxycycline. On necropsy, 75 percent demonstrated persistent infection using culture, immunofluorescence, and PCR techniques. In a separate trial of the same study, the researchers infected monkeys and treated them at the early stages with four weeks of oral doxycycline. Persistent infection was demonstrated by xenodiagnosis: uninfected ticks allowed to feed on these monkeys then exhibited *Bb* in their midguts.[43]

In a follow-up study, Embers exposed monkeys to ticks carrying *Bb* and four months later treated them with doxycycline orally for twenty-eight days at a dose proportional to that used in humans. Living *Bb* spirochetes were found in multiple organs after treatment. "It is apparent from these data that *B. burgdorferi* bacteria, which have had time to adapt to their host, have the ability to escape immune recognition, tolerate the antibiotic doxycycline, and invade vital organs such as the brain and the heart."[44]

Emir Hodzic and colleagues injected mice with *Bb* and treated them with ceftriax-one injections for thirty days. At twelve months, all the mice were positive for persistent infection based on xenodiagnosis—positive PCR for *Bb* in ticks that fed off the mice.[45]

This is just a sampling of the hundreds of articles in the medical literature that demonstrate persistent infection with the Lyme spirochete.[†] Dr. Keith Berndtson extensively reviewed the evidence of persistent infection and documented that the Lyme spirochete can "remain infective in humans and animals despite aggressive antibiotic challenge." In this article he also reviewed the mechanisms by which *Borrelia* spirochetes evade immune defenses and survive treatment with antibiotics.[46]

HOW DO THE LYME BACTERIA EVADE THE IMMUNE SYSTEM AND RESIST ANTIBIOTICS?

Microbes have developed a wide range of strategies to adapt to their environment, and employ a number of survival tactics that can lead to persistent infection. *Bb*, as well as other bacteria, fungi, viruses, and protozoa, can hide in biofilms—gelatinous polysaccharide (starchy) matrices that protect organisms from immune defenses and antibiotic therapy.[47] Dr. Eva Sapi and colleagues studied a patient who died after sixteen years of extensive antibiotic treatment for Lyme. On autopsy they found culture positive spirochetes, i.e. live bacteria, demonstrating that "*B. burgdorferi* can persist in the human body, not only in the spirochetal but also in the antibiotic-resistant biofilm form, even after long-term antibiotic treatment."[48]

Bb are pleomorphic, which is a fancy way of stating that they are shape-shifters. A host's immune system may be on an active search-and-destroy mission to target Lyme spirochetes, but under stress these corkscrew-shaped bacteria can morph into cysts, which the immune system is not pursuing.[49] Different antibiotics are necessary to treat *Bb* in their cystic morphology.

Bb has other means of hiding in plain sight. The Lyme disease spirochete can continually change a major surface lipoprotein and thereby evade immune recognition.[50] These outer-surface proteins are what trigger the immune system's radar and direct its attack. It's as if the police have issued an all-points bulletin to nab a thief with a black jacket, but the suspect keeps changing his outerwear. And *Bb* can actually cloak itself in the host organism's own proteins so the immune system doesn't recognize the presence of a foreign invader.[51] Lab researchers using electron

---

microscopy have observed spirochetes entering a cell, then exiting wrapped up in some of the host cell membrane—a stealth bomber.

These microbes have found other strategies in order to hide. Following treatment with antibiotics, *Bb* can be found within parts of the body where they can evade immune detection, often in areas that antibiotics don't access. These include fibroblasts,[52] tendons and ligaments,[53] endothelial cells,[54] joints,[55] and the central nervous system.[56]

Bb can sabotage immune function. The complement pathway is one mechanism by which the immune system targets invaders. Although *Bb* infection will activate the complement pathway, it is also capable of deceiving this immune response to avoid being killed. Some other documented methods of immune subversion include differential gene expression and co-opting a tick salivary protein that protects it from antibody destruction.[57]

Antibiotics employed to kill *Bb* inevitably leave a small population of surviving bacteria. These are referred to as persister cells, variants that neither grow nor die in the presence of antibiotics. These persisters can activate and give rise to chronic infection.[58] Much of the latest research on antimicrobial regimens for treating chronic Lyme is directed at targeting these persister cells.

Finally, and of critical importance, are co-infections. Ticks are a veritable cesspool of microbes, and many ticks carry multiple pathogens.[59,60,61] The presence of multiple infections entirely changes the clinical picture, increasing the severity and duration of illness. LLMDs have found that almost all patients with chronic Lyme disease have one or more co-infections, leading to the more precise label of "Lyme disease complex." This issue will be discussed in greater detail in subsequent chapters.

RETREATMENT STUDIES THAT DOCUMENT POSITIVE OUTCOMES

Dr. Daniel Cameron performed a randomized, double-blind, placebo-controlled trial of eighty-four patients with persistent symptoms following treatment for acute Lyme disease. Fifty-two patients received oral amoxicillin for three months and thirty-four received a placebo. Forty-six percent of the treated patients experienced significant improvements in quality of life as measured by the SF-36 questionnaire as compared with 18 percent of the untreated patients.[62]

In 1997, Dr. Sam Donta reported on 277 patients treated with tetracycline for one to eleven months. According to Donta, 20 percent were cured, 70 percent improved, and 10 percent failed.[63] Dr. P. Wahlberg and colleagues treated one hundred patients with different combinations of oral and IV antibiotics. They concluded that while short courses of antibiotics are generally ineffective, over 80 percent of patients improved with IV ceftriaxone followed by one hundred days of oral antibiotics, either amoxicillin or cefadroxil.[64] Dr. J. Oksi and colleagues reported on thirty patients with disseminated Lyme disease treated with either oral cefixime for one hundred days or IV ceftriaxone for fourteen days followed by oral amoxicillin for one hundred days. Ninety percent experienced excellent to very good responses without a difference between the two treatment protocols.[65]

Meanwhile, researchers at Johns Hopkins are now reconsidering the role of persistent infection in patients with PTLDS. In a study published March 28, 2019, Zhang and colleagues demonstrated persistent infection in mice inoculated with *Bb* that were resistant to single drugs but responded to a three-drug cocktail.[66]

WHAT CAN WE CONCLUDE?

Western medicine adheres to the principle of evidence-based medicine (EBM) as the standard of care. According to Dr. David Sackett, considered the father of EBM, "EBM is the integration of clinical expertise, patient values, and the best research evidence into the decision making process for patient care. Clinical expertise refers to the clinician's cumulated experience, education, and clinical skills. The patient brings to the encounter his or her own personal and unique concerns, expectations, and values. The best evidence is usually found in clinically relevant research that has been conducted using sound methodology."[67]

As the medical community has adopted EBM, Sackett's emphasis on "clinical expertise and patient values" has been lost. The current misapplication of EBM by the IDSA and the medical establishment amounts to a dictatorial system that encourages doctors to practice within established guidelines that may be based on poor research, individual bias, and conflicts of interest, and punishes them for using their clinical judgment in concert with the patient's considerations.

It is clear that further research is needed to delineate optimal diagnostic and treatment modalities. However, the majority of medical trials are predicated on isolating a single variable. This model is not easily applicable to a cohort of chronically ill patients who have multiple confounding factors manifesting in a complex spectrum of illness.‡ Despite the difficulties of accurately assessing

---

‡   Dr. Dale Breseden, who has performed primary research on the pathogenesis of Alzheimer's, developed a multifocal treatment strategy that delineates the multiple sources of inflammation, toxicity, and hormone and nutrient imbalances that result in neuronal death in patients who develop dementia. In his book *The End of Alzheimer's* (New York: Avery, 2017), Breseden describes multiple case studies documenting the efficacy of his multipronged approach. He also describes his inability to secure an IRB (Investigational Review Board) approval to conduct a controlled study because the IRB committees insisted there only be one variable difference between the treated patients and controls who receive placebo. This is the same issue that exists with research on Lyme disease complex, which, not coincidentally, involves similar imbalances that Breseden documents in patients with dementia.

treatment outcomes in these patients, several conclusions can be drawn from the existing data.

A significant percentage of patients who have been treated for Lyme disease continue to have persistent symptoms. Many of these patients have chronic, persistent infections.

- The longer patients go between initial infection and treatment, the more difficult they are to treat.
- *Borrelia burgdorferi* has adapted many strategies for persistence of infection despite treatment with antibiotics. The presence of co-infections seriously complicates the clinical picture.
- While the IDSA maintains that there is no evidence of persistent infection after a short course of antibiotics, there are numerous animal and human studies that document persistent infection even after aggressive antibiotic treatment.
- There is no evidence that three weeks of antibiotics cures all cases of acute or chronic Lyme disease. There is strong evidence that patients with chronic symptoms benefit from long-term treatment with antibiotics

Paraphrasing Sackett, we have developed expertise based on well-designed studies as well as the accumulation of a vast amount of clinical experience in the diagnosis and treatment of patients with Lyme disease complex. Most people get better, even if they have been ill for decades.

Section Two

MEET THE BUGS

The intention of this book is to give a working knowledge of how to diagnose and treat Lyme and its co-conspirators that have made a home in blacklegged ticks (a.k.a. deer ticks) across the United States. The microbes other than *Bb* that populate the deer tick menagerie are termed co-infections. That sounds as if they play a subordinate role in making people sick. But on the contrary, these bugs are often more virulent and cause more suffering than *Bb*. There are tick-borne pathogens that are not included here because their prevalence is much lower than the ones I detail in this book and they are not associated with Lyme disease.

Patients often ask why it is not possible to give a two-week course of antibiotics to clear these infections. Would that it were so. The next chapter details the many complications associated with these microbial invaders. But it is important to realize that once these bugs become chronic homesteaders, they don't cause infection the way we normally envision. Instead of destroying hardware by invading tissue resulting in local inflammation and damage to cells, they confound our software.

Think of the Sorcerer's Apprentice. When the apprentice puts a spell on the broom to clear the workspace, it initially works well. But then the broom goes wild and destroys the premises. Similarly, inflammation is an essential metabolic process in our bodies, fighting infection as well as errant cells that can become cancerous. But if inflammation is unchecked, we have a problem—and that is what happens with these infections. It appears that some people with Lyme disease are genetically predisposed toward what amounts to an autoimmune issue when infected with *Bb*.[1,2]

This variation on the normal infectious process makes treatment much more difficult. The immune system is dysfunctional, and in addition to the hyper-inflammatory response, the normal boundary-containment function of the immune system is not working properly—immune suppression.[3] Think of an army with too many soldiers in the field, but disorganized and attacking randomly . . .

and sometimes shooting at one another. Also, consider the fact that the immune system is not an isolated player in the body, but rather is part of a network that includes endocrine and nervous systems as well as other vital functions, all of which often become dysregulated.

It is important that we see every patient as a whole person. But to understand their illness, we first need to assemble the historical narrative, the physical examination, and the laboratory data. Only then are we able to differentiate the patterns of the different infections as well as the disparate physiological imbalances. Only then can we integrate these overlapping and interacting patterns into the whole patient who sits before us.

Chapter 4

It's Complicated

I am frequently asked how I treat Lyme disease. My answer is that I don't—I treat people, and they are all different. There is no cookbook, even for treating early or acute Lyme disease. Ideally patients should avoid any practitioner who uses a "one size fits all" approach. Treating Lyme patients effectively is complicated. This chapter will explain why.

ISSUES WITH ACUTE LYME DISEASE

Acute Lyme disease would seem to be straightforward. A recent infection should be easily diagnosed and treated. But it often isn't. Here's why.

- Many people, perhaps most, do not observe a tick attachment.
- A rash is often absent, missed, or ignored.
- The early symptoms of acute Lyme disease may be absent or mild, or self-diagnosed as the flu, and therefore ignored by the patient.
- The diagnosis of acute Lyme disease is often missed by medical practitioners.
- The standard treatment recommended for acute Lyme disease is inadequate for eradicating the infection in many people.[1]
- Infection with the Lyme bacteria is frequently accompanied by co-infections that require different antibiotics as well as more aggressive treatment.
- Some patients who present with acute Lyme are, unwittingly, suffering from chronic tick-borne infections that were acquired at some time in the past.
- *Borrelia burgdorferi* can suppress the immune system, resulting in persistent infection.[2,3]

- Although acute Lyme disease is characterised as being localized to the skin, *Borrelia burgdorferi* can spread systemically by the time the rash appears.[4]

The previous chapter highlighted the several ways in which *Bb* has evolved to evade the immune system and resist antibiotics. In addition, not all *Bb* bacteria are the same; there are multiple strains of *Bb,* each with varying degrees of virulence and an affinity for different organs.

CHRONIC INFECTION IS MORE COMPLICATED

Chronic infection is a different ball game altogether. The majority of patients with chronic illness do not just have a long-term infestation with *Bb*. Rather, their Lyme disease complex* often includes other tick-borne infections, referred to as co-infections. Multiple studies have confirmed that ticks are veritable cesspools of microbes, and a single tick may harbor a handful of different bacteria. For example, a collection of 286 ticks in upstate New York revealed that 64 percent had *Bb*, 20 percent had *Anaplasma* and 20 percent had *Babesia*; but 17 percent had *Bb* and *Babesia*, 16 percent had *Bb* and *Anaplasma*, and 5 percent had all three. One of the ticks had four pathogens: *Bb, Babesia, Anaplasma,* and *B.miyamotoi*.[5] In fact, co-infection of ticks is the rule rather than the exception.[6] Dr. Joseph Burrascano refers to these ticks as "nature's dirty needles."†

The presence of combined infections typically causes more severe symptoms than *Bb* by itself. The immune suppression from *Bb* infection is compounded by co-infections, and polymicrobial infections are more difficult to treat.[7,8] Virtually all patients with Lyme disease complex are co-infected,[9] and treatment of persistent infection with *Bb* will be unsuccessful unless therapy is also directed at these co-infections. Many additional complications have been associated with Lyme disease complex:

- Chronic inflammation associated with chronic infection results in many imbalances throughout the body. These will be discussed in detail in subsequent chapters.
- Detoxification pathways get overloaded and fail to metabolize and excrete toxins efficiently. (See Chapter 19.)

---

*   I will be referring to long-term infection with only *Bb* as chronic Lyme disease. But when referring to chronic infection with Lyme and co-infections, I will refer to the complex of issues as Lyme disease complex.
†   Personal communication.

- Adrenal glands, which work hard to compensate for the ongoing stress, lose their reserve and in time become overtaxed, resulting in adrenal insufficiency. This not only induces fatigue, but also contributes to immune dysfunction. (See Chapter 15.)
- Hypothyroidism is common—even people with normal thyroid gland function can present with symptoms of hypothyroidism. They often are converting too much of their T4 hormone to reverse T3, a form that blocks thyroid action at the cellular level, rather than making the usable form of the hormone. (See Chapter 15.)
- Insulin resistance leads to elevated insulin levels, resulting in increased inflammation, fatigue, and immune suppression. (See Chapter 15.)
- The autonomic nervous system, which regulates the body's automatic activities such as breathing, pulse, and body temperature, becomes destabilized. The resulting dysautonomia can cause chaotic manifestations: unstable blood pressure, both racing and slow pulse rates, difficulty breathing, heat and cold intolerance, anxiety, plus a host of other symptoms. (See Chapter 17.)
- Immune imbalances may result in the development of food sensitivities, particularly to gluten. Some people also develop multiple chemical sensitivity syndrome (MCS). People with MCS react to low-dose exposures of chemicals such as perfumes, cleaning agents, and exhaust fumes, many of which are unavoidable in our current environment. (See Chapters 16 and 18.)
- Immune dysregulation often results in autoimmunity, in which the immune system attacks its own cells.[10]
- Suppression of immune function from multiple tick-borne infections can lead to activation of microbes that were previously dormant. Many patients with Lyme disease complex experience reactivation of viral infections such as Epstein-Barr virus (EBV) and human herpesvirus 6 (HHV6).[11] (See Chapter 21.)
- People with chronic tick-borne infections seem particularly susceptible to complications from mold. Mold exposure is normally associated with respiratory symptoms such as congestion, sinus problems, and asthma; but reactions can also be systemic, resulting in migraine headaches, fatigue, joint pains, cognitive dysfunction, and depression. In other words, mold exposure can cause the same symptoms as Lyme disease complex. Complicating issues further, those molds most commonly associated with indoor water damage also excrete poisonous mold toxins. The symptoms of mold toxin exposure overlap with those of chronic

infection, often resulting in severe inflammation and hormonal dysfunction, particularly suppressing the pituitary gland. (See Chapter 19.)

- Histamine reactions, either due to increased release of histamine into the circulation, decreased metabolism of circulating histamine, or heightened sensitivity to histamine, can add to inflammatory symptoms. This condition is referred to as mast cell activation syndrome (MCAS). (See Chapter 18.)

- *Bb* has an affinity for the nervous system, resulting in an array of neurological issues. A common problem is cognitive dysfunction, or brain fog, which, among other things, compromises the patient's capacity to make good therapeutic choices and follow through on treatment regimens. This issue is exacerbated by sleep disorders. (See Chapter 17.)

- *Bb* and its co-infections, particularly *Babesia* and *Bartonella*, often cause neuropsychiatric disorders, particularly anxiety, depression, and irritability.[12] Symptoms can be severe, resulting in panic attacks, suicidal ideation (and successful suicides), and rage episodes. It is important to realize that these problems are not only a secondary response to illness, they can be a direct result of infection causing neuroinflammation and neurotransmitter imbalance. (See Chapter 17.)

People have very different physiologies, and their constitutions differ considerably. Genetic differences can impact detoxification, allergic dispositions, and autoimmune reactivity. There are also differences in each person's immune system, impacting their individual capacity to contain and eliminate infections.

By definition, people with Lyme disease complex have been sick for a long time. Many have been ill for years or decades before they receive a diagnosis, let alone find a practitioner willing to treat them. They often become weak and fragile, losing the rebound capacity of otherwise healthy people. As stated at the outset of this chapter, treating those with Lyme disease complex is complicated.

RISK FACTORS OF CHRONIC ILLNESS

Prior or ongoing exposures to mold and mold toxins, heavy metals, and chemical volatile organic compounds (VOCs) vastly impact a person's capacity to fight infection.

People also have enormously different tolerances to different antimicrobial agents, both herbal and pharmaceutical. Some patients have great difficulty taking any antimicrobials at all because they cannot tolerate the "die-off," also known as a Herxheimer reaction.

A history of emotional trauma can result in immune dysfunction and difficulty fighting infection.[13] Social and emotional support structures have been shown to enhance emotional well-being and boost immune competence. Lack of support adds an extra hurdle to treatment. (See Chapters 1 and 2.)

Physicians are taught in medical school, "When a patient presents with multiple symptoms, search for the common denominator that explains everything." This axiom applies well to acute illness: if a person has been healthy until two weeks ago and then develops fever, muscle aches, abdominal pain, nausea, and diarrhea, all these symptoms can be explained by a single pathogen.

Although Western medicine has done a good job of addressing acute illness, it has not been nearly as successful in addressing chronic disease. The "single-common-denominator" paradigm of illness no longer applies; there are usually multiple confounding issues. It takes detective work to uncover the assorted imbalances and restore people to good health.

Awareness of these tick-borne infections is critical; equally essential is recognition that every patient is unique. The seed is important, but understanding the soil is equally relevant. Lyme disease complex is complicated. It takes a persistent sleuth to help people get better.

TAKE-HOME POINTS

1. Everybody is different, and treatment needs to be individualized.
2. The diagnosis of acute Lyme disease is often missed for multiple reasons.
3. Co-infections and toxic exposures increase the severity and duration of illness.
4. *Bb* and co-infections may suppress immune function.
5. Most people with Lyme disease complex have co-infections.
6. Downstream issues of chronic infection complicate the clinical picture; endocrine, immunological, neurological, and gastrointestinal issues are common.
7. Emotional stress can make recovery more difficult while social support can promote healing.

Chapter 5

Acute Lyme Disease

Michael was fifty-one years old when he was driving back to Denver after visiting his mother in Pennsylvania. He and his girlfriend stopped in Indiana, where they took a walk in the woods. Two days later he removed a tick that had attached under his right shoulder blade, and two days after that he developed a bull's-eye rash. When he saw me a week later his main complaint was fatigue.

THE PRESENTATION OF ACUTE LYME DISEASE

In medical terminology, *acute* means recent onset; it does not refer to the severity of illness. According to standard textbooks, Lyme disease has a well-documented and clear presentation. Here is a rendition of what you will read in the textbooks:

Acute Lyme disease can occur three to thirty days after a tick attachment, but usually occurs within five to seven days. According to experts, the tick needs to be attached thirty-six to forty-eight hours for disease transmission to occur. An erythema migrans (EM), or bull's-eye rash, readily identifies infection with Lyme.

Flu-like symptoms occur three days to three weeks after the rash, but typically after one week. Symptoms include fever, fatigue, headache, muscle aches, joint pains, neck pain, and stiffness. Less often there is respiratory congestion or gastrointestinal upset.

If untreated, acute Lyme disease will progress into early disseminated Lyme, which occurs weeks after the tick bite. It is associated with the spread of the *Borrelia* bacteria in the bloodstream. Early disseminated Lyme disease may result in the following:
• Multiple EM rashes

- Bell's palsy or other cranial neuropathies (problems with nerves that originate in the brain)
- Meningitis
- Radiculopathies (shooting pains from infected spinal nerve roots)
- Carditis (heart inflammation), usually with conduction defects, particularly heart block
- Joint pain and swelling

Disseminated infection can be self-limited or may transition directly into late-stage Lyme disease. However, *Bb* are unaware of the textbook descriptions. In reality, the diagnosis of acute Lyme disease is often missed. This can occur for a variety of reasons:

- Nymphal ticks, which transmit the majority of infections, are quite small (~2 mm) and easily overlooked. In clinical experience only about 15 percent of people recall being bitten prior to becoming ill.
- It does not take thirty-six to forty-eight hours to transmit infection. Ticks "spit into" their hosts as they attach. Their saliva contains anticoagulants (to keep the site open), immune suppressants, and analgesics (which eliminate any sensation of attachment). The saliva can also contain *Bb*—ticks harbor bacteria in their salivary glands as well as in their mid-guts, and therefore have the potential of transmitting infection during the very act of attachment. This is well documented with other tick-borne illnesses; for example, *Rickettsiae* and Powassan virus infections are transmitted within minutes of the tick attachment.[1] And despite what the "textbook experts" say, transmission of *Bb* with less than twenty-four hours of attachment has been documented.[2]
- Only about 50 percent of patients develop a rash at the site of the tick attachment. When an EM rash does occur, the most common presentation is an oval, salmon-colored solid rash; fewer than half look like the signature bull's-eye with a single or multiple rings around a pale center.[3] The EM rash is usually flat, and only occasionally painful or itchy.
- Blood cultures performed on patients with early Lyme disease and EM rashes have grown *Bb*, suggesting that distribution through the bloodstream occurs early in the infective process.[4]
- Flu-like symptoms occur only about one third of the time. Anyone with flu-like symptoms in the warmer months should be particularly suspicious of Lyme; influenza does not occur in the summer. Both the rash and the flu-like symptoms resolve without treatment.

- Antibody testing within two weeks of the onset of infection is usually negative. [5, 6]
- Antibody testing will also be negative if antibiotics are begun within the first two weeks of attachment, as treatment will negate an antibody response. Early treatment will also result in false negative tests at a later date. In other words, early treatment of Lyme is recommended, but lab tests will not demonstrate Lyme antibodies in the future. [7]
- The routine Lyme ELISA screening test has up to 60 percent false negativity. [8]
- Early Lyme symptoms of rash and flu-like illness can be delayed up to a month after exposure. [9] This can make it difficult to associate symptoms with a previous trip to Cape Cod or a walk in the woods.
- People who don't live in an area where Lyme is common are not as aware of the symptoms as those who live in endemic regions such as Connecticut. Neither are their physicians.
- Ticks slow down in the winter but are not totally dormant, and are not killed by freezing temperatures. [10] People living in New England have observed active movement of ticks in sub-zero weather.
- Late-stage or chronic Lyme disease can occur long after a tick bite even in those who never experienced the symptoms and signs of acute Lyme disease. Many people develop late-stage or chronic Lyme weeks, months, or years after a tick bite of which they were unaware. [11]

TREATMENT OF ACUTE LYME DISEASE

The most widely recommended antibiotic to treat acute Lyme disease is doxycycline, which has the advantage of also treating some co-infections: *Ehrlichia*, *Anaplasma*, and *Rickettsiae*. Doxycycline also has activity against *Babesia*, *Bartonella*, and *Mycoplasma*, although it is not as effective against these common co-infections.

There are also disadvantages to doxycycline. It often causes severe indigestion or nausea, even when taken with food. Most people develop sun sensitization and therefore burn easily; it is not uncommon to see second-degree burns in patients who are lax about covering up and using sunscreen. Doxycycline needs to be taken separately from dairy products and mineral supplements, since these will inhibit its absorption. Patients also need to avoid lying down for thirty minutes after taking doxycycline; if the pill is still in the esophagus, it can erode the lining and cause an ulcer resulting in severe chest pain.

Doxycycline taken at the recommended dose of 100 mg twice daily is a static drug. This means that it will inhibit the bacteria from replicating but it will not kill them. Bacteriostatic antibiotics depend on an intact immune system to completely eradicate an infection. Higher doses of doxycycline are required for it to have cidal, or killing, activity. Most LLMDs recommend 200 mg twice daily, which, unfortunately, increases the likelihood of indigestion issues.

There are other good choices to treat acute Lyme disease. In general these cause less gastrointestinal distress than doxycycline, but they will not treat co-infections. Antibiotic options include the macrolide class—azithromycin and clarithromycin; beta lactams—amoxicillin and amoxicillin-clavulanate; and cephalosporins— cefuroxime and cefdinir. Please see Table 5–1 below.

COMMON ANTIBIOTICS IN THE TREATMENT OF ACUTE LYME DISEASE			
Generic Name	Brand Name	Adult Dose	Children's Dose
Azithromycin	Zithromax	500 mg 1x/day	10 mg/kg 1x/day
Clarithromycin	Biaxin	500 ng 2xday	7.5 mg/kg 2x/day
Amoxicillin	Amoxil	1500 mg 2x/day	25 mg/kg 2x/day
Amoxicillin Clavulanate	Augmentin	875/125 mg 2x/day	25 mg/kg 2x/day
Cefuroxime	Ceftin	500 mg 2x/day	15 mg/kg 2x/day
Cefdinir	Omnicef	300 mg 2x/day	14 mg/kg 2xday
Doxycycline	Doryx, Vibramycin	200 mg 2x/day	>8 years old 2.2 mg/kg 2x/day
Minocycline	Minocin	100 mg 2x/day	>8 years old 2.0 mg/kg 2x/day

Table 5–1. Common antibiotics in the treatment of acute Lyme disease. These doses are general recommendations only; they need to be adjusted for each individual circumstance, and higher doses are often prescribed.

Simultaneous treatment with an anti-yeast agent, such as Nystatin, as well as a probiotic to maintain healthy gut flora, should always accompany antibiotic use.

The IDSA recommends treating acute Lyme disease with ten days to three weeks of antibiotics. The failure of this treatment course for a significant percentage of patients is well documented.[12] It is also fairly easily explained: antibiotics are most effective during cell replication, yet *Bb* has one of the the longest replication cycles of any known bacteria, up to four weeks. Therefore, six weeks of oral antibiotics is generally effective for an uncomplicated infection.

When the infection reaches the early disseminated phase, IV antibiotics should be considered instead of oral antibiotics, particularly in the following situations:

- Acute carditis with atrio-ventricular heart block
- Acute meningitis
- Acute synovitis with high white blood cell count (WBC) in the joint fluid

Tzohar is my granddaughter. She moved to Israel with her parents when she was two years old. Just before leaving she had been playing in the backyards of her great-grandparents, in both New Jersey and Long Island. Four weeks after arriving in Israel she complained of right knee pain. She refused to walk and had to be carried. She had a fever and her knee was swollen.

Her parents took her to Hadassah Hospital, where doctors took fluid out of her knee joint. The joint fluid had a high white blood cell (WBC) count of 50,000, indicating infection. However, cultures were negative—there was no clear indication of which microbe was causing the infection. The doctors had started Tzohar on IV antibiotics to treat a staph infection, the most common cause of septic arthritis, but she was not responding.

Tzohar did not have a good reason to have a staph infection in her knee, and the culture failed to detect staph. However, the timing was perfect for Tzohar to have had an unseen tick attachment before takeoff, and go on to develop Lyme arthritis when the infection disseminated. I advised the doctors at Hadassah Hospital to administer appropriate treatment with IV ceftriaxone, and Tzohar had a complete recovery.

TESTING OF TICKS

Testing of the tick is advised if a tick is available. However, in my experience, this testing has poor sensitivity. There are many examples of a tick analysis failing to detect a tick-borne pathogen when it clearly transmitted an infection. I have witnessed a handful of examples of tick analysis failing to pick up co-infections that were documented in the patients. It is also possible there were additional tick attachments that were not detected or infection from a previous tick bite.

ALWAYS SUSPECT CO-INFECTIONS

Since testing the tick can be inaccurate, often the best option is to test the person. It is always important to test for the presence of co-infections even if the diagnosis of Lyme is self-evident by the combination of tick attachment and EM rash. Sources such as the Centers for Disease Control and Prevention (CDC) state that the distribution of co-infections in the United States is maintained within clearly defined geographic boundaries. This, unfortunately, is not the case; they have a wide distribution, and are always suspect when there is evidence of Lyme. Many of the symptoms experienced by people diagnosed with chronic Lyme disease can be attributed to co-infections as well as *Bb*. For this reason, all patients diagnosed with acute Lyme disease should have the following tests:

- Complete blood count (CBC). Low WBC and platelet counts suggest a co-infection with *Ehrlichia*, *Anaplasma*, or *Rickettsiae*. Evidence of hemolytic anemia (destruction of red blood cells) suggests babesiosis.
- Urinalysis. *Babesia* can cause hemolytic anemia, which in turn can lead to the presence of free hemoglobin in the urine. This will result in a urine dipstick that tests positive for hematuria but negative for red blood cells. This is an uncommon finding, but when present it strongly suggests babesiosis.
- Co-infection titers measure antibodies to co-infections. These should be drawn at least two weeks after the tick attachment. Unfortunately, some of these tests have a low sensitivity, and the provider should always search for diagnostic clues in the history, physical exam, and other labs. Co-infection testing is discussed in subsequent chapters.

WHAT HAPPENS WHEN LYME IS SUSPECT BUT NOT CLEAR?

Abby was seven years old when she returned to Denver from visiting her grandparents in New Hampshire. Her grandmother did daily tick checks and never saw a bite. Four days after returning to Colorado, Abby's mom noticed that her daughter's cheeks were flushed and the left side of her neck had a one-inch oval red rash. Two small red circular rashes appeared on Abby's right forearm within the next week, each perhaps a half inch in diameter. None of the rashes had a pale center, but the one on her neck persisted for three weeks—it initially had small vesicles, then became scaly. There were no other complaints.

On examination, Abby's cheeks still appeared flushed. The left anterior cervical lymph nodes (on her neck under her jaw) were slightly enlarged, and the skin on her legs was mottled.

I informed Abby's mom that she might have Fifth's Disease (sometimes called Slapped Face Syndrome), which is caused by a parvovirus; this often results in flushed cheeks. But given her exposure in New Hampshire, I also considered Lyme. In addition, I was also suspicious of an infection with Bartonella due to the small vesicles and scaly appearance of the rash, as well as the palpable lymph nodes and mottled skin. It was unclear if Abby had tick-borne infections, but I decided to start her on antibiotics, cefdinir for Lyme and sulfmethoxazole-trimethoprim (Bactrim) for Bartonella, while lab results were pending. When the tests came back Abby tested positive not only for Lyme, but also strongly positive for Mycoplasma *and* Babesia. *Flushing is not uncommon with* Babesia *infection.*

Abby's story demonstrates how suspicious providers need to be when making a Lyme diagnosis, how important a thorough history is to the clinical picture, and how easy it is to miss co-infections. Abby's symtoms weren't suggestive of Lyme, yet she turned out to probably have four tick-borne infections with high potential for causing future problems. Abby's pediatrician had refused to even test her for Lyme.

> *Lisa was forty-two years old when she had the sudden onset of severe nausea and vomiting lasting twenty-four hours. There was no abdominal pain or diarrhea, and no one else at home was ill. She was otherwise fine until three days later, when she noticed a two-inch oval rash inside her right elbow. I suggested she get a CBC and, after waiting an additional week, be tested for Lyme. Her CBC was normal but the Lyme Western blot was strongly positive.*
>
> *However, Lyme doesn't present with nausea and vomiting, nor would systemic symptoms from Lyme precede the rash, so I started Lisa on treatment for bartonellosis, the most likely co-infection to cause gastrointestinal symptoms, as well as for Lyme. When the co-infection profile returned, it turned out she also had babesiosis.*

An important take-home lesson is that symptoms preceding an EM rash are most likely caused by a co-infection. It is interesting that Lisa also had *Babesia*, even though she did not experience the classic symptoms of this infection—headache, night sweats, and shortness of breath or air hunger, a sensation of not getting enough oxygen that usually occurs at rest.

DURATION OF TREATMENT

The recommended six weeks of antibiotic treatment for uncomplicated Lyme disease is inadequate when one or more co-infections are present. The length of treatment should then be guided by patient response. If a patient with Lyme and co-infections promptly becomes asymptomatic, treatment is generally extended to two to three months, usually with the addition of herbal extracts to complement treatment. With patients such as Abby, endpoints are particularly hard to determine; she had three confirmed infections (*Bb, Babesia, Mycoplasma*) and symptoms were suspicious for a fourth (*Bartonella*). In fact, there is a wide divergence between the published IDSA treatment guidelines for Lyme and actual practice. In one survey, the median length of treatment for an EM rash was four weeks.[13]

Follow-up is essential to determine that the patient has fully recovered. Follow-up testing in uncomplicated, asymptomatic patients is not generally necessary. However, a provider should consider the possibility of a missed co-infection as well as extending or changing treatment if the patient continues to be symptomatic. Follow-up testing in these patients may show persistent IgM in the Lyme Western blot rather than seroconversion to IgG, which suggests persistent infection. See Chapter 7 on testing for Lyme disease.

HERBAL ANTIMICROBIALS

Several reports have demonstrated the effectiveness of herbal antimicrobials, although these are based on in vitro laboratory studies, which do not always translate to in vivo effectiveness.[14,15,16] Researchers at Johns Hopkins have reported that several essential oils also have activity against *Bb*.[17] Clinically, many LLMDs have observed consistent benefits from nonprescription herbal antimicrobials, at times used alone but usually to complement pharmaceutical antibiotics. Some of the most commonly available herbal products used as antimicrobial regimens for Lyme disease are listed below. Succeeding chapters will discuss treatment of co-infections in more detail, and include information on both herbal and prescription antibiotics.

- Nutramedix: Samento and Banderol treats Lyme in both spirochetal and cyst form, and is also effective against biofilms;[18] Banderol is also active against *Bartonella*
- Researched Nutritionals: BLt is active against *Bb* and *Bartonella*
- Byron White: A-L Complex
- Beyond Balance: MC BB-1

It is important to note that there are several other companies that offer herbal antimicrobials. The ones listed above have a long track record of use by integrative LLMDs, who have had extensive positive clinical experience with these extracts.

LYME MYTHOLOGY

It is worthwhile pointing out several fallacies that have prevented people from getting properly diagnosed:

- If you don't recall a tick bite, it is unlikely you have Lyme disease.
- The tick has to be embedded thirty-six to forty-eight hours to transmit infection.

- If you don't have a bull's-eye rash, you don't have Lyme disease.
- If you don't have arthritis, you don't have Lyme disease.
- If you have a negative Lyme test, you don't have Lyme disease.
- If you live in _____ (fill in a state other than those in the Northeast, Great Lakes region, or Northwest), you don't have Lyme.
- Ticks are dormant in the winter.
- Antibiotics taken for ten days to three weeks cures Lyme disease. If you are still sick after that, it is something else.

SOME PATIENTS WITH ACUTE LYME DISEASE ALSO HAVE CHRONIC TICK-BORNE INFECTIONS

Michael, whose case was described at the beginning of this chapter, clearly had acute Lyme disease. But a complete history revealed that he had suffered from anxiety and depression since a young age. Additional long-term symptoms included poor memory, light and sound sensitivity, and allodynia—simple touch to his skin felt like fire. Michael had lived in Pennsylvania, Maine, and Massachusetts, as well as Colorado. He was an avid camper and hiker.

Michael's case will appear again in subsequent chapters; in addition to acute Lyme, he also had chronic infections with *Bb* and *Bartonella*. It illustrates how people who present with acute Lyme disease can also have previously acquired yet undiagnosed chronic tick-borne infections. Many people with chronic mood problems, joint pains, fatigue, sleep disturbance, and other problems blame their symptoms on lifestyle, aging, or "something else." It takes a physician willing to put the pieces of the puzzle together to recognize that these can be the result of long-standing untreated tick-borne infections.

There are presently no tests available to prove eradication of any of these microbes from the body. However, clinical experience shows that the sooner treatment commences, the better the outcome. Therefore, Lisa and Abby will do quite well, but Michael will likely require long-term treatment; he not only has acute Lyme disease, but he also has suffered for decades with Lyme disease complex: chronic infection with *Bb* and *Bartonella*.

It cannot be emphasized enough: treating people with tick-borne infections requires delving below the surface. And this is just the beginning of the story.

TAKE-HOME POINTS

1. Most patients with acute Lyme disease do not notice a tick attachment, and only a minority have a bull's-eye rash.
2. Treatment for acute Lyme disease with antibiotics for ten to thirty days may not eradicate *Bb*. Six weeks of antibiotics is recommended for an uncomplicated acute infection.
3. All patients with acute Lyme disease need to be screened for co-infections.
4. There is most likely a co-infection if systemic symptoms precede a rash.
5. Longer antibiotic courses are necessary to treat Lyme disease complicated by co-infections.

Chapter 6

Presentation of Chronic Lyme Disease

C hronic Lyme disease patients can be classified in two categories—those who know they previously contracted Lyme disease and those who don't. Patients in the first group who received prior antibiotic treatment are presently labeled as having post-treatment Lyme disease syndrome (PTLDS), implying that there is no evidence of ongoing infection despite their ongoing symptoms. The second group has no knowledge of prior tick-borne infection; people in this group either never experienced or didn't take note of the signs of early Lyme disease, yet they developed late-stage or Lyme disease complex weeks, months, or even years after the unnoticed tick attachment. This latter group of patients is not in the medical literature, because at this point of time there is no official case definition of chronic Lyme disease. However, LLMDs estimate that there are millions of people who fall into this category.

Ned was well into his mid-thirties when he developed increasing attention and memory issues, fatigue, a random cough, and chest pain. He would wake at night with anxiety and panic attacks, sweating and gasping for air. His symptoms multiplied over the next decade, and grew to include headaches, paresthesias (pins and needles sensations), and blurry vision.

Ned consulted physicians at the Mayo Clinic, where he went through myriad tests and was given the diagnosis of generalized anxiety disorder (GAD); this did not feel satisfactory nor correct to him. Ned continued to seek out answers; subsequent doctors diagnosed him with chronic fatigue syndrome (CFS).

Ned was forty-six years old when I first met him on a camping trip. He shared that he had quit his job because of his CFS, and when I heard more of his history I suggested he be tested for Lyme disease. I met Ned again two years later at a social gathering and he said he hadn't gotten tested because he didn't want to get his hopes up. However, after he revealed more of his symptoms, I told him that the likelihood of Lyme was quite high; and he agreed to testing.

Ned's story is distressingly familiar. Not nearly as commonplace is that Ned was eventually properly diagnosed and treated, leading to a full recovery. It is incredibly sad that there are millions of people who are diagnosed with CFS, fibromyalgia, anxiety, depression, and autoimmune disorders—all of which are increasingly prevalent—who never get diagnosed and treated for the real cause of their symptoms: tick-borne infections.

COMMON SYMPTOMS OF CHRONIC LYME DISEASE

By far the most prominent symptoms of chronic Lyme disease are musculoskeletal and neurological complaints. However, tick-borne infections can affect every system in the body, and the list of possible symptoms is quite long. Not all of these are easily identified as related to a tick bite, but when the downstream effects of chronic infection such as endocrine disruption, immune imbalance, and nervous system dysregulation are factored in, there's a lot that can go wrong.

Think of it like driving a car when a tire goes flat. If you keep driving, eventually the rim will get bent, then the tie-rods will bend, and perhaps an axle will break. Replacing the tire will no longer fix the problem. People who have been ill for years, or even decades, are out of balance on many fronts. Just replacing the tire won't fix the problem.

Symptoms often wax and wane with good days and bad days. Sometimes there is a clear-cut cycle with symptom flares every month or so; both Lyme and *Babesia* are famous for these cycles. In premenopausal women, these flares usually coincide with menstruation. Here are the most common complaints:

- **Fatigue**—often associated with weakness. Patients should note if the fatigue is above the neck or below the neck: the former is sleepy fatigue— the need to close one's eyes and take naps; the latter is body lethargy— being too tired to walk down the stairs and do the laundry. Lyme can cause both, but when folks are sleepy, also be on the lookout for issues like sleep apnea, food sensitivities, and insulin resistance. Fatigue is rarely the only presenting symptom. Post-exertional malaise (an increase in fatigue after activity) is common. Adrenal and thyroid function should always be evaluated when fatigue is a presenting symptom.

- **Joint pains** (arthralgias)—usually without swelling, most commonly affecting the large joints like knees, hips, and shoulders, but often smaller joints as well. This type of joint pain tends to migrate—one day the knee is sore, the next day the elbow. If swelling occurs it is officially "Lyme arthritis," but this only occurs in about 10 percent of patients. This is different from rheumatoid arthritis (RA), which usually attacks small joints first, is consistent day to day, and is accompanied by severe morning stiffness. Stiff joints may also occur with Lyme, but usually not to the same degree as with RA.

- **Muscle aches** (myalgias)—common in the neck, arms, legs, and sometimes the back, often accompanied by stiffness and usually worse after exertion. Patients with this complaint are often diagnosed with fibromyalgia.

- **Sleep issues**—difficulty falling asleep, waking frequently, waking unrefreshed, or hypersomnia (sleeping excessively). It is imperative to treat sleep problems aggressively because if a person does not get a good night's sleep, not only does it contribute to fatigue, it will also impact immune and endocrine function and interfere with the ability to fight infection.

- **Cognitive dysfunction**—often referred to as "brain fog," including attention and focus issues, short-term memory problems, confusion, and difficulties with executive function (the ability to organize and execute tasks). When severe, it results in outright confusion and disorientation. This can result in major disability. Simple math problems become enormously difficult. Patients have been known to get lost in their own neighborhoods.

- **Mood disorders**—anxiety, often with panic attacks; depression, potential suicidality; and irritability that can manifest with episodes of rage. Many Lyme disease complex patients, like Ned, end up with psychiatric diagnoses. These infections can even result in bipolar disorder and other psychoses. Children often present with oppositional defiance disorder (ODD) and uncontrollable tantrums.

Tables 6–1 to 6–6 list the various manifestations of the above issues. But these are not the only symptoms that can occur; Lyme can attack other parts of the body, as described later in this chapter.

MUSCULOSKELETAL MANIFESTATIONS OF LYME DISEASE		
Muscle pains, stiffness	Muscle twitching	Degenerative spine disease
Joint pains, stiffness	Muscle spasms	Myositis (muscle tissue inflammation)
Neck pain, stiffness	Temporomandibular joint dysfunction (TMJ)	Bursitis
Back pain, stiffness	Bone pain	Enthesitis
Arthritis (joint swelling, pain and redness)	Carpal tunnel syndrome	Degenerative spine disease
Chest pain	Herniated disc	Bursitis
Chronic tendonitis	Muscle twitching	

Table 6–1. Musculoskeletal Manifestations of Lyme Disease

NEUROLOGICAL CONDITIONS ASSOCIATED WITH LYME DISEASE		
Condition	Symptoms	Illnesses, conditions, and medications that cause similar symptoms
Cranial nerve palsies	(See Table 6–4)	Viral infections ALS (Lou Gehrig's disease) Multiple sclerosis Brain tumors
Radiculoneuropathy	Shooting pains Weakness Numbness Tingling	Herniated disc Shingles Sciatica Various spinal disorders
Neuropathy	Numbness Tingling Loss of sensation Pain, burning Increased sensitivity to touch Clumsiness/ coordination difficulties Weakness Creepy, crawling sensations Vibration sensation	Diabetic neuropathy Alcoholic neuropathy Guillain-Barré syndrome Shingles Epstein-Barr virus Cytomegalovirus Various spinal disorders

(Table continued on next page)

Condition	Symptoms	Illnesses, conditions, and medications that cause similar symptoms
Meningitis	Headache Neck pain, stiffness Nausea, vomiting Memory & concentration impairment Confusion	Bacterial meningitis Viral meningitis Fungal meningitis
Headaches	Pain	Migraines Tension headaches Brain tumors Allergies
Transverse myelitis	Weakness Balance difficulties Difficulty walking Loss of sensation Loss of bladder/bowel control Clumsiness/coordination difficulties	Viral infections Multiple sclerosis Spinal cord injury/tumor
Dysautonomia	Erratic or rapid heart rate Fluctuating blood pressure Light-headedness Passing out Headache Sexual dysfunction Bowel abnormalities Bladder abnormalities Light sensitivity Heat/cold intolerance	Viral infections Chronic fatigue syndrome Adrenal insufficiency Anxiety Allergies Multiple sclerosis Shy-Drager syndrome
Encephalopathy	Memory and concentration impairment/dementia (see Table 6–3) Psychiatric disease (see Table 6–5) Fatigue/malaise Stupor/coma Learning disabilities ADD/ADHD	Chronic fatigue syndrome Heavy metal toxicity Alzheimer's disease Liver failure Kidney failure Drug toxicity Substance abuse Chemical toxicity Mold toxins Allergies Lupus Depression Mental illness Syphilis

Condition	Symptoms	Illnesses, conditions, and medications that cause similar symptoms
		Other infections Multiple sclerosis Hypothyroidism Menopause
Encephalomyelitis	Visual difficulties Weakness Paralysis Sensory abnormalities Talking difficulties Personality changes Psychosis Memory and concentration impairment/confusion Visual and hearing loss Learning disabilities ADD/ADHD	Multiple sclerosis Viral infections Stroke Spinal cord injury Mental illness Spinal cord injury/tumor Mental illness Other infections Vasculitis (e.g. lupus)
Eye disorders	Impaired vision Blindness Floaters Difficulty focusing Dry eyes Flashing lights Loss of depth perception Light sensitivity Irritation/itching/redness Discharge Double vision Tunnel vision Swelling around eyes Pressure in or behind eyes Color vision abnormality Droopy eyelids	Multiple sclerosis Stroke Migraine headache Brain tumor Autoimmune illnesses Diabetes Bacterial conjunctivitis Myasthenia gravis Graves' disease
Movement disorders	Tremor Chorea (Involuntary movements) Catatonia Myoclonic jerks Tourette's disease (tics) Torticollis (neck spasm)	Parkinson's disease Rheumatic fever Huntington's chorea Mental illness Liver, kidney, or lung disorders Allergies Drug toxicity

(Table continued on next page)

Condition	Symptoms	Illnesses, conditions, and medications that cause similar symptoms
Motor neuron disease	Weakness Difficulty walking Difficulty talking Difficulty swallowing Muscle cramps Fine trembling Motor neuropathy with block	ALS (Lou Gehrig's disease) Heavy metal toxicity
Seizure disorders	Grand mal seizures Partial-complex seizure disorder Focal motor seizures	Epilepsy Other brain infections Brain tumors Hypoglycemia
Benign intracranial hypertension	Headache Impaired vision/blindness Memory and concentration impairment Balance difficulties Depression Nausea/vomiting Sleep disorder	Brain tumor Vitamin A toxicity Oral contraceptives Medications-tetracyclines Steroid withdrawal
Stroke	Weakness Paralysis Sensory abnormalities Balance difficulties See symptom list for Encephalomyelitis	Cerebrovascular disease Vasculitis (e.g. lupus) Aneurysm Oral contraceptives Synthetic hormone replacement

Table 6–2. Neurological Conditions Associated with Lyme disease and their Differential Diagnosis. Note that co-infections, particularly Babesia and Bartonella, can also be responsible for these neurological conditions.

COGNITIVE DYSFUNCTION ASSOCIATED WITH LYME DISEASE	
Concentration and focus issues—new onset ADD	Visual-spatial difficulties—e.g. trouble finding things, directional impairment—getting lost in familiar places
Short-term and working memory difficulties	Auditory processing disorders
Comprehension issues	Visual processing disorders
Word finding, word generation, and communication difficulties	Sensory integration disorders
Confusion, decline in overall intellectual performance—"Brain fog"	Decline in executive functions—planning and organization

Table 6–3. Cognitive Dysfunction Associated with Lyme Disease

CERVICAL NERVE PALSIES ASSOCIATED WITH LYME DISEASE	
Cranial Nerve	**Symptoms**
I. Olfactory	Loss of smell Smells become intense or noxious
II. Optic	Visual impairment Blindness
III. Oculomotor	Eyelids drop Deviation of eyeball—outward Excessive squinting Dilation of pupils Double vision
IV. Trochlear	Deviation of eyeball—upward and outward Double vision on downward gaze
V. Trigeminal	Pain or numbness in face, scalp, forehead, temple, jaw, eye, or teeth Chewing difficulty Jaw deviation
VI. Abducens	Deviation of eye—outward Excessive squinting Double vision
VII. Facial	Bell's palsy—one side or both sides Facial drooping Facial numbness, tingling, hypersensitivity Facial pain Inability to close eye completely Chewing difficulty Dribbling
VIII. Vestibulocochlear	Hearing loss Tinnitus (ringing in the ears) Vertigo, dizziness Light-headedness, loss of balance Nausea, vomiting Ear pain Ear fullness Nystagmus
IX. Glossopharyngeal	Abnormal taste sensations Decreased taste Swallowing difficulty Sore throat

(Table continued on next page)

X. Vagus	Swallowing difficulty
	Talking difficulty
	Drooping shoulders
	Difficulty rotating head
	Palpitations
	Breathing difficulties
	Phrenic nerve palsy with respiratory distress
	Hemi-diagphragm paralysis
	Persistent cough
	Hoarseness, weak voice
	Vomiting
XI. Spinal Accessory	Weakness/paralysis of upper back and neck
	Difficulty tilting or rotating head
	Back spasms
XII. Hypoglossal	Tongue weak or paralyzed on one side
	Speech difficulty
	Swallowing difficulty

Table 6–4. Cervical Nerve Palsies Associated with Lyme Disease

PSYCHIATRIC CONDITIONS ASSOCIATED WITH LYME DISEASE	
Depression	Inappropriate laughter
Agitated depression	Nightmares
Bipolar (manic) depression	Paranoia
Anxiety	Hallucinations—auditory, olfactory, and visual
Panic attacks	Psychosis, hallucinations, delusions
Sleep disorders—insomnia and hypersomnolence	Schizophrenia-like disorder
Post-traumatic stress disorder (PTSD)	Obsessive-compulsive disorder (OCD)
Eating disorder	Attention deficit disorder (ADD)
Personality and behavioral changes	Attention deficit and hyperactivity disorder (ADHD)
Irritability, inappropriate anger, aggression	Learning disorders—e.g., dyslexia
Rage or violent outbursts/Oppositional defiance disorder	Autism
Rapid mood swings	Feeling disconnected

Table 6–5. Psychiatric Conditions Associated with Lyme Disease[*]

---

[*] Dr. Robert Bransfield has authored a comprehensive review of neuropsychiatric manifestations of Lyme disease: Bransfield RC. "Neuropsychiatric Lyme Borreliosis: An Overview with a Focus on a Specialty Psychiatrist's Clinical Practice." *Healthcare (Basel).* 2018 Aug 25;6(3). pii: E104.

LYME DISEASE IN CHILDREN	
Behavioral and personality changes	School phobias
Attention deficit disorder	Academic problems
Attention deficit disorder with hyperactivity	Learning disabilities
Irritability/rage	Oppositional defiance disorder
Eating disorders	Drug abuse

Table 6–6. Lyme Disease in Children May Present with These Conditions

LYME DISEASE IMPACTS MULTIPLE ORGAN SYSTEMS

Borrelia burgdorferi is a spirochete, a helical bacteria. Syphilis is also caused by a spirochete—*Treponema pallidum.* Sir William Osler, considered the father of modern medicine, has been famously quoted as saying "He who knows syphilis knows medicine," because this microbe can cause problems in every organ system. It turns out that *Bb* is exceedingly more complex than *T.pallidum.*[1] One LLMD referred to syphilis as Lyme's dumb cousin. Tables 6–7 through 6–11 list manifestations of Lyme disease in multiple organ systems.

GASTROINTESTINAL CONDITIONS ASSOCIATED WITH LYME DISEASE	
Nausea	Chronic gastritis
Abdominal pain	Chronic duodenitis
Irritable bowel syndrome with diarrhea and/or constipation/gastroparesis	Ulcerative colitis
Hepatic granulomas	Crohn's disease

Table 6–7. Gastrointestinal Conditions Associated with Lyme Disease

EYE CONDITIONS ASSOCIATED WITH LYME DISEASE		
Blurry vision with no objective abnormality	Endophthalmitis	Chorioretinopathy
Frequent changes in visual acuity	Keratitis	Pigment epitheliitis
Floaters	Nystagmus	Episcleritis
Conjunctivitis (pink eye)	Retinal vasculitis	Iritis
Optic neuritis	Retinal vein occlusion	Neuroretinitis
Choiroditis	Scleritis	Double vision
Drooping eyelid	Uveitis	Blindness

Table 6–8. Eye Conditions Associated with Lyme Disease

DERMATOLOGICAL CONDITIONS ASSOCIATED WITH LYME DISEASE		
Erythema migrans	Acrodermatitis chronica atrophicans	Flushing (*Babesia*)
Multiple EM rashes	Erythromelalgia	Livedo reticularis (mottling of the skin—often *Bartonella*
Erythema multiforme	Hives	Subcutaneous nodules (*Bartonella*)
Lymphocytoma	Striae (particularly associated with *Bartonella* co-infections)	

Table 6–9. Dermatological Conditions Associated with Lyme Disease

URINARY CONDITIONS ASSOCIATED WITH LYME DISEASE		
Prostatitis	Urinary frequency	Dysuria—painful urination
Hypotonic bladder with urinary retention	Often concurrent diabetes Insipidus with polyuria	Interstitial cystitis
Urinary incontinence		Testicular pain

Table 6–10. Urinary Issues Associated with Lyme Disease

GYNECOLOGICAL CONDITIONS ASSOCIATED WITH LYME DISEASE	
Chronic pelvic pain	Decreased libido
Menstrual irregularity	Severe PMS
Endometriosis	Vaginitis/vulvodynia
Dyspareunia—painful intercourse	Galactorrhea—breast discharge

Table 6–11. Gynecological Issues Associated with Lyme Disease

THE DOWNSTREAM ISSUES

Over time the chronic infectious process leads to systemic inflammation, which can result in hormone disruption, immune imbalance, and nervous system dysregulation. Every organ system in the body can be impacted. These disruptions may manifest as adrenal insufficiency, pituitary and hypothalamic disorders, thyroid dysfunction, food sensitivities, gluten intolerance, multiple chemical sensitivities, gastrointestinal issues, neuropsychological disorders, and autoimmune syndromes. Each will be discussed in subsequent chapters.

Ned tested positive for Lyme disease. His symptoms of night sweats accompanied by anxiety and shortness of breath suggested a co-infection with Babesia. *In addition, Ned had taken the antimalarial medication Malarone for*

prophylaxis on a trip to Africa, and it had resulted in a Herxheimer reaction. Malarone also targets Babesia, *and his reaction to this drug also supported the diagnosis of babesiosis.*

Most medical journal articles describing Lyme disease do not separate out the impact of co-infections. Admittedly this is a difficult task, since co-infection testing is notoriously insensitive and the symptoms associated with various tick-borne infections overlap. In clinical practice, however, most LLMDs report that essentially all patients who present with chronic Lyme also have co-infections. Subsequent chapters will discuss the clinical assessment of co-infections by history, physical exam, and lab tests.

It is possible that the main difference between the IDSA's stance that Lyme disease can be successfully treated with ten days to three weeks of antibiotics and the reality of persistent *Bb* infection requiring long-term treatment is the presence of co-infections.[2] The presence of multiple infections suppresses the immune system and therefore requires longer, more aggressive treatment.[3]

Nancy lives in western Colorado. When she was thirty-four years old, she visited Williamsburg, Virginia, and then Sacramento, California. She never saw a tick bite or rash, but three months after returning home she experienced the sudden onset of multiple symptoms: fatigue, left facial pain, headaches, visual floaters, palpitations, intermittent racing pulse—heart rate increased to 145 when she stood up, headaches, insomnia, nausea, joint pains, rib pain, numbness and tingling, fevers, night sweats, sole pain, diarrhea, and poor appetite. She lost forty pounds over three months.

Nancy was savvy enough to get tested for Lyme, and the test was strongly positive. She was treated first with Augmentin, then Zithromax and Tindamax, but experienced minimal improvement. She did forty "dives" of hyperbaric oxygen without benefit. She went to the Mayo Clinic, where she was diagnosed with postural orthostatic tachycardia syndrome (POTS)—a form of autonomic dysfunction that causes rapid heart rate and light-headedness upon standing (POTS is discussed in detail in Chapter 17). Over the next three years, her symptoms continued with increasingly severe anxiety, panic attacks, and depression.

I saw Nancy four years after the onset of symptoms. Her husband was clearly skeptical that she had an organic issue—he thought her problems were primarily psychiatric. As it turned out, Nancy was suffering from Lyme disease, babesiosis, bartonellosis, adrenal insufficiency, methylation impairment, and sensitivities to sugar, yeast, and gluten. After two years of treatment she became asymptomatic and has remained well since. Her husband has changed his mind.

HISTORICAL CLUES THAT CAN HELP MAKE A DIAGNOSIS

It is important that a provider investigate the patient's previous response to treatment with antibiotics for an intercurrent illness such as sinusitis. Was there improvement in symptoms or was there a flare in symptoms, i.e. a Herxheimer reaction? In 1895, Dr. Adolph Jarisch first described a marked increase in symptoms when patients initiated treatment for that other spirochetal illness, syphilis. Dr. Karl Herxheimer later described similar experiences, and they postulated that the exacerbation in symptoms was associated with toxins released by the bacteria when they were killed.

Modern researchers suspect that the die-off mechanism is related to cellular components of the microbe that stimulate a cytokine cascade—i.e. a severe inflammatory reaction.[4] Whatever the mechanism, the phenomenon is quite real and occurs in most patients being treated for Lyme and co-infections. Ned's experience when taking the antimalarial Malarone when he went on safari, in which there was an exacerbation in symptoms and subsequent improvement, is a classic sign of babesiosis in a patient with Lyme.

Another question that merits investigation is what happens when the patient is at high altitude. The Lyme spirochete is a facultative anaerobe, a technical way of saying that it grows better in low-oxygen environments. In other words, when oxygen levels drop, the bugs come out and party. People with *Bb* infection often feel worse upon traveling to places like Denver or Boulder at 5,000 feet, or Santa Fe at 7,500 feet above sea level. Many more will experience a flare in symptoms in places such as Vail or Aspen, with altitudes approximating 8,000 feet. Some people with Lyme will even notice they are worse after a long flight, since travelers on airplanes experience a significant reduction in oxygen saturation.[5] For those who are particularly sensitive to these changes, the ability to take oxygen during air travel can make a big difference in how they feel.

Likewise, patients treated with corticosteroids for conditions such as poison ivy or asthma will often have an adverse reaction. High-dose steroids like prednisone or a Medrol Dose-pak suppress the immune system, again allowing the bugs to party. Although steroids may temporarily decrease inflammation, resulting in fewer symptoms, this decrease is often followed by a flare. In addition, patients previously treated for chronic Lyme often experience a relapse after having surgery, since steroids are routinely administered intravenously during general anesthesia to decrease nausea and vomiting. Note that patients with Lyme who are planning surgery with general anesthesia can request that they be given an alternative to corticosteroids.

As illustrated by the case studies in this chapter, it is quite common for people with chronic Lyme to visit multiple physicians prior to obtaining a correct diagnosis. Many patients who have been to the Mayo Clinic and other academic centers come away disappointed, if not downright angry; most of these institutions share the IDSA's narrow view of Lyme. However, Lyme should always be part of the differential diagnosis (see below) if a patient has chronic symptoms—particularly musculoskeletal and neurological ones—and has been to dozens of doctors, or has been diagnosed with CFS, fibromyalgia, an autoimmune disorder unresponsive to treatment, or a psychiatric condition.

Dr. Joseph Burrascano did the Lyme community a colossal favor when he wrote "Advanced Topics in Lyme Disease: Diagnostic Hints and Treatment Guidelines for Lyme and Other Tick-Borne Illnesses." He updated it sixteen times, most recently in 2008, and offered it for free on the Internet, where it is still available. The Burrascano guidelines provided a stepping-stone for many LLMDs when they were getting started. It includes a symptom checklist; a revised version can be found in Appendix B, and is recommended for anyone who suspects he or she may have chronic Lyme.

THE DIFFERENTIAL DIAGNOSIS

The differential diagnosis is the process of distinguishing one disease or condition from other illnesses that present with similar signs and symptoms. Any provider formulating a differential diagnosis that includes tick-borne infections needs to account for the multi-systemic nature of these infections: they cause multiple symptoms in multiple organ systems. There is also the possibility that tick-borne co-infections can present in a similar fashion to Lyme disease in the absence of infection with *Bb*.

Viral infections, *Chlamydia*, and *Mycoplasma* as well as endocrinopathies, multifocal neurologic disease, autoimmune disorders, syphilis, HIV, tuberculosis, subacute bacterial endocarditis, hepatitis, sarcoidosis, Ehler-Danlos syndrome, porphyrias, toxin-induced illness, and any multi-systemic illness that can evolve over time all need to be kept in mind and considered in the differential diagnosis. Note that these conditions can be concurrent with Lyme disease.

While Lyme often results in endocrine disturbances, and can stimulate an autoimmune response, these problems also occur independent of an infective cause. Any fixed neurologic symptom or deficit could also be caused by a tumor. Both fibromyalgia and CFS are diagnoses of exclusion; all other disorders that can generate fatigue and pain need to be ruled out before making these diagnoses. My professional experience is that the majority of patients with fibromyalgia and CFS have Lyme disease.

The diagnosis of Lyme disease and co-infections is primarily based on taking a thorough history. Many symptoms can be missed during a perfunctory intake, while a comprehensive one will often uncover facts that, taken together, weave a tapestry that supports the diagnosis. The physical exam can be helpful, and laboratory testing can support or confirm the diagnosis, although it is important to remember that negative tests cannot rule out this diagnosis. But the first and most important requirement is an in-depth history.

TAKE-HOME POINTS

1. There are two categories of patients with chronic Lyme disease. One category includes patients with ongoing symptoms after treatment for acute Lyme disease. The second includes people previously undiagnosed with Lyme presenting months to years after a seen or unseen tick bite.
2. People need not have seen a tick bite or a rash or have been aware of a previous infection with *Bb* to present with chronic Lyme disease months or years later. The diagnosis of Lyme should be considered if a person has multiple unexplained symptoms.
3. Symptoms primarily impact musculoskeletal and neurologic systems, often fluctuate from day to day, and may cycle on a regular basis. Joint pains are often migratory.
4. Additional clues to diagnosis include reactions to antibiotics and corticosteroids in the past, and flares in symptoms at higher altitudes.
5. The vast majority of chronic Lyme disease patients have co-infections, and while negative tests cannot rule them out, a systematic approach is necessary for proper diagnosis.
6. Suspect Lyme disease when there has been a failure to diagnose after multiple consultations.

Chapter 7

Laboratory Evaluation of Lyme Disease

Diagnostic tests for Lyme disease are an important tool; however, it is important to note that they are not accurate or sensitive enough to pick up the presence of Lyme disease in all patients infected with *Bb*. The most commonly utilized tests fall into two main categories: indirect and direct. The former measures the body's immune response to infection, mainly via antibodies. The latter actually looks for the presence of the bacteria, either for the entire bug or for some of its parts. In addition, there are tests that measure *Bb*'s impact on the immune system as well as on the brain.

INDIRECT TESTS

The most commonly used tests for Lyme are antibody tests, which fall under the category of indirect tests. Antibodies, also known as immunoglobulins, are proteins that recognize foreign agents in the body, attach to them, and target them for destruction and elimination. There are specific antibodies for each foreign germ. For example, an antibody to influenza won't fight a strep infection or, unfortunately, Lyme disease. Here are the most commonly used indirect tests:

Lyme ELISA
The IDSA and the CDC recommend that doctors use the Lyme ELISA test as a first-line screening test for the diagnosis of Lyme disease. ELISA stands for Enzyme-Linked Immunosorbent Assay, and it is a widely used test to look for antibodies. In this case, the ELISA test uses enzymes to detect antibodies that specifically target Lyme spirochetes. It may measure IgM and IgG (see below) separately or together.

Supposedly, a screening test is a highly sensitive test that casts a wide net, like fishermen trawling for tuna. By dragging a huge net, they haul in virtually all the tuna in their path, but they also pick up some other fish they don't want and have to throw back. Similarly, the ELISA test, in theory, is designed to catch nearly everyone with Lyme, but will pick up a few without Lyme as well—those are false positives. Although lacking specificity, this should make it a good screening test. But is it?

By definition, a screening test should have at least a 95 percent sensitivity. This means that five out of one hundred people with Lyme will be incorrectly told that they don't have the infection. Ninety-five percent is considered "acceptable" accuracy, although those five might not agree. However, in one study, the ELISA test missed 56 percent of Lyme diagnoses, as compared with the investigators' diagnoses.[1] This means the ELISA test missed fifty-six out of one hundred people with Lyme disease. This is not acceptable by anyone's standards. Imagine a pregnancy test with that level of sensitivity!

Other studies have demonstrated even worse results. M. G. Golightly and colleagues found that the ELISA test missed over 70 percent of people with early Lyme disease and up to 46 percent with late manifestations of Lyme.[2] In a later study, the American College of Pathologists sent samples to 516 laboratories nationwide. They reported that 55 percent of the laboratories could not accurately identify blood samples from Lyme disease patients. They concluded that "currently used screening tests for Lyme disease are not adequate . . . The current methodologies need to be improved to adequately screen samples for confirmatory testing."[3] The big net that the ELISA test casts in search of Lyme has some really large holes, i.e. false negatives.

However, the CDC continues to recommend the Lyme ELISA as a first-line screening test. It may not be clear, at first glance, why they haven't revised this recommendation given the growing body of evidence of its poor sensitivity, but more than research appears to play a role. In fact, it is worth asking who holds the patents on the test kits and who makes the guideline recommendations.

Lyme IFA

Another quantitative antibody test that has been used as a screening tool is called IFA, for immunofluorescent assay. Results from this test are roughly as reliable as the ELISA, but it is still offered in some laboratories.

C6 Peptide ELISA

Commercial ELISA and the IFA tests use a whole-cell preparation of the *Bb* spirochete; by comparison the C6 Peptide ELISA test for Lyme uses a single antigen. Although research has yielded varying results, in practice it has not been found to be a sensitive indicator of *Bb* infection,[4] as it does not appear to have reliable sensitivity.

Western Blot

The Western blot is another antibody test, but is more specific than the ELISA. This means it is more like fishing with hooks that can snag only tuna, leaving the other fish alone. The Western blot differentiates between, and then reports, antibodies of particular classes. Although antibodies are unique for different germs, they also fall into distinct classes. Two of these are particularly relevant to testing for infectious disease: IgM and IgG.

Antibodies in the IgM class are the first to respond to infection. In theory, IgM levels are detectable within one to two weeks of the onset of infection, peak at four weeks, then gradually decline. Meanwhile, the IgG class of antibodies are slower to respond. Levels of IgG antibodies begin to rise three to four weeks after an infection. A person's body continues to produce IgG for the duration of the infection and beyond, often for years or even a lifetime. Thus the presence of IgM antibodies should establish that there was recent exposure, while testing for IgG antibodies should be able to determine if there was prior exposure or illness, although it cannot differentiate whether the infection is still active.

In reality, however, people with long-term *Bb* infection are just as likely to have circulating IgM antibodies (the "early" responders) as IgG antibodies (the "late" responders) on a Western blot test. It is as if their immune systems keep encountering *Bb* as a new infection over and over again. There are several studies documenting the persistence of IgM antibodies to *Bb* in chronically infected people.[5,6] In clinical practice, most patients with Lyme disease complex, including those who have been ill for years or even decades, have IgM positivity disproportionate to IgG positives prior to treatment. Those who choose to consult with an infectious disease physician rather than an LLMD are usually told that the positive IgM must be a "false positive" because they have not had a recent infection. *However, a positive IgM is consistent with a persistent infection as well as a recent infection.*

IgM positivity tends to decline as treatment progresses, while IgG positivity increases. IgG declines in some patients in parallel with symptom improvement, but IgG antibodies are likely to persist after successful therapy. If all antibodies become negative, the patient is usually in remission. This does not mean that *Bb* is completely eradicated from their body; as touched on previously, *Bb* has developed sophisticated mechanisms for persistence. Some people in remission may relapse in the future, particularly if they experience any immune compromise. Currently there is no test that definitively proves eradication of *Bb* from the body.

So how does the Western blot work? The test kit is made from the Lyme spirochete itself, which is broken down by ultrasound and a detergent is used to disperse the bacterial fragments on a gelatin-like strip of paper. Then an electric current is applied, causing the pieces of Lyme spirochetes to migrate to discrete places along the strip of paper. The degree of migration occurs according to weight; the lighter the fragment, the further it moves; protein antigens of specific weights migrate a specific distance. When a patient's serum is added to the paper, any antibodies to *Bb* that are present will bind to the protein pieces of spirochetes on the paper. A reagent is then added, causing a color change at those places where antibodies are bound.

The result will show up visually as bands of dark color, with each band corresponding to a different antibody adhering to a particular spirochete fragment. The more bands that "light up," the more types of antibodies are present in the person's serum. This means that the Western blot not only differentiates between IgM and IgG antibodies, it also can identify antibodies to particular proteins in the bacteria—each will create a separate band.

If antibodies are present, theoretically that should provide definitive proof of exposure. Out of the twenty-five possible bands performed in Western blot testing, some are antibodies that cross-react with other germs, and some are of unclear significance. Table 7–1 contains a list of the bands and their meanings. You can see in this table, however, that certain bands are fairly specific for Lyme. These are 23–25, 31, 34, 39, and 83–93. The 31 and 83–93 bands can also be generated by some viruses. One laboratory that specializes in testing for tick-borne infections, IGeneX, offers a further epitope test, in which DNA collected from band 31 is amplified, to determine whether or not it is definitively from Lyme.

INTERPRETATION OF THE WESTERN BLOT BANDS	
23–25 kDa	Specific for *Bb*, outer-surface protein C (OspC)
28 kDa	Unknown
30 kDa	Unknown
31 kDa	Specific for *Bb*, outer-surface protein A (OspA) but cross-reacts with some viruses
34 kDa	Specific for *Bb*, outer-surface protein B (OspB)
39 kDa	Specific for *Bb*, major protein of *Bb* flagellin
41 kDa	Specific for all *Borrelia* but not specific for *Bb*; major protein of *Borrelia* flagellin, usually the first to appear after *Bb* infection.
45 kDa	Cross-reactive for all *Borrelia*, not specific to *Bb*
58 kDa	Unknown
66 kDa	Cross-reactive for all *Borrelia*, common in other bacteria
83–93 kDa	Specific for *Bb*, probably a cytoplasmic membrane but cross-reacts with some viruses

Table 7–1. Interpretation of the Western blot. kD is a unit of distance, marking the migration of the Bb antigen along the gel-strip of paper when an electric current is applied.

Prior to 1994, any positive Lyme-specific band on the Western blot was considered diagnostic. However, in that year a political decision was made at the CDC's Dearborn conference. As with many areas of medicine, monied interests came into play and were prioritized over accuracy. The "problem" was that the Western blot was a more sensitive test than the ELISA when using the criteria that any single Lyme-specific band was diagnostic. Those with a vested interest in the ELISA found this unacceptable; their test would no longer be in demand. They devised a way to make the Western blot a less sensitive test by imposing strict interpretative guidelines on it.* This move allowed the Lyme ELISA test to continue to be recommended as a first-line screening test.

Thus, since 1994 the CDC's published guidelines for the laboratory diagnosis of Lyme disease state that a patient must have either two of the following IgM bands present: 23–25, 39, 41; or five of the following IgG bands present: 18, 21, 28, 30, 39, 41, 45, 58, 66, 93; to receive a positive diagnosis.[7]

This is the irrational rationale behind the two-tier testing recommendation that came out of the Dearborn Conference. Per those guidelines, providers should first use the Lyme ELISA test as a screen. Any positive finding should be confirmed with the more specific Western blot test, since the ELISA can produce a false positive result. However, evaluation of this protocol reveals its limitations. The sensitivity of the two-tier testing is limited by the first test, the Lyme ELISA, which has a roughly 40 percent sensitivity. The sensitivity of the Western blot is further limited by the restrictive criteria the CDC imposed on interpretation of the Western blot. Therefore, by employing the CDC recommended two-tier testing with the Lyme ELISA as a screening tool and following any positive results with the restrictive Western blot criteria, there is only a 22 percent chance that a *Bb* infection will be detected.[8]

In a recent review of the CDC guidelines, a group of researchers from Rutgers, Yale, and Harvard as well as the Food and Drug Administration (FDA), National Institutes of Health (NIH), and CDC concluded that "The 1994 serodiagnostic testing guidelines predated a full understanding of key *B. burgdorferi* antigens and have a number of shortcomings."[9] When the CDC cites data documenting over 400,000 new cases of Lyme disease annually, they are basing this figure on positive results that satisfy their two-tier criteria. If these criteria only diagnose one in four to five people with Lyme, then there are over 1.6 million people who get Lyme disease in the United States each year.

---

* The explanation for this recommendation was related to me by Dr. Sam Donta, who resigned in protest at Dearborn when this decision was made. I asked Sam why so much false information continues to be disseminated about Lyme disease in medical journals, and he answered, "Never before in medicine have I witnessed so few people having so much influence and been so wrong."

At one time the CDC made it clear that their two-tier criteria were meant for epidemiologic reporting only. Specifically, they said, "This surveillance case definition was developed for national reporting of Lyme disease; it is not intended for use in the clinical diagnosis."[10] In other words, the CDC directive to physicians was not to use these criteria to make or dismiss the diagnosis of Lyme disease in their practices. But that is exactly what happens in doctors' offices all over the country, and, significantly, these criteria are also used by insurance companies.

Rather than two-tier testing, the Western blot should be the first recommended step in the laboratory evaluation of a patient suspected of Lyme disease. However, not all Western blot results reported by different laboratories yield similar results. Steven Luger and Elliot Krauss sent blood from each of nine patients with a history of Lyme disease to nine clinical labs, including national, university, state, and local hospital laboratories. They found huge variability from lab to lab, with results ranging from eighteen of eighteen specimens positive on the IgG measurement in one university lab (100 percent detection) to only eight of eighteen specimens reported as positive in a state lab (44 percent detection). IgM detection was worse: the results ranged from two of eighteen positive to ten of eighteen positive.[11]

IGeneX Laboratory provides a Western blot assay that is superior to those offered at standard commercial labs. This statement is made without any personal or financial interest in the company. Their results are more accurate for a number of reasons:

Most commercial labs testing for Lyme Western blots (like Quest or LabCorp) target one laboratory strain of *B.burgdorferi*, B-31. The IGeneX Western blot test targets two strains of *Bb*: B-31 and 297.[12]

- Most labs only report the bands requested by the CDC surveillance criteria, and don't report other bands that could potentially be useful in the diagnosis. In particular, they exclude Band 31 (OspA) and Band 34 (OspB), both of which are fairly specific for Lyme. The commercial labs claim that including these bands will result in more false positive results, as 31 and 34 will be positive in patients previously vaccinated for Lyme. This is a small population who could readily report that they had the Lyme vaccine (LYMErix, which was taken off the market in 2002); inclusion of bands 31 and 34 can provide essential diagnostic information.
- While the 31 band usually reflects the presence of an antibody to a *Bb* outer-surface protein, it can also be a response to some viral infections (the cross-reactivity discussed above). IGeneX offers the 31 epitope test that can determine whether this antibody is indeed from a *Bb* infection.
- A machine does not read the Western blot at IGeneX; the test strip is visually evaluated by technicians. IGeneX is dedicated to testing only for

tick-borne infections and has highly trained technicians. Sometimes a technician will see a faint positive band that does not quite meet the criteria for positivity (i.e. is not as strong as the positive control). IGeneX will report it as IND—indeterminate. The experience of LLMDs, many of whom have inspected thousands of test reports and then followed the patients, is that IND bands are true positives.

As a result of these advantages, IGeneX tests have greater than 90 percent sensitivity compared with 46 percent sensitivity in standard commercial labs. Even so, physicians need to understand how to interpret the test.

Remember Ned? After fifteen years of suffering and being diagnosed with CFS and anxiety, here is what his Western blot showed:

Band	IgM	IgG
18 kDa	-	-
23–25 kDa	IND	-
28 kDa	-	-
30 kDa	+	-
31 kDa	++	+++
34 kDa	IND	-
39 kDa	IND	IND
41 kDa	++	++
45 kDa	-	+
58 kDa	+	++
66 kDa	-	-
83–93 kDa	IND	-

If Ned's tests were interpreted using the CDC criteria, with indeterminate bands not considered positive, both his IgG and IgM would be reported as negative. Even if the IND are accepted as indicating antibody presence, his IgG would be CDC negative. However, by looking at the Lyme (mostly) specific bands (18, 23–25, 31, 34, 39, 83–93) and interpreting IND bands as indicative of antibody presence, this is a positive test.

Observe that the indeterminates are all in Lyme-specific bands; this is usually the case. Also note that the IgM positivity is in someone who has been sick for years. Positive IgM is evidence of persistent as well as recent infection. And here is a clinical pearl: bands 31 and 34 do not turn positive for either IgM or IgG until a minimum of one year after exposure. Finally, antibodies do not prove active infection—the patient's symptoms must be taken into account. A person who has a positive test but is asymptomatic may have an infection that is dormant or even cleared. In Ned's case his symptoms are compatible with Lyme disease and other diagnoses had been ruled out, so his Western blot was a diagnostic slam-dunk.

Remember Abby, the seven-year-old I described in Chapter 7 with a rash that she got when visiting her grandmother in New Hampshire? Here is what her Western blot looked like:

Band	IgM	IgG
18 kDa	+	+
23–25 kDa	IND	-
28 kDa	-	-
30 kDa	+	-
31 kDa	IND	-
34 kDa	-	-
39 kDa	IND	-
41 kDa	+++	++
45 kDa	-	-
58 kDa	++	+
66 kDa	-	-
83–93 kDa	++	-

This Western blot is negative by CDC surveillance criteria, but it is clearly positive when Lyme-specific Band 31 and the multiple bands marked IND are taken into account. Abby also tested positive for *Babesia* and *Mycoplasma*.

While proper interpretation of an IGeneX Western blot yields a 90 percent sensitivity of detecting Lyme, there are still 10 percent of symptomatic patients whose tests are negative for Lyme. Here are some reasons for false negatives:

- The Lyme spirochete is a stealth pathogen, and can elude detection by the immune system.
- The Western blot will not reliably pick up all strains and species of *Bb*, some of which are unlike B31 and 297.
- The person may have a depressed immune system because of an illness such as AIDS, leukemia, or another chronic ailment, and therefore not be capable of an antibody response; remember, this is an indirect test for antibodies, not a direct test for the organism. There is also evidence that Lyme disease itself can depress immune function, especially when paired with a co-infection.
- Medications such as corticosteroids or chemotherapy may be suppressing the antibody response.

- All of the person's antibodies may be bound to bacteria, and no free antibodies available to be picked up by the tests.
- The body's immune system may be using mechanisms other than antibodies to fight the infection.
- Treatment with antibiotics early in the course of illness may reduce or prevent an antibody response, even if the infection persists or is reactivated.
- If a test is performed too soon after exposure, not enough time will have elapsed for the production of antibodies. It can take two weeks after infection to detect an antibody response.
- The lab is using an inferior test kit or poor procedure for analysis. The accuracy of the test is dependent on the quality of the laboratory and the experience of the testing personnel.

When clinical suspicion is high but the test is negative, clinicians have the option of doing an antibiotic provocation. *Bb* is a shape-shifter—when under stress the bacteria can convert from its active spirochetal form to a relatively dormant cyst. The antibiotic metronidazole (brand name Flagyl) will attack the Lyme cysts, forcing them back into the spirochetal form, which theoretically will stimulate an antibody response. Typically metronidazole is prescribed for five days, and the Western blot then repeated in a month. A Herxheimer response to the antibiotic is also helpful diagnostically, but it needs to be differentiated from a drug reaction.

Lyme Immunoblot Assay

IGeneX also offers a Lyme immunoblot test that is a more specific and sensitive assay than the IGeneX Western blot. The difference is that they have created pure recombinant proteins for use as the test antigens, rather than using proteins from cultures of lab strains. This results in less cross-reactivity with viruses and non-*Borrelia* bacteria. Another advantage is that the recombinant proteins include all *Borrelia*-specific antigens covering North American and European strains of *Bb*, not just B31 or 297. What this means is that the immunoblot assay detects antibodies to other *Borrelia* species included in the category of *Borrelia burgdorferi sensuo lato (Bbsl)*.[13] *Bbsl* includes *Borrelia* species in other parts of the world that cause Lyme disease, not only *B. burgdorferi*. (See Chapter 13.) Note, however, that *Bbsl* does not include the *Borrelia* relapsing fever group.

IGeneX considers the IgM immunoblot positive if two out of the five bands of 23, 31, 34, 39, and 41 kDa are present, and the IgG immunoblot positive if two out of the six bands of 23, 31, 34, 39, 41, and 93 kDa are present. Note that if band 31 is positive in the immunoblot test, this is 100 percent specific for *Bbsl*.

The Lyme immunoblot assay's sensitivity has increased enough that it can detect antibodies closer to the onset of infection. While it is standard to delay antibody testing until two weeks after a known tick attachment or one week after an EM rash, the immunoblot has been shown to be positive as early as the onset of the rash. The Lyme immunoblot test may make the standard Western blot test obsolete, but it is also more expensive.

Lyme IgXSpot

When the immune system encounters *Bb,* there is both a humoral response (i.e. antibodies) and a cellular response, which involves cytotoxic T-cells. (See Chapter 18 for a description of the immune system's response to infection.) This cellular immune response occurs earlier than humoral activation in most patients with Lyme disease. The Lyme IgXSpot offered by IGeneX is an enzyme-linked assay that detects human T-cells reactive to *Bb*-specific antigens. The IgXSpot can detect Lyme disease early after infection, before antibodies are detectable. In addition, the IgXSpot can detect *Bb* infection in patients who have a poor humoral response, particularly those who are quite ill after long-term persistent infection.[†]

DIRECT TESTS

An alternative to indirect testing for the presence of Lyme disease is the direct detection of the Lyme spirochete.

PCR—Polymerase Chain Reaction

The most frequently used direct test for Lyme is polymerase chain reaction (PCR). A PCR test identifies the DNA of a pathogen, and as such is highly specific. A positive Lyme PCR from a reputable laboratory indicates bacterial presence, although the IDSA considers Lyme PCR testing "experimental." This is curious since PCR testing is widely used in other infections such as HIV and hepatitis C. PCR testing can be done not only on blood but also on cerebrospinal fluid (CSF), serum, urine, joint fluid, breast milk, and umbilical cord blood at delivery.

Unfortunately, while PCR testing is highly specific for *Bb,* it is subject to contamination, which can result in false positives. In addition, the sensitivity of serum PCR testing in Lyme disease is only about 20 percent. After initial infection, Lyme bacteria leave the bloodstream fairly rapidly and head for lower-oxygen environments such as soft tissues and the inside of cells, which would account for the difficulty of finding their DNA in blood. This also explains why the sensitivity of PCR testing in the CSF and synovial fluid is somewhat higher.[14]

---

†   ArminLabs in Germany also offers the immunoblot and the Elispot, a test that detects cellular response to infection.

Urine PCR testing for *Bb* as well as for co-infections is available at IGeneX. The specificity of this testing should be high, but the community consensus sensitivity is around 20–30 percent. Some physicians will pretreat patients with antibiotics for five days before collecting specimens, which may increase recovery in the urine.

Lyme Culture

Many infections are detected by doing cultures, but this process is dependent on the ability of a lab to create the proper environment for the organism to grow. *Bb* is technically difficult to culture, and Lyme culture was not available in commercial labs until Dr. Eva Sapi developed a technique for Advanced Laboratory Services. They claimed 94 percent sensitivity if the specimens are held for three months.[15] IGeneX purchased Advanced Laboratory Services and are in the process of obtaining state and federal certification as of this writing.

However, there are a number of drawbacks to culture testing. These include the wait time, as patients need to be off antibiotics for two months before the blood draw; the long wait for results, which can take two to three months; and the potential of *Bb* hiding in protected tissues and therefore not present in the blood. It is impossible to know accurately how sensitive this test is since there is currently no "gold standard" with which it can be compared.

Lyme Dot-blot Assay

Another direct test is the urine Lyme Dot-blot Assay (LDA) offered by IGeneX. The LDA test detects fragments of *Bb* by using anti-*Bb* antibodies. IGeneX claims this test has a 42 percent sensitivity and an 89 percent specificity. Taking antibiotics prior to obtaining the urine sample can enhance sensitivity, since killing the bacteria can lead to bacterial fragments being excreted in the urine. There are several different provocation protocols using a range of antibiotics.

INDIRECT IMMUNE TESTS

CD57 Lymphocyte Test

Although chronic infection with *Bb* is associated with immune abnormalities, there are no immunologic markers that have been specific and sensitive for this infection. Ray Stricker and Ed Winger published a study which suggested that people with chronic Lyme have a decrease in the CD57 lymphocyte subset, while those with acute infection and patients with HIV have normal values.[16] However, many LLMDs have found that CD57 counts vary markedly over time irrespective of clinical course, and are not consistently low in people with active *Bb* infection. Nonetheless, the CD57 test can still be diagnostically useful because my clinical experience has shown that very low CD57 values (less than 20 by LabCorp) are usually associated with active *Babesia* infection.

BRAIN SCANS

Brain scans often show abnormalities in patients with Lyme, but none of the demonstrated abnormalities are specific for Lyme disease.

MRI Scan

MRI scans depict physical structure and inflammatory abnormalities in the brain. People with Lyme disease often show hyperintensities or flairs consistent with inflammation. These flairs are also present in other central nervous system infections as well as in multiple sclerosis, and they may also be present in otherwise healthy aging adults, so this is not a specific finding. An MRI scan is indicated in patients with fixed neurologic findings in which a tumor needs to be ruled out.

SPECT Scan

Single-photon emission computerized tomography (SPECT) scans demonstrate circulatory abnormalities in the brain. Patients with Lyme disease may exhibit inadequate blood supply to specific areas of the brain, and sometimes throughout the brain. This lack of normal blood flow would account for the severe cognitive dysfunction that is so common in people with Lyme disease complex. Dr. Sam Donta reported that 75 percent of patients with Lyme disease had abnormal SPECT scans.[17] Dr. Brian Fallon has suggested that different patterns of abnormal SPECT scans can distinguish between primary neuropsychological disorders and Lyme disease.[18]

PET Scan

Positron-emission tomography (PET) scans monitor sugar metabolism. In one small study, 75 percent of patients with Lyme disease had evidence of slowed metabolism in the brain, particularly in the temporal lobes.[19]

MAKING THE DIAGNOSIS

The first step in the diagnosis of Lyme disease is taking a careful history. Laboratory tests can *only* support or confirm the diagnosis, but cannot rule it out.

TAKE-HOME POINTS

1. Skip the Lyme ELISA test and go straight to the Western blot. The Lyme Immunoblot test is more sensitive and offers increased sensitivity over the Western Blot.

2. I recommend IGeneX laboratory over other commercial labs in the United States.

3. Anyone infected outside the United States should request the IGeneX Lyme immunoblot assay. ArminLabs in Augsburg, Germany, is a resource for patients in Europe.

4. The Lyme (mostly) specific bands are: 18, 23–25, 31, 34, 39, and 83–93.

5. The presence of specific antibodies to *Bb* is consistent with exposure to *Bb*, but does not prove active infection.

6. IgM positivity is consistent with both recent and persistent infection.

7. The presence of bands 31 and 34 indicates that the patient was exposed to *Bb* at least one year previously, or else had the LYMErix vaccine prior to 2002.

8. Additional direct detection techniques include PCR testing and the Lyme Dot-blot assay. IGeneX is about to make a culture available.

9. If CD57 counts are less than 20, consider active infection with *Babesia*.

10. All patients with chronic infection with *Bb* need to be evaluated for co-infections. In Appendix C I list blood tests that I request on most new patients.

11. If the diagnosis is unclear, consider a therapeutic trial of antimicrobials.

Chapter 8

Treatment of Chronic Lyme Disease

Patients with chronic Lyme disease have been sick for a long time, and typically present with multiple issues that complicate the clinical picture. It is important for patients to understand that when treating chronic Lyme disease, the tortoise beats the hare—this process is a marathon, not a sprint. Starting a number of interventions at once often leads to confusion, making it difficult to determine what is helping and what is hurting. Given the heterogeneity of patients with Lyme disease complex, it is necessary to take treatment in steps and individualize recommendations.

WHERE DO WE START?

This chapter will describe treatment of *Bb*, while subsequent chapters will address treatment of co-infections as well as the multiple chronic issues delineated in Chapter 4. When chronic Lyme disease is complicated with co-infections and the downstream issues of chronic inflammation, my preferred nomenclature is Lyme disease complex. Note that Lyme disease complex cannot be fully treated with antibiotics alone; it is important to address infrastructure (diet, detox, food sensitivities, yeast issues, digestive problems, endocrine balance, etc.) either prior to or simultaneous with antimicrobial therapy.

Let's return to Ned from Chapters 6 and 7:

Ned had been diagnosed with CFS and anxiety, and was taking two medications—Ritalin for attention deficit disorder and zolpidem for sleep—at the time he came in for Lyme testing. Ned had elected to do some traveling after his increasing fatigue and cognitive dysfunction caused him to stop working. By the time his positive Western blot test results were in, he was in Colombia, South America.

It's no secret that getting pharmaceuticals south of the border is a lot easier than in the United States. We decided to take advantage of his location, and arranged through physicians in Colombia to start Ned on intravenous ceftriaxone at 2 gm daily. Within two weeks Ned was improving. His symptoms of nighttime sweats, air hunger, and anxiety indicated a co-infection with Babesia, *and his Herxheimer reaction when he took Malarone while on safari confirmed this diagnosis. We took advantage of his having a PICC line and added clindamycin 900 mg IV every twelve hours to treat* Babesia.*

Soon Ned relayed that his energy was better, his cognition had improved, he was sleeping better, and he was less irritable and more social. His doctors in Colombia would not continue the IV after two months, so they stopped it and started him on oral doxycycline 100 mg twice daily. Within six weeks Ned's symptoms had relapsed. I convinced the physicians to stop the doxycycline and start Ned on clarithromycin 500 mg and cefuroxime 500 mg twice daily. After two weeks Ned was feeling better again.

ORAL ANTIBIOTICS FOR LYME

We'll come back to Ned, but first let's talk about initial antibiotics for Lyme disease. Doxycycline ("doxy") is often heralded as the drug of choice. Its pros and cons for treatment of acute Lyme disease were catalogued in Chapter 5. How does it fare for those with Lyme disease complex? Dr. Joseph Burrascano tested the blood levels of doxy in his patients with Lyme disease and found that the majority of those taking the typical dosage of 100 mg twice daily did not have therapeutic levels in their blood.[1] Based on these findings, many LLMDs began prescribing doxy at higher doses, most often 200 mg twice daily, although even this dose may be insufficient to reach therapeutic blood levels. However, the higher doses do significantly increase the potential side effects.

Another strategy used by LLMDs is to combine an antibiotic that works inside the bacteria (interfering with protein synthesis) with one that attacks the cell wall, respectively referred to as intracellular and extracellular antibiotics. The intracellular antibiotics include the tetracyclines (doxycycline being one) and the macrolides, while the extracellular antibiotics are usually beta lactam antibiotics and cephalosporins. While this generally works well, it is prudent to add only one medication at a time for several reasons:

- It is easier to ascertain how well a patient is tolerating an intervention by changing only one variable at a time.
- Patients starting any antimicrobial, whether an herb or a drug, may experience a Herxheimer ("Herx") response. Not only can these reactions

be exceedingly uncomfortable, the inflammatory reaction can set the person back in their recovery. It doesn't make sense for someone to be Herxing on two agents simultaneously.

- A Herxheimer reaction yields diagnostic information—it allows the provider to clearly ascertain which agent is precipitating the reaction. Starting two medications simultaneously confounds the picture.

A typical treatment plan for most chronically ill patients will be to start an antibiotic at half dose and increase it to full dose after a week if there is no Herx, or if a Herx has subsided by that time. If the patient is stable and no longer Herxing after an additional week on the full dose, they can start the second agent, following the same process. It is important to emphasize to patients that if they are Herxing they should not increase the dose or add another agent. If the flare continues unabated, the best strategies are to either decrease the dose or consider stopping the drug entirely and try another medication after the Herx has remitted. If a Herx is severe, the antibiotics should be stopped immediately.

Some physicians claim that treating with half doses can result in antibiotic resistance, but this has not been borne out in clinical practice nor in research studies.[2] (Antibiotic resistance is discussed in greater detail in Chapter 24.) Treatment of Herx reactions is detailed below. Table 8–1 lists the most commonly employed oral antibiotics to treat Lyme disease.

ORAL ANTIBIOTICS USED TO TREAT LYME DISEASE				
Action	**Class**	**Drug**	**Adult Dose**	**Child Dose**
Intracellular	Tetracycline	Doxycycline	200 mg 2x/day	2.2 mg/kg 1x/day
		Minocycline	100 mg 2x/day	2.0 mg/kg 1x/day
		Tetracycline	500 mg 2x/day	N/A
	Macrolide	Azithromycin	500 mg 1x/day	10 mg/kg 1x/day
		Clarithromycin	500 mg 2x/day	7.5 mg/kg 2x/day
Extracellular	Beta Lactam	Amoxicillin (Probenecid will increase blood levels)	1500 mg 2-3x/day	25 mg/kg 2x/day
		Amoxicillin Clavulanate	875/125 mg 2x/day	25 mg/kg 2x/day
	Cephalosporin	Cefuroxime	500 mg-1000 mg 2x/day	15 mg/kg 2x/day
		Cefdinir	300 mg 2x/day	14 mg/kg 2xday

Table 8–1. Oral antibiotics commonly used to treat Lyme disease. An intracellular and extracellular antibiotic can be combined for increased efficacy. Doses will vary from patient to patient on the basis of clinical response and tolerance.

HERBAL ANTIMICROBIALS FOR LYME

Pharmaceutical antibiotics are not the only option when addressing the infection. There are many herbal extracts that have been used to treat Lyme disease. While they do not have controlled studies to document effectiveness in patients with Lyme disease, some do have proven efficacy in vitro.[3,4,5] On the basis of extensive clinical experience, some have clearly demonstrated *in vivo* effectiveness as well. The herbal remedies in Table 8–2 below are not the only ones available, but are some of the more commonly used by LLMDs in integrative practice.

HERBAL ANTIMICROBIALS USED TO TREAT LYME DISEASE		
Product	Company	Comments
MC-BB1	Beyond Balance	Mild—starting point for sensitive adults and children
MC-BB2	Beyond Balance	Stronger than MC-BB1; used to progress treatment when at full dose of MC-BB1
Samento	Nutramedix	Effective single remedy but often combined with other Nutramedix remedies, especially Noni and Banderol
A-L Complex	Byron White	Particularly powerful

Table 8–2. Common herbal antimicrobials used to treat Lyme disease. Doses are up to 15–25 drops in water twice daily for all of the above.

NEW DRUG POSSIBILITIES: DISULFIRAM

In March 2016, Dr. Jayakamur Rajadas from Stanford University published a research paper of great interest. His group had tested the effect of 4,366 drugs against *Bb* in the laboratory, and published their top twenty hits.[6] They ranked disulfiram as number one in activity.

After Alexandra Cohen developed Lyme disease, she and her husband established the Cohen Lyme Disease Tick-Borne Initiative, a division within their philanthropic organization that sponsored the First Annual Lyme Disease in the Era of Precision Medicine Conference in October 2016. One of the speakers was Kim Lewis, the leader of Northeastern University's Antimicrobial Discovery Center. He slso presented data on the relative effectiveness of different antibiotics against *Bb* in his laboratory.[7] Lewis found that disulfiram was the most effective drug they had tested against the Lyme bacteria. It completely sterilized their cultures, eradicating all persisters.

Disulfiram blocks acetaldehyde dehydrogenase, which converts acetaldehyde, the breakdown product of alcohol, to acetic acid.

$$\text{Alcohol} \xrightarrow{\hspace{3cm}} \text{Acetaldehyde} \xrightarrow{\hspace{3cm}} \text{Acetic acid}$$
$$\text{Alcohol dehydrogenase} \qquad \text{Acetaldehyde dehydrogenase}$$

The accumulation of acetaldehyde results in severe hangover effects, and this medication has been prescribed for decades to alcoholics as a deterrent to consuming alcohol. It had not been prescribed previously as an antibiotic.

The effectiveness of a medication in the laboratory does not always translate to its success in people, and there have been no controlled animal or human studies that have researched the efficacy of disulfiram in the treatment of Lyme disease. But a patient of Dr. Ken Liegner's of Pawling, New York, saw the lecture by Dr. Lewis on YouTube and asked to be treated with disulfiram. This patient had been infected in May 2008 and diagnosed with both Lyme disease and babesiosis. After nine years of treatment the patient had improved substantially, but any attempt to decrease or discontinue his antibiotics resulted in a relapse of his multi-systemic symptoms within two weeks.

Liegner prescribed disulfiram 500 mg daily and discontinued the previous antibiotic regimen. After four months the patient declared himself cured, stopped the disulfiram, and has remained well for over three years at the time of this writing. Dr. Liegner has reported the successful results of treating his first three patients with disulfiram in the journal *Antibiotics*.[8] These results as well as Liegner's experience with subsequent patients suggest that disulfiram may be an extremely powerful drug to treat Lyme disease as well as babesiosis. Since disulfiram has been shown to kill *Plamodium falciparum* (malaria) in the laboratory,[9] it is not surprising that it would also be effective against *Babesia,* which is a protozoa sensitive to antimalarial medications.

Brian Fallon at Columbia University has initiated a controlled trial using disulfiram in well-characterized patients with Lyme disease. Despite the lack of controlled trials, but based on the laboratory studies and anecdotal reports, I and a number of physicians have begun recommending disulfiram for patients with Lyme disease complex.

At the time of this writing, I have treated over 100 patients with disulfiram. My clinical experience is that it appears to be the most powerful drug in our armamentarium against *Bb* and *Babesia.* But as with any medication, there are also risks, and it is not for everyone.

The first issue is Herxheimer reactions, and for that reason I start patients on 31.25 mg (⅛ of a standard 250 mg tablet) every three days. If the Herxheimer reaction is severe or prolonged, then the dose of disulfiram should be decreased. I advise my patients to never advance the dosage if they are still Herxing, and to check in with me by email every two weeks. Some patients do not tolerate extremely low doses of disulfiram because of severe Herxheimer reactions, and need to stop the drug.

Of greater concern is the potential for neurotoxicity. At times this can be difficult to distinguish from a Herxheimer reaction. These neurotoxic reactions typically occur at higher doses, often soon after a dose increase, but some patients experience neurotoxicity at low doses. If symptoms of pins and needles, numbness, stabbing, shooting, or burning pains develop, this could represent disulfiram-induced neuropathy. If symptoms of brain fog/impaired cognition, headache, mood changes, or vision issues develop, this could represent toxic encephalopathy, which is brain toxicity. If the disulfiram dose is lowered or if the drug is stopped within days of the onset of neurotoxic symptoms, they will usually remit quickly.

One of the mechanisms of neurotoxicity appears to be activation of copper, which promotes peroxidation of lipid membranes resulting in neuropathy.[10] Therefore, I recommend taking supplemental zinc, which will depress copper levels. I also suggest adding alpha lipoic acid (ALA), melatonin, and vitamin C, which can be neuroprotective.[11,12] Even with neuroprotection, some patients cannot take disulfiram without experiencing toxic neuropathy, and need to stop the medication.

The maintenance or target dose is based on weight *but also tolerance*: Target doses approximate 4–5 mg/kg, which is 250mg for someone who weighs 130 pounds. Patients continue the target dose for six to ten weeks then stop. However, this target dose strategy does not work for many patients. Because of Herxheimer reactions or neurotoxicity, many patients cannot progress their doses to the target level based on weight. Nevertheless, some patients have significant resolution of symptoms at lower doses and we simply maintain these patients on lower doses for an extended period.

Obviously, patients on disulfiram must avoid alcohol. This includes any topical products that contain alcohol such as some lotions and shampoos. Any tinctures that are alcohol based should be put in hot water for ten minutes to allow the alcohol to evaporate. Sugar and fermented foods need to be avoided including vinegar, kombucha, soy sauce, pickles, olives, and sauerkraut. Green tea can interact with a disulfiram metabolite and cause toxicity and should be avoided. Yeast can also produce acetaldehyde, and patients with yeast overgrowth issues must follow a strict yeast-free diet and take appropriate antifungals.

There are a host of minor side effects that occur in some patients that are usually not severe. These include constipation and bloating, acne, bad breath, body odor, nausea, weight gain, metallic taste, mood issues, headaches, and fatigue. Appendix D is a handout I give to all patients who are taking disulfiram.

There are reports that disulfiram can cause hypertension and even psychosis, as well as irritation of the liver. It is important to get blood tests regularly to monitor liver function.

Most of my patients are already on antimicrobials when they begin disulfiram. If they stay on these, the Herxheimer reactions are more severe. Therefore, when Herxheimer reactions are an issue, I taper the antimicrobials as I increase the dose of disulfiram. I am aware that some other physicians maintain their patients on disulfiram on additional antimicrobials, but many of my patients do not tolerate that level of polypharmacy.

It is too soon to claim that disulfiram is curing Lyme disease or babesiosis, but many patients are having sustained remissions off all treatment. And other patients who cannot progress the dose of disulfiram to the target level sometimes have significant benefit at lower doses. We are still on a steep learning curve regarding the use of disulfiram in the treatment of Lyme disease complex. Hopefully future research will elucidate disulfiram's antimicrobial action, the best method of delivery, and ways to decrease neurotoxicity. In the meantime, disulfiram appears to be a breakthrough in the treatment of Lyme disease for some patients.

NEW DRUG POSSIBILITIES: DAPSONE

Dr. Richard Horowitz has been recommending dapsone to treat persistent Lyme infection, citing evidence that it is effective at treating persister forms of *Bb* bacteria that survive regardless of antibiotic treatment.[13] Horowitz and Friedman have described the results of treating three patients with double-dose dapsone combination therapy (DDD-CT) for 7 to 8 weeks, and a retrospective review of an additional 38 patients. They described improvements in 98% with 45% remaining in remission for a year or longer.[14]

The combination therapy included tetracycline, rifampin, nystatin, hydroxychloroquine, and cimetidine (a gastric acid inhibitor and antihistamine that also can modulate immune function). While this regimen deserves further study, it should be noted that it is potentially quite toxic and should only be administered with careful surveillance.

STARTING ANTIMICROBIAL THERAPY

Where should patients with Lyme disease complex start treatment? It appears best to target *Bb* first. Even though a co-infection may be causing the more severe symptoms, *Bb* can suppress the immune system. Once the *Bb* bacterial load has been lessened, the patient's immune system has an improved capacity to take on the other microbes.

The choice of which antimicrobial to start first is always a toss-up. If a patient has *Candida* issues or seems fragile, generally the best option is to begin with an herb so as not to flare the yeast issues. Beyond Balance MC-BB1 is the most gentle herbal preparation for most people. But everyone is different; some tolerate the more powerful agents better than ones considered milder. Many patients who tolerate pharmaceuticals fairly well cannot tolerate any of the herbal extracts, even at low doses. Some patients tolerate IV antibiotics better than oral medications or herbs.

Some physicians routinely rotate antibiotics to prevent resistance, although most LLMDs have not found this to be necessary and prefer to stay with a regimen that is effective and is well tolerated. Another strategy that has been employed to treat Lyme disease complex is cyclic therapy. The theory underlying this approach is that stopping all antimicrobials temporarily will induce Bb into their growth phase. The patient will notice a flare in symptoms after a number of days off therapy, and will then restart aggressive treatment with a full dose regimen. This on-again-off-again treatment is repeated until the symptoms no longer return, at which time medications are discontinued. Laboratory studies have documented the success of this strategy in eradicating persister cells,[15] but the Herxheimer reactions can be severe.

That said, most LLMDs prescribe continuous dosing of medications, starting with fairly low doses of pharmaceutical antibiotics and gradually increasing the dose based on tolerance as described above. Once patients are stable on the antibiotics, herbal antimicrobials can be added one at a time, as the herbs appear to complement the effectiveness of the drugs.

The approach of "starting low and gradually increasing dosage" applies to the herbal extracts as well as to pharmaceutical medications. This can mean taking as little as one drop in water twice daily, and increasing the dose by one drop every four days. The individual patient's response is used as a guide; if there is a bad Herx reaction, the dose is decreased by one drop and held at that dose until symptoms resolve before increasing the dose or adding another agent. If there is a mild Herx reaction that resolves in a few days, the patient can continue increasing the dose; if there is a strong Herx, the patient should stay on the lower dose. By utilizing this method, the ideal dose for the individual can be ascertained. It is not uncommon, for example, for a patient to feel better on ten drops twice daily, but eleven drops consistently causes a bad flare, and therefore the patient should stay on the ten-drop dose.

INTRAVENOUS ANTIBIOTICS FOR LYME

Intravenous antibiotics result in higher blood levels, deeper cellular penetration, and more killing power than oral therapy. There are important considerations to address prior to initiating IVs:

- Have co-infections been identified?
- Has a thorough endocrine workup been performed?

- Is the patient's body performing appropriate detoxification?
- Are mold issues present?
- Has there been exposure to heavy metals?
- What about chemical/xenobiotic exposures?
- Are other allergens contributing to inflammation?
- Are there diet or GI issues? These may include food sensitivities, parasites, malabsorption, or small intestinal bacterial overgrowth (SIBO).
- Is there evidence of excess histamine activation?
- Does the patient have adequate emotional support?
- Does the patient have adequate physical support?
- What is their insurance coverage?

The majority of people with Lyme disease complex do not require IV antibiotics. However, it is generally accepted that aggressive IV antibiotic therapy deserves consideration in those presenting with the following conditions:

- Meningitis with elevated WBC and protein in the cerebrospinal fluid
- Acute disseminated infection in the first trimester of pregnancy
- Acute carditis, usually with third degree atrio-ventricular heart block
- Acute synovitis with high WBC in the joint fluid
- Motor neuron disease/ALS
- Failure of oral therapy
- Gastrointestinal intolerance of oral antibiotics

There are a number of IV drug options; those in Table 8–3 below are the most commonly employed agents. These can be started at lower doses than listed in the table to ensure tolerance. When weighing the risks versus benefits of IV therapy, it is prudent to remember that a severe Herxheimer reaction can potentially be fatal in a severely compromised patient, such as one with ALS.

IV ANTIBIOTICS MOST COMMONLY USED IN LYME DISEASE		
Drug	**Dose**	**Special Considerations**
Ceftriaxone	2 gm IV/day or pulse: 2 gm IV 2x/day, 4 days on, 3 days off	Risk of biliary sludge; co-administer ursodiol
Cefotaxime	2 gm IV every 8 hours	Monitor for liver toxicity
Doxycycline	400 mg IV/day	Requires central line
Azithromycin	500 mg IV/day	Requires central line

Table 8–3. Most commonly utilized IV antibiotics. Doses can vary.

In addition to the agents listed in Table 8–3, other antibiotics may be prescribed when patients are not responding adequately. These include vancomycin, daptomycin, meropenem, Primaxin, and Unasyn. IV antibiotics are rarely necessary if all co-infections and co-morbidities are being addressed.

INTRAMUSCULAR ANTIBIOTICS FOR LYME

There is another option when oral antibiotics are not doing the job: intramuscular (IM) antibiotics. These sometimes work as well as the IVs and do not require intravenous access, nor do they carry the risks of an indwelling central line or PICC line used by the majority of patients receiving IV therapy. As with all antibiotics, it is best to start IM antibiotics slowly to determine patient tolerance.

Bicillin L-A (penicillin G benzathine) is administered in doses up to 2.4 million units IM every other day. Ceftriaxone is given 1 gm intramuscularly daily; depending on pain at the injection site the dose can be increased to 2 gm daily.

ANTIBIOTICS TO TREAT THE CYSTIC FORM OF LYME

Lyme is a shape-shifter. Under stress, such as antibiotics, *Bb* can morph from the active spirochetal form to a relatively dormant cyst. Not only are the cysts resistant to the common antibiotics in Table 8–1, they also hide from immune detection. Alternative antibiotics are therefore employed to address this non-spirochetal, persistent form of *Bb*. The effectiveness of these antimicrobials has largely been demonstrated in the laboratory, which does not always translate to what occurs in the body.

The most commonly employed antimicrobial "cyst busters" are metronidazole (Flagyl)[16] and tinidazole (Tindamax).[17] However, other agents have demonstrated killing power in the laboratory: these include grapefruit seed extract[18] and the combination of Samento and Banderol by Nutramedix.[19] Hydroxychloroquine has also been recommended,[20] but clinical practice has not borne out its effectiveness in treating Lyme cysts. It is, however, helpful as an anti-inflammatory agent and intracellular alkalanizer (see below).

There are quite a few protocols on how to employ the different anti-cyst agents. Some doctors will prescribe the usual antibiotics five days a week, and on the remaining two days will prescribe metronidazole or tinidazole. Others will treat with the usual Lyme antibiotics, then add the cyst busters when the patient has clinically improved. Still others will treat with all antibiotics at once from the get-go.

This is one instance where the herbal extracts appear to have an advantage over the pharmaceutical options. Metronidazole causes severe side effects in a significant number of patients. Although tinidazole is much better tolerated, especially

once patients have stabilized, grapefruit seed extract can be used for the dual pur-
pose of addressing the cystic form of *Bb* and keeping yeast in check. In addition, the
combination of the Nutramedix products Samento and Banderol has demonstrated
effectiveness against both spirochetal and cystic forms of Lyme per in vitro studies;
adding this natural regimen to any treatment addresses the Lyme cysts as well. If
symptoms are not well controlled, then a trial of tinidazole should be considered.

BIOFILMS

It is now well established that most chronic infections exist in biofilm communities.
Dentists have long been aware of this issue in the form of dental plaque, the presence of which results in dental decay and gum disease. Biofilms are typically composed of groups of organisms—bacteria, fungi, protozoa, viruses, etc.—in which
the cells stick to one another within a slimy matrix of proteins, polysaccharides,
and DNA. In other words, the bugs are not floating freely in tissues or blood, but
rather existing within biofilm communities called quorums, where they are relatively protected from both antibiotics and immune detection.

There are several agents that appear to interrupt these matrices and make the
bugs more vulnerable. The most common are listed in Table 8–4.

AGENTS THAT COMBAT BIOFILMS	
Agent	**Considerations**
EDTA	Can be administered IV, orally, and via rectal suppository
	Often used for heavy metal detoxification
Boswellia	Also an anti-inflammatory agent
NAC	Assists liver detox and is a component of glutathione
Serrapeptase	Inexpensive and effective in vitro
Nattokinase	Also decreases coagulability
Lumbrokinase	Expensive but powerful; decreases coagulability
Samento and Banderol	Also effective against Lyme spirochetes and cysts and *Bartonella*

Table 8–4. Agents That Combat Biofilms.

TRANSFER FACTORS

Transfer factors are a class of messengers that provide cell-to-cell communication
in the immune system. As might be inferred from their name, transfer factors
essentially transfer the ability to express cell-mediated immunity from one place
to another, and this is not limited to one organism; they can transfer this ability
from immune donors to nonimmune recipients. What this means in practice is

that humans can receive immune system proteins that target disease from others—including animals.[21] Mothers download transfer factor to their newborns in their colostrum. Transfer factors specifically strengthen the Th1 immune response, as described in Chapter 18.

The company Researched Nutritionals distributes Transfer Factor Lyme-Plus, which boosts cellular immunity to *Bb* and its co-infections, with the exception of *Mycoplasma*. It also promotes immune reactivity to *Chlamydia pneumonia* and some viruses including EBV, CMV, and HHV6. This product is derived from the egg yolk of chickens that have been exposed to these pathogens. Transfer factors can cause Herxheimer reactions, so they should be started slowly in fragile patients.

CANDIDA ISSUES

Patients often present with yeast problems in the form of candidiasis sensitivity syndrome (CSS) even before starting antibiotics. (See Chapter 16 for a more complete discussion on CSS.) Use of pharmaceutical antibiotics will only exacerbate this problem. In this case, antimicrobial treatment should start with herbs while the patient works on getting the *Candida* issues under control with diet and antifungals. Even those people without prior *Candida* issues may experience an overgrowth of *Candida* in the intestines if taking antibiotics without concurrent use of anti-yeast agents and probiotics. This is because the beneficial bacteria such as lactobacilli that are normally present in the intestines produce lactic acid, which suppresses the growth of yeast. *Candida* overgrowth issues occur more often in women because female hormones favor yeast growth.[22]

Probiotics are essential. Patients on antibiotics should take 50–100 billion colony-forming units daily, and sometimes more. This can be taken in one dose, away from antibiotics but always with some food—otherwise, the unbuffered hydrochloric acid in the stomach will destroy the beneficial bacteria. In addition, it is a good idea to take *Saccharomyces boulardii*, a probiotic known as "yeast against yeast." *Saccharomyces* not only inhibits *Candida* growth, it also supports the immune system of the gut, and is reputed to be the best probiotic to control antibiotic-induced diarrhea with *Clostridium difficile* because it binds with *C. diff* toxins.[23]

All patients who are taking antibiotics should concurrently take an anti-yeast agent. Grapefruit seed extract (GSE), usually 500 mg twice daily, is highly recommended.[24] As previously noted, this is not only an antifungal, it also attacks *Bb* in its spirochetal and cyst forms.[25] GSE comes in capsules as well as a liquid extract; most people prefer the former since the latter tastes terrible. In addition, most women (and some men) benefit from taking Nystatin, 500,000 unit tablets, one to two tablets twice daily, to keep *Candida* at bay—Nystatin works in the gut only; it is not absorbed. There are a handful of other anti-yeast agents available over the counter, such as caprylic acid, undecylenic acid, and olive leaf and oregano extracts. If yeast issues appear more serious, then systemic agents such as fluconazole (Diflucan) may be needed.

HYDROXYCHLOROQUINE

Hydroxychloroquine (Plaquenil) has long been recommended as an anti-inflammatory agent for patients with rheumatoid arthritis and lupus. Since it is an antimalarial drug, it would seem be an effective agent to add to a regimen when treating babesiosis. However, in clinical practice it does not seem to be an effective anti-*Babesia* agent.

On the other hand, hydroxychloroquine often does help Lyme patients, both due to its anti-inflammatory action and because it alkalinizes the interior of the cell, thus making the intracellular antibiotics more effective. For these reasons, Dr. Sam Donta has suggested adding it to antibiotics such as doxycycline, azithromycin, and clarithromycin.[26] It has now become common practice among LLMDs to add hydroxychloroquine to many antibiotic regimens; note that the name brand Plaquenil is often better tolerated and more effective than the generic hydroxychloroquine; unfortunately, it is difficult to get insurance coverage for the brand name option. The usual dose is 200 mg twice daily.

Important: Patients on long-term treatment with hydroxychloroquine can develop retinal problems, which, if left unchecked, can lead to loss of vision. This is rare, but all patients should still have a baseline eye exam and repeat evaluations every six months if they are going to take hydroxychloroquine for a year or more.

HERXHEIMER REACTIONS

The flare in symptoms upon initiating treatment appears to be caused by a cytokine cascade—i.e. an inflammatory reaction—probably triggered by a release of cellular components in the microbes.[27] The dose of the antimicrobial should be reduced or the drug stopped altogether if the Herxheimer reaction results in significant distress. Herx reactions are not good for patients, and measures should be taken to mitigate them, although to some degree they are unavoidable. Table 8–5 lists interventions that usually lessen the severity of Herxheimer reactions.

COMMON INTERVENTIONS FOR HERXHEIMER REACTIONS		
Alkalinizing agents	Water with lemon	3+ liters/day
	Tri-Salts	½ tsp or 3 caps 3x/day
	Alka Seltzer Gold	2 tabs in water 3x/day
Detoxification support	Charcoal	2–6 caps 2x/day away from food, meds, and supplements
	Bentonite	2–4 Tbsp 2x/day away from food, meds, and supplements
	Nutramedix Burbur-Pinella	20–30 drops in water 3-4x/day; can increase to hourly if necessary
	Pekana Apo-Hepat, Renelix and Itires	Homeopathic drainage remedies that address liver, kidneys, and lymphatics respectively; 30 drops in water 3x/day
	Hot baths with 6 cups each of baking soda and Epsom salt	Hot baths are not always well tolerated, especially if there is severe dysautonomia
	Glutathione	Oral and/or intravenous
Anti-Inflammatory agents	Curcumin	Active ingredient in turmeric
	Boswellia	Inhibits 5-lipoxygenase, an enzyme responsible for inflammation
	Hemp oil CBD	Anti-inflammatory and pain reduction; works best if taken regularly
Analgesic agents	Pain medications	OTC and/or by prescription

Table 8–5. Common interventions for Herxheimer reactions.

THE OVERALL STRATEGY

It is already clear that everyone is different. When treating the patient with Lyme disease complex, there are often other issues that need to be addressed such as mold exposure, gut problems, and severe methylation problems. However, steps in the overall strategy are the same for the majority of patients:

- Provide infrastructure support (as detailed in following chapters). For example, if a patient has low adrenal and thyroid function, these deficiencies will not only contribute to fatigue but will also undermine immune competence. If yeast overgrowth and sensitization are an issue, address these before initiating antibiotics. Patients who are fragile and more ill often require infrastructure support before antimicrobial treatment.

- Begin antibiotics one at a time. Only progress the doses as tolerated.
- Add herbal extracts one at a time while maintaining the prescription antibiotics.
- If the patient remains stable and in remission, withdraw antibiotics one at a time and monitor (see below).

While it is great to have a general strategy, the fact is that it won't work for all people. Some patients simply don't tolerate any prescription antibiotics but respond well to herbal antimicrobials. Some have the opposite experience: herbal antimicrobials cause severe Herxheimer reactions at low doses, but pharmaceutical antibiotics work well. Every patient is different, and it is crucial to respect their biochemical individuality.

Some doctors practice a more aggressive approach and initially start chronically ill patients on three antibiotics at full doses. Their patients may suffer severe Herxheimer reactions, and either stop the regimen or fail to improve after a year of treatment. Upon review, the clinical picture is muddied; is is unclear which agent caused the die-off reaction and which may have benefited the patient. Any resumption of treatment means, in essence, starting from scratch. *It is essential to stagger interventions to determine how well a drug is tolerated and whether it is helping.*

The introduction of disulfiram allows for an alternative strategy. In Dr. Liegner's report, his first three patients had all been on years of multiple antibiotics, and two of them on intermittent intravenous antibiotics. They have all maintained sustained remissions after a few months of disulfiram and off all other treatment, although one had to undergo retreatment with disulfiram. At present we are recommending treatment for six to ten weeks after reaching the target dose.

HOW LONG TO TREAT?

After patients with Lyme disease complex have been treated and are free of symptoms, are they cured or are they in remission? The word "cure" suggests the bugs have been eradicated from the person's body. However, studies in animals and humans have demonstrated persistence of *Bb* even after aggressive IV antibiotics.[28] In addition, there are no tests that can determine if the bacteria are truly gone, and experience shows that some of these patients relapse. Therefore the word "remission" is more accurate than "cure." (The recent results of disulfiram in the laboratory and among some patients holds promise that *Bb* can effectively be eradicated in some patients.)

Once a patient's symptoms go into remission, the herbal regimen should be maintained while the pharmaceutical medications are discontinued one at a time. The antibiotics should be stopped cold turkey rather than tapered. A relapse in symptoms will necessitate restarting antibiotics; if a patient relapses, usually *Bartonella* is the first infection to recur.

Everyone who has lived with Lyme disease complex and then worked to achieve remission hopes that their immune system has recovered enough to keep the bugs in check effectively over the long term. After all, each of us has trillions of microbes in our bodies. One option is to do what Ned did—he went off all pharmaceutical antibiotics and then discontinued the herbal extracts. He has remained asymptomatic on diet and endocrine support. But he has also remained vigilant against the return of previous symptoms.

Another option is to stay on the antimicrobial herbs indefinitely. They keep the bugs at bay and also support the immune system, so this option affords some added insurance, although ongoing vigilance is still important.

There are some people whose symptoms are in remission while they are taking antimicrobial herbs and drugs, but who relapse whenever the antimicrobials are withdrawn. Persister cells may be the cause of recurrent relapses, but this situation necessitates investigating other factors that may still be in play. These include mold exposure, heavy metals, viral infections, undiagnosed co-infections, and emotional stress, which are discussed in greater detail in subsequent chapters.

WHAT ARE THE RISKS OF LONG-TERM ANTIBIOTICS?

A frequent question is whether antibiotics are harmful over time. It is always important to weigh the risks of treatment to the risks of withholding treatment; untreated infections clearly pose a more serious threat than antibiotics. The most common problem associated with prescription antibiotics, but not with most herbs, is disruption of the gut microbiome. Maintenance of probiotics and use of anti-yeast agents deals with some of this issue. Disturbance of the microbiome by antibiotics can lead to activation of *Clostridium difficle,* a bacteria which colonizes up to 3 percent of normal adults. *C. difficile* toxin can trigger a serious bout of colitis, and needs to be addressed quickly. This complication does not occur often, perhaps because most patients are taking *Saccharomyces boulardii*, which binds with the *C. difficile* toxins.[29] If a patient develops abdominal pain and diarrhea, antibiotics should be withheld while the patient is tested for *C. difficile*.

Antibiotics do not suppress the immune system as some websites allege, although some antibiotics are anti-inflammatory. The risk of injury to the liver and kidneys is low, but patients on antibiotics should have routine lab tests to monitor these issues.

One potential issue is that prolonged antibiotics may cause fatigue in some patients by compromising mitochondrial function.[30] A patient whose symptoms resolve with the exception of fatigue should consider stopping antibiotics and supporting mitochondrial function, as described in Chapter 21.

WHY DO PATIENTS RELAPSE?

Patients undergoing treatment for Lyme disease complex usually have a bumpy course. Gradually most start having more good days and fewer bad days, and eventually just feel well. But sometimes everything goes south—symptoms return, seemingly out of nowhere. What happened? Here are some possibilities:

- An increase in the dose of an antimicrobial has resulted in a Herxheimer reaction.
- The patient has stopped one or more antimicrobials.
- The patient had a mold exposure.
- The patient had an intercurrent infection such as a virus.
- The patient experienced significant emotional stress.
- The patient fell off his or her diet, particularly with sugar or alcohol.
- The patient took corticosteroids for poison ivy or asthma, or was given steroids during general anesthesia for surgery.
- The patient experienced physical trauma, particularly a bump to the head.
- The patient had another tick bite and a new infection.
- The patient went to a high-altitude location where the partial pressure of oxygen is decreased; this includes long-distance air travel.
- The patient had a vaccine, which resulted in systemic inflammation.

EDUCATION AND SUPPORT

It can easily feel overwhelming to patients when the multitude of issues that need attention are outlined at their first appointment. It is helpful if patients bring a family member or friend to take notes, and patients should also consider recording the session. It is crucial to proceed one step at a time, with the reassurance that even though the road will be bumpy, most of their issues are reversible. The odds are that they will get better; about 90 percent of patients treated as outlined in this book will improve 80 to 100 percent. But LLMDs do not have all the answers, and some Lyme disease complex patients have remained quite ill despite careful and thorough treatment. Most often these patients have immune function that is in overdrive—they react to almost all interventions, even at extremely low doses, and they often have autoimmune issues. (See Chapter 25.)

When health practitioners assume the responsibility of treating people with Lyme disease complex—the vast majority of whom have experienced neglect and often disdain from mainstream physicians—it is incumbent on them to be available on a timely basis to answer inevitable questions that arise during treatment—e.g. "When I added X, I felt Y. What should I do?" The practitioner should be available by phone or e-mail for problems that require immediate attention. I inform my patients to expect a response within twenty-four hours.

When patients embark on treatment, it is important that they know what to expect. It is common for those initiating treatment to describe small windows of feeling better, or more normal. Over time these windows get clearer and stay open longer. It is sometimes helpful for new patients to be in touch with other Lyme patients who are willing to share their own experiences and offer counsel and support. A well-run support group can be a blessing, but a poorly run one can dissolve into complaints rather than support. The Internet can also be a mixed bag; not all the information is accurate, and the people who are blogging their personal stories are often disproportionately sicker than the general population of Lyme patients— that's why they are indoors on their computers instead of getting on with their lives. Pamela Weintraub's book *Cure Unknown*[31] is an excellent resource for patients; Pam is a science journalist who has done an exceptional job describing the science and politics of Lyme disease.

Patients must have hope. That starts with education about the disease and the treatment process, and the knowledge that the vast majority of Lyme sufferers recover when their problems are addressed systematically and comprehensively.

TAKE-HOME POINTS

1. Infrastructure issues such as endocrine disruption and *Candida* sensitivity syndrome need to be addressed early in the course of treatment. This may need to occur before beginning antimicrobials, especially in a very ill patient.
2. Effectiveness and tolerance of antibiotics differs from patient to patient.
3. Lyme disease is best treated with a combination of intracellular and cell-wall agents.
4. Antimicrobial herbs can be quite effective, especially when paired with pharmaceutical antibiotics.
5. All antimicrobials should be introduced in a staggered fashion.
6. Disulfiram holds great promise as a well-tolerated agent against *Bb*.

7. The gut microbiome must be protected with probiotics and anti-yeast agents.
8. Consider treating with anti-cyst agents and biofilm busters.
9. Education, support, and hope are essential.

Chapter 9

Babesia

I f we were to prepare a Venn diagram with symptoms of the different tick-borne infections, 90 percent of symptoms would overlap. All these infections can cause fatigue, muscle and joint pains, sleep problems, and cognitive issues. However, a careful history can often tease out symptoms that suggest a particular infection.

Remember Ned's complaints of waking with night sweats, shortness of breath, and anxiety? Those are indicative of infection with *Babesia*. Remember the initial symptoms I had—high fever, shaking chills followed by drenching sweats, muscle aches, and headaches? Those are also indicative of babesiosis. Lyme by itself does not cause high fevers and drenching sweats.

WHAT IS *BABESIA*?

Babesiosis, also known as piroplasmosis, is a parasitic infection caused by a bug similar to *Plasmodium falciparum*, the protozoa responsible for malaria. *Babesia* has long been known as the cause of common infections in free living animals worldwide, but it wasn't until 1957 that this parasite was found to cause disease in humans. Some bio-theologians, those who study the synthesis of biology and religious doctrines, contend that this microbe caused the plague on the Egyptians' cattle described in the book of Exodus. Now it appears to be a partner in another plague.

There are several different strains of *Babesia*. Human babesiosis in North America is most often caused by *Babesia microti*, typically referred to as *B. microti*. In 1993, a second type of *Babesia* was identified in the state of Washington, initially dubbed *Babesia WA1*. It was believed that this strain was limited to the West Coast until doctors on the East Coast started testing for it. *Babesia WA1* has been renamed *Babesia duncani*. Note that patients can be infected simultaneously with both species of *Babesia*.

As far as we know, *Babesia* are spread primarily through blacklegged tick bites, but can also be spread via some wood ticks. There is evidence in animals that it can be transmitted orally and through sexual relations, as well as transplacentally from mother to fetus—a sobering thought. *Babesia* has also been transmitted through blood transfusions, and in May 2019 the FDA began recommending that agencies begin screening all blood donations for evidence of *Babesia*.[1]

Human infection with *Babesia* was first described in Europe, where it is caused by a different strain, *Babesia divergens*. *B. divergens* results in a more virulent disease, one that is often lethal. But infections in Europe have been rare, and most of the victims have had some prior compromise in their immune systems such as AIDS, leukemia, the removal of their spleens, or being very old or very young. Unfortunately this experience has led American physicians to believe that babesiosis in the United States is similar—specifically, that it is uncommon and only a problem for those who are immunosuppressed. However, the population at risk is much larger than they suspect.

Studies have shown that a co-infection of *Babesia* with *Bb* results in higher numbers of spirochetes. It is also likely that *Bb* enhances infection with *Babesia*. What is clear from clinical experience is that co-infections with other tick-borne pathogens results in more severe illness that is more difficult to treat.[2]

How common is *Babesia*? In one study of 192 individuals living on Nantucket (off Cape Cod), Block Island (near Rhode Island), and southeastern Connecticut, 39 percent of people with Lyme also had co-infections, mainly babesiosis.[3] Richard Horowitz, a physician in Hyde Park, New York, found *Babesia* in 43 percent of thirty ticks that he had analyzed from his county in upstate New York. He also took blood samples from 192 patients suspected of having Lyme and had them analyzed; 66 percent showed evidence of *Babesia*.[4] Clearly, babesiosis, like Lyme, is gaining ground. The CDC reported a twenty-six-fold increase in cases of babesiosis in Wisconsin between 2001 and 2015.[5]

ACUTE BABESIOSIS

Babesiosis, like all the tick-borne infections, is an emerging illness. What this means is that both researchers and clinicians are still on a steep learning curve and don't fully understand all the ways this protozoa can cause problems. It appears that infections can be asymptomatic and self-limited, but they can also result in a severe malaria-like illness with high fevers, chills, sweats, muscle aching, and fatigue. Acute infections can cause gastrointestinal symptoms such as nausea, vomiting, loss of appetite, and abdominal pain. *Babesia* sometimes trigger hemolytic anemia, a condition in which red blood cells are destroyed. Complaints of cough and shortness of breath are not uncommon.

Since these early symptoms usually coincide with Lyme disease, it is virtually impossible to tell which is the culprit. However, high fevers with shaking chills should immediately make one suspicious of babesiosis, particularly if these symptoms are recurrent. My own history, in which high fevers, bed-shaking chills, and drenching sweats returned each week and my spleen was enlarged was, in retrospect, classic for babesiosis. This infection can be fatal in people who are immunocompromised, particularly those who have had their spleens removed.

CHRONIC BABESIOSIS

Once babesiosis reaches a chronic stage it causes a wide array of additional symptoms similar to Lyme. Symptoms particularly suggestive of infection with *Babesia* include the following:

- Fevers, chills, flushing, and sweats; particularly night sweats that may be drenching
- Heat and cold intolerance
- Shortness of breath, often described as air hunger; cough
- Headaches and neck pain; often migraine headaches
- Cyclical nature to the symptoms, often with symptom flares every one to two weeks
- Exacerbation of underlying Lyme disease symptoms; particularly increased fatigue, joint aches, and cognitive dysfunction
- Sleep disorders
- Neuropathic pain: sharp, shooting, burning
- Neuropathic sensations: numbness, pins and needles, vibration, electric shocks, "creepy-crawlies"
- Exacerbation of mood disturbances, particularly anxiety and depression
- Dysautonomia, often with postural orthostatic tachycardia syndrome (POTS) and/or neurally mediated hypotension (NMH). (Dysautonomia is described in detail in Chapter 17.)
- The physical exam doesn't offer much else in the way of distinguishing clues, but enlargement of the liver and spleen, usually in recent infection, are more common in babesiosis than with Lyme disease alone.

DIAGNOSIS OF BABESIOSIS

Acute babesiosis can cause hemolytic anemia, which results in the release of bilirubin into the blood and may cause jaundice. Patients may notice a dark color to their urine and urinalysis may show evidence of hemoglobin and protein. People with severe cases can develop renal failure. Fragments of red cells may be visible on blood smears, which may also show *Babesia* parasites inside the red cells, but laboratory technicians need special expertise to accurately identify these microbes. The majority of cases go undetected by routine blood examination.

Laboratory testing for babesiosis, like Lyme, is far from foolproof. The most sensitive test is antibody detection: IgM and IgG to *B. microti* and *B. duncani*. However, in clinical experience these tests will still miss the diagnosis in nearly half of all patients with babesiosis.

One direct test is the PCR, a DNA test. However, this test has about 20 percent sensitivity, so it will miss the diagnosis four out of five times. Another is the FISH test, offered by IGeneX, which detects RNA specific for *Babesia*; this also has a sensitivity of about 20 percent.

As with testing for Lyme, the different *Babesia* tests often fail to indicate infection even when active illness is present. However, the chances of finding the infection are significantly improved when all available tests are combined. For example, I had two negative antibody levels and four negative PCRs on six different blood specimens before a seventh blood test detected a positive PCR.

Antibody tests for *B. microti* and *B. duncani* are not cross-reactive; this means that each must be ordered separately. A few labs, such as IGeneX, offers both IgG and IgM antibody tests for *Babesia duncani*, while Quest Diagnostics and LabCorp only offer the IgG.

Some clues on routine lab tests should raise suspicion of babesiosis. For example, elevations in liver enzymes, anemia, and a decrease in platelet count are common in people with recent *Babesia* infection. The white blood cell count may also be low, although this is more typical of *Ehrlichia*, *Anaplasma*, and *Rickettsia* infections.

If routine *Babesia* antibody tests are negative but the history is strongly suggestive—night sweats, air hunger, headaches—there is benefit to empirically treating for *Babesia*; the response to treatment often confirms the diagnosis. *Babesia* has become so prevalent that everyone who has Lyme disease should be evaluated for this infection even in the absence of classic symptoms. Abby and Lisa in Chapter 5 were positive for *Babesia* although they were asymptomatic at the time.

If the diagnosis of babesiosis is still unclear after history, physical exam, and lab tests, consider an A-Bab challenge. A-Bab is an herbal combination made by Byron White Formulas, Inc. Byron White is an herbalist in northern California who has created multiple herbal remedies for treating tick-borne and other infections. The most salient feature of these extracts is that they are both powerful and specific. A-Bab will work on *Babesia*, but will not touch the other infections like *Bb* and *Bartonella*. Therefore, in clinical experience, a Herxheimer reaction to A-Bab confirms babesiosis.

The recommended challenge is one drop of A-Bab in water twice daily for three days, then five drops twice daily for three days, then ten drops twice daily for three days, then fifteen drops twice daily for three weeks. There are three possible outcomes. The first is a Herxheimer reaction, which can occur on as low a dose as one drop. If that happens, patients are instructed to stop the challenge immediately, as they have their diagnosis. The second possibility is that nothing happens, even after three weeks on the last dose. This suggests, with 90 percent certainty in my experience, that infection with *Babesia* is not an issue. The third possibility occurs rarely—there is no Herxheimer reaction, but after three weeks the patient reports feeling much better. Some people just don't Herx, but the improvement suggests that the A-Bab was in fact treating a *Babesia* infection.

TREATMENT OF BABESIOSIS

As with Lyme disease, the sooner the treatment commences, the better the outcome, although it is now well accepted that *Babesia* can persist after treatment and cause recurrent symptoms.[6] This knowledge has led to the recommendation that anyone who has suffered from babesiosis should never donate blood.[7]

Treatment of acute babesiosis is essentially the same as for chronic babesiosis, although the duration of treatment will be shorter. The only good news about infection with *Babesia* is that there are many treatment options; all antimalarial drugs and herbs are active against this protozoa. Prior to the year 2000, the recommended treatment was a combination of clindamycin and quinine; however, many patients who were prescribed this duo of medications became so ill from the quinine that they could not complete the treatment. In 2000, Krause and colleagues described treatment with a combination of azithromycin (Zithromax) and atovaquone (Mepron), and this regimen has become the standard treatment recommendation.[8] The macrolide antibiotics, including azithromycin and clarithromycin (Biaxin), have some anti-*Babesia* activity, and paired with atovaquone, help prevent resistance to treatment. The most common pharmaceutical regimens to treat *Babesia* are listed in Table 9–1.

Patients differ in which treatment regimens are most effective and best tolerated. Malarone is a combination of two antimalarials—atovaquone and proguanil—while Mepron (atovaquone) is a single drug suspension. Malarone appears to be tolerated better than Mepron for many though not all patients. A patient with acute babesiosis who was previously healthy may start on a full dosage, but the chronically infected patient is advised to start slowly and increase the dose only as tolerated. For example, rather than the recommended dose of Malarone of two tablets twice a day, the chronically ill person may start Malarone at one tablet daily or even one tablet every other day, and increase gradually. Herxheimer reactions are the norm.

Once stable on a medication regimen, antimicrobial herbs can be slowly introduced to increase effectiveness. Most herbal extracts are added at one drop twice

MEDICATIONS TO TREAT BABESIOSIS				
Brand Name	Generic	How Supplied	Dose	Considerations
Mepron	Atovaquone	750 mg/5 cc suspension	5 cc 2x/day	Paired with a macrolide
Malarone	Atovaquone + proguanil	250/100 mg tablets	2 tabs 2x/ day	May be paired with a macrolide
Lariam	Mefloquine	250 mg tablets	1 tab 3x/ week	Can cause nightmares, psychosis, depression, and anxiety—I don't prescribe it
Coartem	Artemether/ lumefantrine	20/120 mg tablets	4 tabs 2x/ day for 3 days	May repeat every 1–3 weeks; can cause severe Q-T prolongation
Cleocin	Clindamycin	300 mg tablets	1–2 tabs 3x/ day	No longer paired with quinine due to side effects, but often useful as adjunct treatment
Doryx	Doxycycline	100 mg capsules	2 caps 2x/ day	Usually combined with malarone and hydroxychloroquine

Table 9–1. Medications to treat babesiosis. Dosages are average for adults, and will vary based on tolerance and effectiveness.

daily, then increased by one drop every four to five days as tolerated. Artemisinin and *Mimosa pudica* are started at one capsule per day, then slowly increased to full dosage. If at any point a patient Herxes, the dose should be cut back to previous levels and sustained at that dose for a week or more before trying to progress again. Table 9–2 lists the most common herbs used in the treatment of babesiosis.

Artemisinin merits special mention. In 2015 the Nobel Prize for medicine went to Professor Youyou Tu for her work isolating artemisinin from *Artemisia annua*. Artemisinin became the treatment of choice for malaria resistant to the quinolone-based antimalarial drugs. The result was a wholesale decrease in malaria deaths; from 2000 to 2012 the global death rate dropped an incredible 42 percent.[9] In 2019 the *Lancet* reported an increase in artemisinin-resistant malaria in southeast Asia,[10] but resistance has not been documented with *Babesia*.

Artemisinin stimulates the cytochrome enzymes in the body. These enzymes function to metabolize many drugs, including artemisinin itself. Any medication which stimulates the cytochrome pathway, whether pharmaceutical or herbal in origin, has the potential to lower circulating levels of other drugs also metabolized by the cytochrome enzymes, and thereby decrease their effectiveness. This is why it is often recommended to pulse artemisinin four days on, three days off—doing

HERBAL EXTRACTS USED TO TREAT BABESIOSIS			
Product	**Company**	**Dosage**	**Comments**
A-Bab	Byron White	Up to 25 drops 2x/day	Powerful, can cause severe Herx reactions
MC-Bab1	Beyond Balance	Up to 25 drops 2x/day	Mild for most people; active against *B.microti*
MC-Bab2	Beyond Balance	Up to 25 drops 2x/day	Mild for most people; active against *B.duncani*
MC-Bab3	Beyond Balance	Up to 25 drops 2x/day	Mild for most people; active against both strains of *Babesia*
Artemisinin	Allergy Research Group; Researched Nutritionals and others	Up to 200 mg 2x/day, 4 days on and 3 days off	Active component of *Artemisia*; stimulates cytochrome enzymes
Mimosa pudica	Hopkinton Pharmacy	Up to 3 caps 2x/day	Asian antimalarial herb
Cryptolepis	Woodland Essence, Infuserve, Researched Nutritionals (Crypto-plus)	Up to 1 tbsp 3x/day	African antimalarial
Quina	Nutramedics	Up to 25 drops 3x/day	Mild for most people

Table 9–2. Herbal extracts used to treat babesiosis. Dosages vary according to tolerance.

so gives the cytochrome enzymes a chance to normalize. Alternatively, artemisinin can be taken every other day. In addition, eating grapefruit or taking grapefruit seed extract capsules as well as silymarin (milk thistle) is recommended, as these suppress the cytochrome enzymes and thereby counter the stimulatory effect of the artemisinin. The antibiotic clarithromycin will also suppress the cytochrome enzymes.

> *Let's return to Ned, who received IV antibiotics followed by oral antibiotics in Colombia, and has now returned to the United States. I added the antimalarial drug Malarone to Ned's regimen to treat babesiosis, and he continued to improve. The next steps were adding Byron White's A-L Complex for Lyme then A-Bab for babesiosis; the latter caused a mild Herx but he was able to progress to the full dosage quickly.*
>
> *Once Ned was feeling much better, he became aware that ingesting carbohydrates, alcohol, or caffeine resulted in fatigue and grogginess, so he maintained a low-glycemic diet. Laboratory workup also revealed genetic*

mutations in his methylation pathways (homozygous for MTHFR C677T) and endocrine issues including low DHEA, elevated reverse T3, and diabetes insipidus. These issues will be addressed in subsequent chapters.

After a few months Ned stopped the antibacterial and antimalarial medications and only took the extracts; he continued to feel well. After a few more months he stopped the extracts and has remained asymptomatic.

The general strategy is to start on pharmaceuticals, then add herbal extracts, then stop the pharmaceuticals and later stop the extracts. But general strategy does not work for everyone. Some patients do not tolerate the pharmaceuticals at all, yet do well on the herbs. Surprisingly, there are many patients who do well on the pharmaceuticals but don't tolerate herbs. There are also a small percentage of patients who tolerate neither; they need to consider alternatives like ozone, Rife machines, and low-dose immunotherapy, options described in Chapter 23.

There is always the question of when to stop treatment. A rule of thumb used by many LLMDs when they began treating patients with Lyme disease complex was to treat for two additional months after a patient became asymptomatic. Sadly, lots of people have relapsed, even after being asymptomatic for months or even years. A more practical approach has evolved, that of discontinuing use of pharmaceutical medications after symptoms have resolved, but considering the option of staying on the herbs for long-term maintenance.

DISULFIRAM

In Chapter 7, I described the experience of treating Lyme disease with disulfiram both in the laboratory as well as in patients. In 1979, Scheibel and colleagues found that disulfiram inhibits the human malaria protozoa *Plasmodium falciparum*.[11] It therefore comes as no surprise that disulfiram is also effective against *Babesia,* and that was the experience of Ken Liegner when he treated patients with disulfiram with both Lyme disease and babesiosis.[12] Treatment with disulfiram for most of my patients begins at 31.25 mg (⅛ of a 250 mg tablet) every three days, and increased every two weeks as tolerated. Occasional patients have to lower the starting dose because of Herxheimer reactions. The average adult target dose depends on weight but also drug tolerance. Patients stay on the target dose for about six to ten weeks before stopping the medication. Chapter 7 provides additional details on the use of disulfiram. While disulfiram has been effective in many patients with babesiosis, its use has been limited by Herxheimer reactions and neurotoxicity.

At the time of this writing, there are no studies on the treatment of *Babesia* with disulfiram, although the Stanford group that found disulfiram to be extremely powerful against *Bb*[13] are planning to study the effect of disulfiram against *Babesia* in their laboratory.* In the meantime, several practitioners including this author are having early, yet promising, success with this treatment.

TAKE-HOME POINTS

1. *Babesia* is a common co-infection. Suspect it in everyone who has Lyme.
2. There are symptoms strongly suggestive of babesiosis—such as night sweats, air hunger, and headaches—but some people do not have this classic presentation.
3. Laboratory tests for babesiosis are not sensitive. Consider an A-Bab challenge or a therapeutic trial of anti-*Babesia* medications if a patient is not responding to treatment for Lyme.

---

* Personal communication, Jayakumar Rajadas and Venkata Raveendra Pothineni.

Chapter 10

Bartonella

R emember Mike from Chapter 5? He developed a bull's-eye rash and fatigue when he was fifty-one years old, after taking a walk in the Indiana woods. But on close questioning he also described having chronic symptoms since childhood, chief among them anxiety and depression. This was not a mild mood disorder; he was disabled owing to their severity. He also had neuropathic symptoms. It turns out that in addition to acute Lyme, he had Lyme disease complex since he was young with a *Bartonella* co-infection, which is notorious for causing psychiatric disorders and neuropathy.[1]

WHAT IS *BARTONELLA*?

Bartonella henselae is the cause of cat scratch disease (CSD), an infection transmitted through either a cat's scratch or a wound in the skin that is exposed to cat saliva. On a disquieting note, the *Bartonella* microbe is typically carried in flea feces, which can be found under the nails of the cat. Biting insects such as sand flies, lice, and fleas can also transmit *Bartonella*. Of particular interest here, *Bartonella* can be tick-borne.[2]

In September 2001, Eugene Eskow and colleagues described four patients with histories of tick bites and Lyme disease.[3] The patients had not responded appropriately to aggressive antibiotic therapy for Lyme and were suffering from severe nervous system problems including seizures. Laboratory testing for other tick-borne infections (babesiosis and ehrlichiosis) was negative, but Eskow had read a report from the Netherlands that found evidence of *Bartonella* infection in 70 percent of ticks tested.[4] When Eskow tested the blood in these four patients, he found they all had antibodies to *Bartonella*. In addition, analyses of cerebrospinal fluid revealed positive PCR for *Bartonella*. The patients went on treatment with appropriate antibiotics for *Bartonella* and they recovered.

Since then *Bartonella* has been increasingly recognized as a tick-borne pathogen. Unfortunately, testing for *Bartonella* is notoriously poor, and it's impossible to accurately determine how many people with Lyme are co-infected with this bacteria. However, its prevalence in ticks is high. A 2004 survey of deer ticks in New Jersey revealed *Bb* in 34 percent, *Babesia* in 8 percent, *Ehrlichia* in 2 percent, and *Bartonella* in 35 percent.[5] In the population of patients with Lyme disease complex, it is estimated that more than half are clinically diagnosed with *Bartonella*; overall, it may be the most common tick-borne pathogen.

There are over two dozen known species of *Bartonella*, although not all of them cause infection in humans. *Bartonella henselae* causes CSD and *Bartonella quintana* is the cause of trench mouth. Some people infected with *Bartonella* are completely asymptomatic. The medical literature states that 90 percent of people with CSD recover without antibiotic treatment. But when combined with *Bb* as a tick-borne microbe, *Bartonella* regularly causes severe pain and suffering. *Bartonella* can infect the endothelium or inner lining of blood vessels, causing vasculitis and circulatory issues; on rare occasions it has caused strokes.[6] It often triggers autoimmune issues,[7] and it has a particular predilection for the nervous system, triggering severe neuropsychiatric symptoms.[8]

CLINICAL PRESENTATION OF *BARTONELLA*

Consider *Bartonella* when someone with acute Lyme disease has an erythema migrans rash that itches, is scaly, or has a blistering vesicular eruption. Also be suspicious if the person has enlarged lymph nodes, complains of gastrointestinal symptoms, or has the sudden onset of anxiety or other neuropsychiatric symptoms.

While *Bartonella* infection can cause the same symptoms as those associated with other tick-borne infections, in particular it causes problems in the nervous system, gastrointestinal system, skin, eyes, and urinary tract. *Bartonella* symptoms are grouped below.

Common systemic symptoms
- Fatigue
- Headaches
- Joint pains
- Muscle aches

Central nervous system symptoms
- Anxiety, agitation, panic attacks
- Depression
- Irritability, rage
- Cognitive dysfunction
- Sleep disorders
- Photophobia (light sensitivity) and/or hyperacusis (sound sensitivity)

- Seizures or seizure-like activity
- Psychosis, bipolar disorder
- Transverse myelitis

Peripheral nervous system symptoms
- Neuropathic pain: sharp, shooting, burning
- Neuropathic sensations: numbness, pins and needles, vibration, electric shocks, "creepy-crawlies"
- Sore soles, especially in the morning, on initial weight-bearing (this can also be a symptom of babesiosis)
- Palsies, weakness

Skin symptoms
- Striae—red streaks that may appear similar to stretch marks but do not follow normal skin planes
- Red papules
- Spider veins
- Skin mottling—livedo reticularis
- Pruritis—itching
- Subcutaneous nodules—erythema nodosum
- Bacillary angiomatosis—small red vascular nodules

Eye symptoms and conditions
- Blurry vision, often with frequent prescription changes
- Difficulty focusing
- Floaters
- Diplopia—double vision
- Conjunctivitis—pink eye
- Retinitis—inflammation of the retina
- Uveitis—eye inflammation
- Choroiditis—inflammation in the choroid, a layer of between the white of the eye and the retina
- Parinaud's Oculoglandular syndrome (POGS)—inflammation of the conjunctivae, eyelid, or adjacent skin with regional lymphadenopathy
- Retinal vasculitis—inflammation of the vascular branches of the retinal artery

Gastrointestinal system symptoms
- Nausea
- Constipation and/or diarrhea
- Abdominal pain
  - Mesenteric adenitis

- o Gastritis
- o Duodenitis
- o Inflammatory bowel disease
- Heartburn
- Liver involvement
  - o Peliosis hepatis—a tumor-like lesion composed of multiple blood-filled cavities
  - o Hypoechogenic/granulomatous lesions
- Spleen involvement
  - o Hypoechogenic/granulomatous lesions

Other symptoms often associated with Bartonella *infection*
- Sore throats
- Lymphadenopathy—enlarged lymph nodes
- Pelvic pain
- Urinary issues—urethritis, interstitial cystitis, neuropathic bladder with difficulty voiding or incontinence

Children
- Oppositional defiance disorder
- Autism spectrum disorders
- Meltdowns, tantrums, rages
- Learning problems
- Attention deficit disorder with or without hyperactivity

Serious Bartonella *issues*
- Vegetative endocarditis—heart valve infections
- Vasculitis, which can result in strokes
- Transverse myelitis
- Psychosis

Mark recalled having an insect bite when was twelve years old, but wasn't certain if it was a tick attachment. He subsequently developed fatigue, depression, anxiety, irritability with rage episodes, headaches, concentration difficulties, joint pains, shooting pains, numbness and tingling, vibration sensation, blurry vision, twitching, tremors, myoclonic jerks, tinnitus, dental pain, nausea, abdominal cramps with diarrhea, heat and cold intolerance, light sensitivity, night sweats, sore throats, and sleep issues. At one point he was diagnosed with H. pylori and treated with amoxicillin, after which his energy, headaches, and cognition partially improved.

> *On physical exam Mark exhibited deep red horizontal stripes on his back;*
> *it looked as if he had been whipped. He thought they were stretch marks,*
> *although he was not overweight. Mark tested positive for Lyme and Babesia,*
> *but the disproportionate neurological symptoms, sore throats, and gastroin-*
> *testinal symptoms suggested concurrent* Bartonella *infection.*

The stripes on his back are known as striae.[9] They are often red or violet in color and are associated with new blood vessel formation. They involve a different level of the dermis than the usual stretch marks that are associated with rapid weight gain, and *Bartonella* striae do not follow normal skin planes. They are often in armpits, thighs, breasts, buttocks, back, and behind knees. As occurs with regular stretch marks, they can turn red, pink, and white over time. While these striae are most commonly associated with *Bartonella*, they have also been seen with *Mycoplasma* infection, and perhaps may occur in other infections as well.

THE PRESENTATION OF *BARTONELLA* IN CHILDREN

Children can acquire *Bartonella* from tick attachments, cat scratches, and perhaps from other biting insects, but they can also get this infection *in utero* from infected mothers (see Chapter 24). Children with *Bartonella* often present with mood, behavioral, and learning issues. A common scenario is that the child began tantruming at age two, which is considered normal, but the tantrums were particularly severe with uncontrollable outbursts of anger, and continued until the child was older, when other symptoms developed such as fatigue, muscle pains, and joint pains. The health of the mother should be investigated whenever a youngster presents with a tick-borne infection, as congenital *Bartonella* infection should always be considered. Teenagers with *Bartonella* may present with severe anxiety, depression, irritability, and eating disorders.

> *Brad's parents brought him to see me when he was eleven years old. He was*
> *different from his older sister from early infancy—he never made eye contact*
> *and never napped. He was always moving and did not want to be held or*
> *swaddled. He was scratched by a cat when he was two years old and devel-*
> *oped enlarged lymph nodes in his neck. As a toddler he began experiencing*
> *episodes of inconsolable crying and rocking. These episodes worsened, and by*
> *the time he was five years old he clearly had focus issues and was not inter-*
> *ested in reading.*
>
> *Brad worsened around age eight. He became agitated and easily over-*
> *whelmed. He had outbursts of anger and rage, and often had to be held by*
> *his father so he didn't destroy the house. Brad described having dark times*

when he had intrusive thoughts such as hurting himself and others. He had severe anxiety and refused to go to school. He had pseudo-seizures, when he would suddenly flop to the ground but be totally conscious. Other symptoms included sharp chest pains associated with shortness of breath; abdominal pain with nausea, constipation and flatulence; knee, neck, and spine pain; light-headedness, sound sensitivity, fatigue, and sugar cravings. Brad's mood issues were so severe that he underwent two psychiatric hospitalizations. His psychiatrist tried several medications, and there was some improvement on Prozac and Trileptal, an antiepileptic drug that is also prescribed as a mood stabilizer.

Brad's psychiatrist was also savvy enough to get him tested for tick-borne infections. The results were as follows:

Lyme Band	IgM	IgG
18 kDa	+	-
23–25 kDa	-	-
28 kDa	-	+
30 kDa		-
31 kDa	IND	-
34 kDa	-	-
39 kDa		+
41 kDa	+	+++
45 kDa	-	-
58 kDa	+	
66 kDa	-	-
83–93 kDa	IND	-

Co-infection testing:
Bartonella henselae IgG   >1:256
Babesia duncani IgG   40

Remember, bands 18 and 39 are quite specific for Lyme. Before Brad had even walked into my office, he was diagnosed with Lyme disease, babesiosis, and bartonellosis. I suspect that Brad had congenital Lyme and babesiosis, and was additionally infected with Bartonella *when he had a cat scratch at age two. Brad's mom clearly had some cognitive issues herself, but has not pursued evaluation.*

TESTING FOR *BARTONELLA*

Bartonella testing is not very reliable, with a high rate of false negative results. Most labs only test for *B. henselae* and *B. quintana*, and some infections are caused by other *Bartonella* species. Serologic testing, i.e. detecting IgM and IgG antibodies, is the most common method to detect *Bartonella*, but my experience is that it is only about 10 to 20 percent sensitive in most commercial labs—it will miss the diagnosis eight to nine out of ten times. IGeneX offers a *Bartonella* Western blot that tests for *B. henselae*, *B. quintana*, *B. elizabethae*, and *B. vinsonii*, yielding higher sensitivity. While IgM positivity suggests active infection, it is not as specific as IgG. Note that a positive IgG test could result from an old resolved infection as well as from a current one.

IGeneX also offers the Bartonella IgX Spot, an enzyme linked immunospot assay, which detects human T cells reactive to *Bartonella* specific antigens. The IgX Spot can provide a diagnosis within a few days of tick attachment, and can detect immune activity against four *Bartonella* species: *B. henselae*, *B. quintana*, *B. elizabethae*, and *B. vinsonii.**

Direct detection via PCR, i.e. DNA testing, is likewise not sensitive, although if positive confirms active infection. Galaxy Diagnostics offers an enhanced PCR test for *Bartonella*. They first use a patented media to culture the serum, which increases the number of bacteria in a sample, then perform specialized PCR testing—they claim this increases sensitivity tenfold. The results can take up to two months. IGeneX offers a different method of direct detection, the *Bartonella* FISH test, which detects RNA rather than DNA. If positive, this is also indicative of an active infection.

One additional test is vascular endothelial growth factor (VEGF). *Bartonella* can induce production of this cytokine, which stimulates the proliferation of endothelial cells that line blood vessels. Though not a sensitive indicator, an elevation in VEGF is strongly suggestive of active *Bartonella* infection.[10]

As with *Babesia*, the more tests that are done, the higher the chance of finding laboratory evidence of infection. However, the patient's clinical presentation will usually raise suspicion. In particular, when neurological symptoms are disproportionately greater than musculoskeletal symptoms, when there are gastrointestinal issues, frequent sore throats, enlarged lymph nodes, or sore soles, then *Bartonella* is likely. The presence of dermatological striae is a big tip-off. If a patient continues to be symptomatic after treatment for other tick-borne infections, consider *Bartonella*.

If uncertain diagnostically, a challenge with A-Bart, similar to the A-Bab challenge described in the previous chapter, can be performed. A-Bart is a Byron White

---

*   The immunoblot and T cell testing is available in Germany at ArminLabs.

herbal formula that is both powerful and specific for *Bartonella*. Patients take one drop in water twice daily for three days, then five drops twice daily for three days, then ten drops twice daily for three days, then fifteen drops twice daily for three weeks. A Herx reaction yields the diagnosis, and the challenge should be stopped immediately if there is a flare in symptoms. Clinical experience is that the A-Bart challenge is 90 percent sensitive.

When I initially saw Mike with acute Lyme disease (Chapter 4), I prescribed cefuroxime and clarithromycin to treat Bb as well as Nystatin and probiotics for the gut. On follow-up he reported that he did not have a Herx, his energy was returning, and he noticed some decrease in his chronic anxiety and depression. I then recommended something I later regretted. Since Mike did not flare at all on the antibiotics, I suspected that he was one of those who simply did not Herx. I suggested he take A-Bart at the dose of fifteen drops twice daily, instead of slowly progressing the dose. Within an hour of taking the first dose he had a severe panic attack. Well, we had our diagnosis, but I apologized to Mike.

BARTONELLA AND AUTOIMMUNITY

Bartonella can induce autoimmune disease.[11] *Bartonella* has been associated with autoimmune thyroiditis,[12] autoimmune hemolytic anemia,[13] juvenile rheumatoid arthritis,[14] IgA nephropathy,[15,16] arthropathies,[17,18,19,20] polyneuropathy,[21,22] Guillain-Barré syndrome,[23] chronic vasculitis,[24] immune thrombocytopenic purpura,[26] transverse myelitis,[27] and Henoch-Schonlein purpura.[28,29] *Bartonella* can trigger anti-neuronal antibodies causing pediatric acute-onset neuropsychological syndrome (PANS).[30] (See Chapter 17 for more information on PANS.) *Bartonella* infection is associated with inflammatory bowel disease as described later in this chapter. It is likely that many of the symptoms associated with *Bartonella* co-infections have an autoimmune pathophysiology.

TREATMENT OF *BARTONELLA* INFECTION

Many antibiotics that are effective against *Bartonella* in the laboratory are not as successful in people. Antibiotics for *Bartonella* that work in culture and are routinely used against *Bb*, such as azithromycin, clarithromycin, and doxycycline, may be ineffective when treating tick-borne *Bartonella* illness in people. Sometimes double or triple antibiotic therapy is needed to treat this infection.[31]

A good antibiotic for *Bartonella* is sulfamethoxazole-trimethoprim (SMZ-TMP, Bactrim, or Septra), a sulfa drug commonly prescribed for urinary infections, sinusitis, and methicillin-resistant *Staphylococcus aureus* (MRSA). SMZ-TMP is generally well tolerated, although it is more likely than other antibiotics to cause allergic reactions. Kidney function needs to be monitored when employed for long-term use.

Another drug of choice is rifampin, an anti-tuberculosis drug. The biggest challenge with this medication is that, like artemisinin, it stimulates a set of enzymes called cytochromes that metabolize many other medications, thereby lowering their levels in the bloodstream and rendering them less effective. (Cytochrome enzymes metabolize artemisinin but do not metabolize rifampin.) For example, giving rifampin to a person taking thyroid replacement can result in the need to increase their thyroid medication dosage because it will be metabolized more quickly. Rifampin will also lower circulating levels of atovaquone, the antimalarial drug often used to treat *Babesia*.

As described in Chapter 9, grapefruit, grapefruit seed extract, and silymarin (milk thistle) have the opposite impact on the cytochrome enzymes, and are therefore recommended to be taken concurrently with rifampin. Clarithromycin, a drug sometimes used to treat Lyme that possesses some activity against *Bartonella,* is a good medication to pair with rifampin because it also has the side effect of suppressing cytochromes. Doxycycline is also often paired with rifampin.

Rifabutin is similar to rifampin, but can be taken with food, while rifampin needs to be taken without food. Another anti-tuberculosis drug that has demonstrated activity against *Bartonella* is pyrazinamide. This drug does not stimulate cytochrome enzymes, and is a good alternative when a patient is on multiple medications.

The most effective antibiotics against *Bartonella* are the fluoroquinolones, particularly ciprofloxacin (Cipro) and levofloxacin (Levaquin). The problem is that these antibiotics have the potential of causing a long list of side effects, some of which, such as muscle and joint pains, can mimic a Herxheimer reaction. More worrisome is that these antibiotics can also cause problems even after they are discontinued. Chief among these is tendonitis, such as tennis elbow and Achilles tendonitis. In severe cases it has led to ruptured tendons. Pretreatment with high doses of magnesium can protect tendons, but this preventive measure is far from fail-safe.[32]

Because of the potential side effects caused by fluoroquinolones, they should be employed only as a last resort and with caution. Patients should take the maximum oral dose of magnesium they can tolerate without causing diarrhea before starting the drug, be advised of tendonitis symptoms, and stop the antibiotic if there is the slightest hint of tendon inflammation. If a patient does develop tendonitis, intravenous magnesium and vitamin C can help; nevertheless, some people continue to have ongoing tendonitis issues.

In addition to the above medications, most patients experience better control of *Bartonella* by adding a cell wall drug such as cefdinir, cefuroxime, amoxicillin, or amoxicillin-clavulanate. These will target *Bartonella* in extra-cellular spaces, as well as adding firepower to the treatment of *Bb*. Table 10–1 lists the most common antibiotics used to treat *Bartonella*.

MEDICATIONS TO TREAT BARTONELLOSIS				
Brand Name	Generic	How Supplied	Dose	Considerations
Bactrim/ Septra	Sulfamethoxazole-Trimethoprim	SS (400/80) DS (800/160)	Up to 1 tab DS, 2x/day	Frequent allergic reactions
Rifadin	Rifampin	150 mg tabs 300 mg tabs	600 mg daily	Many drug interactions; take on empty stomach, turns urine orange
Mycobutin	Rifabutin	150 mg tabs	300 mg daily	Many drug interactions; turns urine orange
Rifater	Pyrazinamide	500 mg tabs	1-2 tabs twice daily	Monitor uric acid
Levaquin	Levofloxacin	500 mg tabs	1 tab daily	Caution: tendonitis
Cipro	Ciprofloxacin	500 mg tabs	1 tab 2x/day	Caution: tendonitis
Biaxin	Clarithromycin	500 mg tabs	1 tab 2x/day	Not potent as a single drug
Zithromax	Azithromycin	500 mg tabs	1 tab daily	Not potent as a single drug
Doryx	Doxycycline	100 mg tabs	2 tabs 2x/day	Not potent as a single drug

Table 10–1. Medications to treat bartonellosis. Dosages are average for adults, and will vary based on tolerance and effectiveness.

To summarize, here are *Bartonella* antibiotic treatment protocols:

- SMZ-TMP + rifampin/rifabutin/pyrazinamide +/- cell wall drug
- SMZ-TMP + macrolide +/- cell wall drug
- SMZ-TMP + doxycycline +/- cell wall drug
- Rifampin/rifabutin/pyrazinamide + macrolide +/- cell wall drug
- Rifampin/rifabutin/pyrazinamide + doxycycline +/- cell wall drug
- Levofloxacin +/- cell wall drug
- Ciprofloxacin +/- cell wall drug

When symptoms are severe or when oral antibiotics are not tolerated, intravenous medications need to be considered. IV Levaquin, Cipro, gentamicin, and vancomycin have all been effective—the usual considerations of using fluoroquinolones still apply. Oral vancomycin, which is not systemically absorbed, has also been effective in treating gastrointestinal *Bartonella* infections. Methylene blue is a recent addition to our armamentarium to treat this infection, but it is unclear at this time if it has advantages over the known alternatives.

Disulfiram was mentioned in both Chapters 9 and 10 as a new treatment for both Lyme and babesiosis. My clinical experience is that it clearly targets *Bartonella*, but it does not appear as effective as it is against *Bb* and *Babesia*. The Stanford group that found disulfiram to be extremely powerful against *Bb*[33,34] are planning to study the effectiveness of disulfiram against *Bartonella* in their laboratory.[†]

As with the treatment of *Bb* and *Babesia*, clinical experience is that patients do better when antimicrobial herbs are added. It is always a toss-up whether to start pharmaceuticals or herbs first, but often patients tolerate the drugs better than the herbs. Either way, always start with low doses because Herxheimer reactions can be severe. Table 10–2 lists herbal extracts that have antimicrobial activity against *Bartonella*. Other companies make extracts that have also been used effectively.

HERBAL TREATMENTS FOR BARTONELLOSIS			
Product	Company	Dosage	Comments
A-Bart	Byron White	Up to 25 drops 2x/day	Powerful, can cause severe Herx reactions
MC-Bar1	Beyond Balance	Up to 25 drops 2x/day	Mild for most people
MC-Bar2	Beyond Balance	Up to 25 drops 2x/day	Add to McBar1
BLt	Researched Nutritionals	Up to 35 drops 2x/day	Active against *Bb* and *Bartonella*
Japanese knotweed a.k.a. Resveratrol	Multiple sources	Up to 2000 mg 2x/day	Also has anti-inflammatory action
Banderol	Nutramedics	Up to 25 drops 2x/day	Usually paired with Samento

Table 10–2. Herbal extracts used to treat bartonellosis. Dosages vary according to tolerance.

The general strategy is to initiate treatment of Lyme disease complex by first treating *Bb*, and address co-infections next. As previously described, treating the *Bb* reduces the overall bacterial load and helps the immune system recover.

---

†   Personal communication Jayakumar Rajadas and Venkata Raveendra Pothineni.

Recall that Nutramedix's Samento and Banderol are effective anti-*Bb* herbs that have umbrella properties, hitting multiple microbes. While Samento preferentially hits *Bb*, Banderol is particularly effective against *Bartonella*—usually a Herx on Samento is from *Bb* and a Herx on Banderol is from *Bartonella*. The Red Root contained in Researched Nutritional's BLt formula is also effective against *Bartonella*.

Always start antimicrobial herbal extracts with one drop in water twice daily, and increase the dose by one drop twice daily every four days to minimize Herxheimer reactions. Cut the dose back if a flare is severe and only progress the dose if no longer Herxing. Never start or increase two antimicrobials at the same time—if a patient has a reaction it is important to know what triggered it and what dose is safe.

Mike started off with a diagnosis of acute Lyme disease described in Chapter 5, but we quickly discovered he also had chronic infections with Bb *and* Bartonella. *Mike continued on clarithromycin and cefdinir to treat his Lyme disease, and since he is allergic to sulfa drugs, started on rifampin. He experienced increasing fatigue and depression when taking only 150 mg daily (one quarter the standard dose), and stopped it. Mike tried the A-Bart at one drop, and still flared. Next he tried Nutramedix Samento and Banderol, but could not tolerate either, even at very low doses. However, after six months on the two antibiotics prescribed for Lyme, he became asymptomatic. His lifelong depression was gone and his anxiety was reduced to situational stress. Even though the only treatment he had for Bartonella was the clarithromycin, I believe that knocking down the Lyme allowed his immune system to recover and keep the Bartonella at bay.*

Bartonella can be particularly difficult to treat. Many patients react like Mike did, and have Herxheimer reactions on low doses of virtually all anti-*Bartonella* antimicrobials. The presumed reason is that attacking *Bartonella* triggers a severe inflammatory reaction, often involving autoimmunity.

Back to eleven-year-old Brad:

The first time I saw Brad in my office he could not sit still in a chair. He was so agitated that he kept popping up and down, and finally his father took him outside for a walk. On physical examination, Brad was clearly overweight and his skin demonstrated extensive mottling. The medical term for this is livedo reticularis, a manifestation of uneven circulation. It is common with Bartonella.

My first recommendation was dietary: no sugar, gluten, or dairy. This was an educated guess based on his gastrointestinal symptoms and sugar cravings. Brad did fairly well on his diet. On one occasion he ate three apples and had a flare of pseudo-seizures. I suspect that the sugar provoked inflammation by feeding yeast, to which he was also sensitive. I also recommended the amino acid theanine, 200 mg three times daily for anxiety, as well as Nystatin and probiotics.

Once Brad's diet and yeast were in check, it was time to address the underlying infections. He started on cefdinir 300 mg once daily for one week, then increased to twice daily. Brad had an increase in his intrusive thoughts, depression, and pseudo-seizures for a few days, then returned to baseline. Next he started on SMZ-TMP single-strength twice daily; he experienced a Herx similar to when he began the cefdinir. But when I saw him two months after his initial visit, he was better overall.

A stool analysis showed elevated fecal fats consistent with pancreatic insufficiency. He added pancreatic enzymes at the end of each meal, fluconazole to suppress yeast overgrowth, and chromium picolinate to curb sugar cravings. Then he began taking Malarone to treat Babesia.

Brad started the Malarone 250/100 at one tablet daily and after two weeks increased to twice daily. He had only mild Herxes with a short-lived increase in agitation. By the time he returned for his next visit he was much improved. His mood was considerably better, his gastrointestinal symptoms were gone, his energy and cognition were good, and other symptoms were minimal. Brad had started school and was getting along well with his friends.

At this point in his care the strategy was to stabilize him by adding antimicrobial herbs to his regimen and then transition him off antibiotics. Brad started on Researched Nutritionals BLt to add to the attack on Bb and Bartonella. With each increase in dose he had some nausea and anxiety that lasted one to two days, then he would stabilize. He worked up to twenty-five drops twice daily, and by then he was totally asymptomatic.

GASTROINTESTINAL MANIFESTATIONS OF *BARTONELLA*

Bartonella is particularly suspect when tick-borne infections are associated with gastrointestinal issues. Dr. Martin Fried has identified *Bartonella* as a frequent cause of abdominal pain and heartburn, and has associated this microbe with gastritis, duodenitis, and mesenteric adenitis.[35] This last condition is inflammation of the lymph nodes in the abdomen, and can cause chronic abdominal pain or can mimic appendicitis. *Bartonella* has also been implicated in inflammatory bowel diseases such as Crohn's disease and ulcerative colitis.[36,37] *Bartonella* can cause hypoechogenic/granulomatous lesions in the liver and spleen, which regress with treatment.[38] A patient in my practice was diagnosed with primary sclerosing cholangitis, a serious condition most often seen in young males that can cause cirrhosis of the liver—it was precipitated by *Bartonella*.[39]

I met Susan when she was eighteen years old. Two years previously she began having nausea, abdominal pain, and headaches, and she saw blood in her stools. A colonoscopy demonstrated patchy inflammation in the colon and ileum, and she was diagnosed with Crohn's disease. Susan was prescribed prednisone, a potent corticosteroid which decreases inflammation but suppresses the immune system. She immediately worsened. Susan was barely able to finish high school and didn't think she was well enough to attend college.

In addition to the GI symptoms, Susan complained of joint pains, mood swings with irritability and anxiety, fatigue, daily headaches, light and sound sensitivity, sore soles worse in the morning, episodic vertigo, burning pains, numbness, frequent sore throats with swollen glands, poor sleep, sweats which were occasionally drenching, flushing, chills and hot flashes, air hunger, poor sleep, and brain fog.

Susan weaned off the prednisone. She went on an elimination diet and experienced little change, although she discovered that she did have more abdominal pain and diarrhea when she ate gluten, and that eating sugar led to abdominal cramping and bloating, indicating probable intestinal yeast overgrowth.

Susan's Lyme Western Blot IgM came back with indeterminate bands 39 and 41; her Lyme Western Blot IgG only showed indeterminate band 41. The CD57 level was eighteen. The remainder of her laboratory was unrevealing, including co-infection testing.

Susan's symptoms suggested infections with Bb, Babesia, and Bartonella. *Her symptoms worsened after taking a corticosteroid that suppressed her immune function, at which point the infections flared. Her Western blot test was not impressive, but prednisone will suppress antibody production resulting in a false negative. A low CD 57 count is particularly common when Babesia is active.*

The first intervention was dietary: Susan strictly stayed off dairy, gluten, sugar, and yeast. She began taking Nystatin to kill intestinal yeast. The next step was to begin treatment for the infections, first addressing the suspected Bb using cefdinir and azithromycin. She began to see improvement.

The next step was atovaquone to treat Babesia. Susan started at a half dose, then progressed to the full 750 mg twice daily. She had a short-lived Herxheimer reaction with headache and nausea, then continued to improve. I suggested Susan begin A-Bart, but at one drop she experienced headaches, bloating, increasing joint pains, vision problems, and worse sleep, so A-Bart was discontinued. She next tried SMZ-TMP, which resulted in nausea and headaches, so it was also discontinued. Next were Samento and Banderol, which caused similar problems.

However, at that point Susan had become asymptomatic, and she decided to stop treatment. Her Bartonella *was never treated other than with the azithromycin, a relatively weak anti-*Bartonella *drug. It appears that treating her Lyme and* Babesia *allowed Susan's immune system to recover and, along with the azithromycin, kept* Bartonella *in check. These bugs are not gone, and Susan will need to stay vigilant in regard to relapsing symptoms.*

When I first met Susan, she felt too ill to begin college. Susan has now graduated from college and plans to start a master's program.

Bartonella is a fascinating and nasty microbe. It appears to cause serious inflammation and may underlie many autoimmune syndromes. Hopefully, better detection tests and treatments will be available in the near future.

TAKE-HOME POINTS

1. *Bartonella* is a frequent tick-borne infection.
2. Some people with *Bartonella* are asymptomatic, but this bacterium can cause a virulent infection with widespread inflammation.
3. In particular, *Bartonella* symptoms include neurological problems, neuropsychiatric disorders, gastrointestinal issues, eye inflammation, and skin rashes.
4. *Bartonella* can trigger systemic autoimmune syndromes.
5. Tests for *Bartonella* have a low sensitivity; diagnosis is often made by clinical presentation and response to treatment.
6. Treatment for *Bartonella* is challenging.

Chapter 11

Mycoplasma

Mycoplasma are small bacteria that have been associated with a long list of chronic ailments including chronic fatigue syndrome, fibromyalgia, Gulf War syndrome, and autoimmune illnesses.[1] *Mycoplasma* is the third most common co-infection I find in patients with Lyme disease complex.

WHAT IS *MYCOPLASMA*?

Mycoplasma are atypical bacteria that lack a cell wall, and are the smallest known free living organisms. There are a multitude of *Mycoplasma* species, but not all of them cause disease in humans. Dr. Garth Nicolson put *Mycoplasma fermentans* on the map when he isolated this microbe in veterans of the First Gulf War in 1990 who were suffering from Gulf War syndrome. Nicolson subsequently studied patients with chronic illnesses such as rheumatoid arthritis, multiple sclerosis, and chronic fatigue syndrome, and concluded that this microbe plays a causative role in most autoimmune and neurodegenerative illnesses.[2] However, the question of whether *M. fermentans* is causative or an innocent bystander in any of these conditions remains controversial. Nicolson also claims that *M. fermentans* and *M. pneumoniae* are frequent Lyme co-infections.[3]

Two other *Mycoplasma* species are *Mycoplasma hominis* and *Ureaplasma urealyticum*. These are often present in polymicrobial infections, and have been associated with pelvic pathologies, from bladder infections to pelvic inflammatory disease and endometriosis. As with *M. fermentans*, these species may be colonizers and not pathogens.

A fourth species, *Mycoplasma pneumonia*, is a common respiratory pathogen. This bacterium causes nasal congestion, sore throats, earaches, and sinusitis, and is a frequent cause of adult bronchitis and pneumonia. Most of the population has been exposed to this common bacterium, and the majority recover without treatment. However, in addition to respiratory illness, systemic infection with *M. pneumoniae* can cause a variety of other issues: neurological disorders such as meningitis, radiculitis, Bell's palsy, and neuropathies; joint and muscle pain; cardiac issues including arrhythmias, heart block, myocarditis, and pericarditis; visual impairment with uveitis and optic neuritis; gastrointestinal symptoms including abdominal pain, nausea and vomiting, diarrhea, and loss of appetite; and skin rashes.[4]

In other words, *Mycoplasma pneumoniae* infection can look like Lyme disease complex. To further complicate the picture, although *M. pneumoniae* is commonly spread through airborne droplets, it can also be transmitted by biting insects such as ticks.[5] Therefore, it is possible that many of the subjects in *Mycoplasma* studies also had undiagnosed *Bb* infections, and vice versa. In people with Lyme disease complex, some likely became co-infected with *Mycoplasma* at the time of tick attachment, while others were previously infected with *M. pneumoniae*, and dormant *Mycoplasma* microbes became active when infections such as *Bb*, *Babesia*, and *Bartonella* suppressed immune function.

CLINICAL PRESENTATION OF *MYCOPLASMA*

Mycoplasma infection associated with Lyme disease does not cause respiratory illness. Rather, it results in an increase in systemic inflammation.[6,7] There are no specific symptoms associated with *Mycoplasma* co-infection—it just makes everything worse. Although not described in the medical literature, the dermatologic striae usually associated with *Bartonella* infection may be evident in patients co-infected with *Mycoplasma*. Also, as with *Bartonella*, *Mycoplasma* can trigger autoimmune inflammation in organs throughout the body, including vasculitis, arthritis, meningitis, and encephalitis.[8,9] In children, *Mycoplasma* can trigger pediatric acute-onset neuropsychiatric syndrome (PANS), discussed in more detail in Chapter 17.[10]

TESTING FOR *MYCOPLASMA*

Sputum PCR and cultures are available for the diagnosis of *M. pneumoniae* respiratory infection, but serum PCR is less sensitive than IgM and IgG antibody detection when testing for systemic *M. pneumoniae*. Antibody testing for other *Mycoplasma* species is not widely available. Clongen Laboratories performs a PCR assay for several *Mycoplasma* species, and Medical Diagnostic Laboratories also tests for *M. fermentans* by PCR. Cold agglutinin autoantibodies are often elevated in acute *Mycoplasma* infection, although this finding is not specific.

It is noteworthy that the *M. pneumoniae* IgM can be falsely positive if another infection is active. By contrast, *M. pneumoniae* IgG is quite specific, but is present in the majority of adults because prior exposure to this microbe is so prevalent. Therefore, one must be careful in the interpretation of these tests. The following guidelines can help:

- If there are high elevations of both IgM and IgG, active infection is likely.
- If IgM is normal but IgG is highly elevated, active infection is likely.
- If IgM is elevated and IgG is normal, a repeat antibody test after four weeks of treatment demonstrating seroconversion of IgM to IgG is consistent with active infection.
- If IgM is negative and IgG is slightly elevated, active infection is not likely; the low-positive serology is more likely from a prior infection.

Finally, since lab testing is not definitive, an herbal challenge can assist in confirming a suspected diagnosis. Byron White Formulas offers A-Myco, an herbal formula specific for *Mycoplasma*. As with *Babesia* and *Bartonella*, a Herxheimer reaction in response to this extract suggests an active *Mycoplasma* infection. The directions are the same as previously outlined with A-Bab for *Babesia* and A-Bart for *Bartonella*: one drop twice daily for three days, then five drops twice daily for three days, then ten drops twice daily for three days, then fifteen drops twice daily for three weeks. Again, patients should stop immediately if symptoms flare, which is consistent with active *Mycoplasma* infection. No response to the challenge suggests that *Mycoplasma* infection is not active.

TREATMENT OF *MYCOPLASMA*

Mycoplasma lack a cell wall. Therefore, antibiotics that attack the cell wall, such as cephalosporins and beta-lactam antibiotics like penicillin, are totally ineffective in treating this infection. Intracellular drugs, which include the macrolides, tetracyclines, and fluoroquinolones, are drugs of choice, as detailed in Table 11–1. While both macrolides and tetracyclines are usually effective in treating respiratory infections with *Mycoplasma*, they are not as effective in treating systemic infection. Adding hydroxychloroquine will increase intracellular alkalinity, enhancing antibiotic efficacy. As with *Bartonella* treatment, the use of fluoroquinolones should be reserved for hard-to-treat cases, and then used with caution.

MEDICATIONS TO TREAT *MYCOPLASMA* INFECTION				
Brand Name	Generic	How Supplied	Dose	Considerations
Biaxin	Clarithromycin	500 mg tabs	1 tab 2x/day	Add hydroxycholoroquine
Zithromax	Azithromycin	500 mg tabs	1 tab 1x/day	Add hydroxycholoroquine
Doryx	Doxycycline	100 mg tabs	2 tabs 2x/day	Add hydroxycholoroquine
Levaquin	Levofloxacin	500 mg tabs	1 tab 1x/day	Caution: tendonitis
Cipro	Ciprofloxacin	500 mg tabs	1 tab 2x/day	Caution: tendonitis

Table 11–1. Medications to treat infection with Mycoplasma. Dosages are average for adults, and will vary based on tolerance and effectiveness.

And, as with the other infections, patients usually do best when pharmaceutical antibiotics are paired with herbal antimicrobials. Table 11–2 lists commonly used extracts that have been effective in treating patients with *Mycoplasma*.

HERBAL EXTRACTS TO TREAT *MYCOPLASMA* INFECTION			
Herb	Company	Dosage	Comments
A-Myco	Byron White	Up to 25 drops 2x/day	Powerful, can cause severe Herx reactions
ENL-MC	Beyond Balance	Up to 25 drops 2x/day	Mild, safe for children
Myc-P	Researched Nutritionals	Up to 35 drops 2x/day	Tolerance varies

Table 11–2. Herbal extracts to treat infection with Mycoplasma

Sandy was fifteen years old and living in Durango, Colorado, when she had the sudden onset of shaking chills, sweats, headaches, and muscle aches, all of which resolved over two days. She was not aware of a tick attachment or a rash. Two months later Sandy experienced fatigue, joint pains, and recurrent colds. A Lyme ELISA test was positive, but her Western blot was interpreted as negative by the physician she saw at the time, and she was not treated for Lyme disease. Her symptoms never really disappeared, and over time they waxed and waned.

When Sandy was in her twenties she lived in a house in Virginia that she suspected was moldy, and her symptoms became noticeably worse. At age thirty a Western blot indicated many positive bands for Lyme disease. She took doxycycline 100 mg twice daily and experienced a Herxheimer reaction, but did not improve, and stopped it after two months.

I initially saw Sandy when she was thirty-one years old. At that time she had the following complaints: fatigue, neck pain and stiffness, ankle and knee pain, cognitive dysfunction with poor memory, mood swings with irritability, anxiety with panic attacks, depression, tinnitus, teeth grinding with temperomandibular joint (TMJ) and dental pain, non-restorative sleep with early awakening, irregular menses, chronic congestion, air hunger, night sweats, excess urination and thirst, lymph node swelling in her neck, sore throats, headaches, light and sound sensitivity, balance issues, light-headedness, nausea, constipation, belching, flatulence, and early satiety (food would sit in her stomach after eating).

Physical examination revealed a blood pressure of 138/90 and pulse of 76 when sitting, with BP 140/96 and pulse 96 upon standing. Romberg sign was present (balance issues when standing with feet next to each other and with

eyes closed). Nothing else was notable on the remainder of the physical exam. Laboratory workup revealed normal CBC, complete metabolic panel (CMP), thyroid tests, and quantitative immunoglobulins (capacity to make antibodies). The following were abnormal:

Test	Result	Normal Range
Vitamin B_{12}	386 pg/ml	211–946
Antidiuretic hormone (fasting/no fluid)	<0.8 pg/ml	>1.0
HHV6 IgM	<1:10	<1:10
HHV6 IgG	13.82	<.76
EBV IgM	51.9 U/ml	<36.0
EBV IgG	>600 U/ml	<18.0
M. pneumoniae IgM	<770 U/ml	<700 U/ml
M. pneumoniae IgG	914 U/ml	<100
B. duncani IgG	1:512	<1:256
Homocysteine	13.9 umol/L	<10.0
MTHFR mutation	A1298C heterozygous	No mutations
Cortisol AM	15 ug/dl	15–20
Salivary cortisol x 4	Normal a.m. cortisol, then low remainder of day	Peaks in a.m., then slowly declines
Other co-infection titers	Negative	Negative

Lyme Western Blot:		
Band	IgM	IgG
18 kDa	++	-
23–25 kDa	-	-
28 kDa	-	-
30 kDa	-	-
31 kDa	+	-
34 kDa	-	+/-
39 kDa	+/-	-
41 kDa	+	++
45 kDa	-	-
58 kDa	+	-
66 kDa	-	-

83–93 kDa	++	+/-

Sandy's case is illustrative of the multi-systemic issues often found in Lyme disease complex patients when *Mycoplasma* is one of their co-infections. Her diagnoses at this point in care were the following:

- Tick-borne infections with *Bb*, *Babesia*, and *Mycoplasma*
  - The Western Blot IgM demonstrated the presence of *Bb*-specific bands 18 and 83–93, consistent with active infection.
  - *Babesia* IgG was strongly positive, and Sandy's initial symptoms of high fevers, rigors, sweats, and headaches, as well as ongoing night sweats and air hunger, were consistent with active *Babesia* infection.
  - *Mycoplasma* IgG was strongly elevated, higher than would be expected from a prior infection; this represented either a co-infection or a reactivation of a dormant infection.
  - *Bartonella* titer was negative, but *Bartonella* infection was still suspected due to her neurologic symptoms such as sound and light sensitivity as well as her neuropsychiatric symptoms.
- Viral activation
  - EBV IgM and IgG positivity indicate active infection; this was likely a dormant infection that became activated when tick-borne infections altered her cellular immunity.
  - The positive HHV6 IgG was likely due to a prior inactive infection.
- Pernicious anemia and hypochlorhydria
  - The B_{12} level, while in a normal range, was much lower than expected, particularly since Sandy ate plenty of meat. This suggests that her absorption of vitamin B_{12} was compromised. Low B_{12}, termed pernicious anemia (even when anemia is not evident on a blood count), can cause neurological problems such as impaired cognition and balance issues, consistent with Sandy's presence of a Romberg sign.
  - Inability to absorb vitamin B_{12} is associated with decreased capacity of the stomach to secrete hydrochloric acid, i.e. hypochlorhydria. This results in poor digestion of protein as well as decreased absorption of minerals (see Chapter 16). Sandy's gastrointestinal symptoms, particularly early satiety, belching, and flatulence, were consistent with low stomach acid.
- Adrenal insufficiency

- o The morning cortisol level was normal, but cortisol levels at noon, late afternoon, and nighttime were low. This was indicative of her adrenal glands working below optimum capacity. Low adrenal function not only results in low energy; it also impacts many metabolic functions and impairs immune function.
- Diabetes Insipidus (DI)
  - o Antidiuretic hormone (ADH) level was undetectable when Sandy was fasting, indicating that her pituitary gland was not releasing this hormone. ADH messages the kidneys to concentrate urine; in its absence the kidneys act as if the person is taking a diuretic. Sandy reported symptoms of excessive urination and thirst, polyuria and polydipsia, consistent with this diagnosis.
  - o Note that DI should not be confused with diabetes mellitus, which is a totally different condition involving sugar and insulin. The term *diabetes* is from Latin and Greek, meaning excessive urination, which is what these entities have in common (also see Chapters 15 and 19).
- Dysautonomia
  - o Sandy's high blood pressure and unstable pulse rate are consistent with dysregulation of the autonomic nervous system. This commonly occurs as a downstream effect of chronic inflammation, and typically results in fluctuations in blood pressure and pulse. (See Chapter 17 for a discussion of dysautonomia.)
- Methylation/detoxification issues
  - o A mutation was detected in the MTHFR gene, indicating reduced cellular capacity to perform methylation, a process crucial for cellular detoxification. (Chapter 19 discusses methylation in detail.)

In addition to the diagnoses outlined above, Sandy's probable exposure to mold raised the question of whether she had an issue with mold toxins. Mycotoxins contribute to immune suppression, hormone dysregulation, and systemic inflammation, making it more difficult to address her infections. Mold toxins often impact pituitary function and have been implicated in diabetes insipidus. (Mold issues are outlined in Chapter 19.)

Sandy's case is fairly typical of patients with Lyme disease complex—i.e., there is a lot going on. The multiple moving parts include genetic issues (MTHFR mutation), previous viral infections (EBV and HHV6), acquired conditions (pernicious anemia with hypochlorhydria), environmental stresses (mold exposure), tick-borne

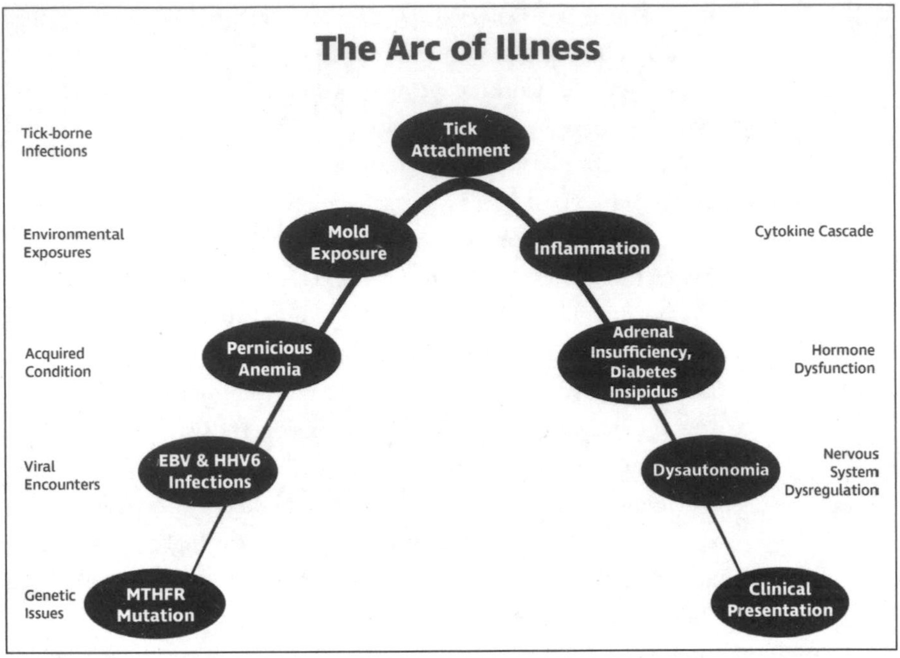

The Arc of Illness

Figure 11–1

infections (*Bb*, *Babesia*, and *Mycoplasma*), and a cytokine cascade of systemic inflammation with downstream issues of adrenal insufficiency, diabetes insipidus, and dysautonomia. The arc of illness is pictured in Figure 11–1.

It is easy to think that people like Sandy become ill when they experience a tick-borne infection. But this event is only one point on a curve, and if patients like Sandy are going to regain full health, all the points on the curve need to be addressed.

> *I address infrastructure issues early, so Sandy began herbs to support her adrenal glands, a pituitary glandular extract to address her diabetes insipidus, and methylated vitamins to bypass the weak enzyme coded for by the mutation in her MTHFR gene. She gave herself vitamin B₁₂ injections, which helped her energy and balance, supplemented her meals with betaine hydrochloride (hydrochloric acid capsules) to improve digestion, and took magnesium at bedtime to help her sleep.*
>
> *Sandy then started taking clarithromycin and hydroxychloroquine to treat Lyme and Mycoplasma. She experienced mild Herx reactions and then minor improvement. She also took probiotics as well as grapefruit seed extract to treat the cyst form of Lyme and keep yeast overgrowth at bay. Next she went on Malarone to treat Babesia, and started having more good days.*

On one occasion, after visiting her in-laws in Virginia who lived in a musty house, Sandy experienced a flare of her symptoms; she suspected this was due to a mold exposure. Sandy also noticed she had symptom flares lasting two to three days in four week cycles, which is classic for Lyme.

Next Sandy added valcyclovir (Valtrex), an antiviral antibiotic, to treat EBV. She had a Herx reaction at 500 mg twice daily, but rapidly improved. However, she had a severe Herx with an outbreak of canker sores when she increased the dose to 1000 mg twice daily, so she went back to the lower dose. By this time Sandy was feeling well most of the time, with the exception of some neck pain and moderate sweats. She did an A-Bart challenge and had no reaction, suggesting that Bartonella was not playing a role.

Sandy began having sugar cravings, athlete's foot, cystic acne, and GI bloating with gas. It appeared that the antibiotics had resulted in yeast over-growth and sensitization despite the grapefruit seed extract and probiotics. She added Nystatin with a mild flare, and then fluconazole with a more severe Herx, and these symptoms resolved.

At this point Sandy added herbal antimicrobials. Mimosa pudica was started at one capsule twice daily and increased to three capsules twice daily to treat Babesia. Then Sandy began A-Bab at one drop twice daily and built up to fifteen drops twice daily, and then added A-L Complex to treat Lyme. Sandy tried to take A-EB/H6, a Byron White formula that addresses viral infections with EBV and HHV6, but could not tolerate the Herx reaction at even one drop. She also could not tolerate A-Myco, the Byron White anti-Mycoplasma formula. I suggested she try the Beyond Balance anti-Mycoplasma herbal formula ENL-MC, which is milder than A-Myco, but she did not follow through. Follow-up blood tests showed reductions in antibodies to M. penumoniae and EBV.

Sandy was feeling well and declined further treatment. She went off all the antimicrobials, both pharmaceutical and herbal, and has continued to feel well. My preference would have been for her to continue treatment while addressing the probable mycotoxin issues, next add more herbal anti-microbials, and only then stop the clarithromycin, hydroxychloroquine, and Malarone. I made it clear to Sandy that the microbes were probably not gone; rather, her immune system had recovered enough to keep down any active infection. I also emphasized that she could relapse in the future if stressed. Sandy promised to contact me if symptoms returned, and three years later she still appears to be doing well.

Environmental doctors often use a beaker metaphor—a low-tech version of the arc of illness (see Figure 11–2). When issues like genetic mutations, nutrient depletion, stress, toxin exposure, allergic reactions, and infection pile up on top of one another, there is a point where they spill over, and the patient becomes symptomatic. In a reverse beaker metaphor, when a handful of the issues are reduced, patients become asymptomatic. However, if the beaker isn't emptied, the remaining residual issues have the potential to cause a recurrence in the future.

Sandy's issues with *Bb*, *Babesia*, *Mycoplasma*, and EBV had clearly improved with treatment. While the antibiotics knocked down these microbes, her immune function and overall constitution also improved, assisted by herbs and glandulars that normalized adrenal and pituitary function, vitamin B_{12} injections that boosted energy and neurological function, betaine hydrochloride supplementation that enhanced digestion, and methylated vitamins that improved detoxification.

The overall clinical picture was a decrease in systemic inflammation, and Sandy went into remission. Would it have been better had she agreed to address her exposure to mycotoxins, metaphorically "emptying her beaker" completely? Perhaps, but if she continues to live a healthy lifestyle and avoids serious mold exposures, it is likely that her immune system will continue to keep her other microbes in check.

There are those who believe that, with treatment, all pathogens are eradicated, but the reality is that microbes have developed brilliant survival strategies. On the

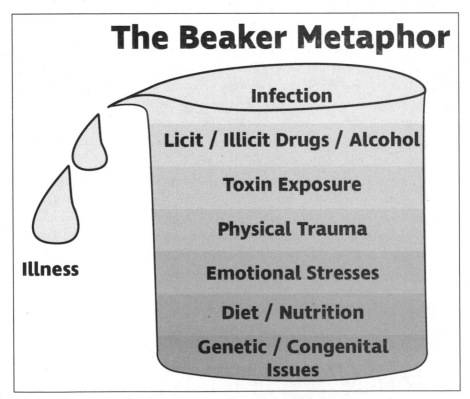

Figure 11–2

other hand, a healthy immune system can keep them at bay, along with the trillions of other microbes with which we coexist.

TAKE-HOME POINTS

1. *Mycoplasma* is the third most common co-infection I see in patients with Lyme disease complex.
2. *Mycoplasma* is a common respiratory pathogen, but can cause serious inflammation in the context of a Lyme co-infection.
3. *Mycoplasma* do not have cell walls and only respond to intracellular antibiotics, not to cell wall drugs.
4. *Mycoplasma* infection may be a tick-borne co-infection, but can also represent activation of a dormant colonizer from a previous respiratory infection.
5. *Mycoplasma* may be an underlying cause of other chronic-fatiguing illnesses and autoimmune disorders.

Chapter 12

Rickettsiales

There has been an extensive and confusing taxonomic reorganization of the bacteria in the Rickettsiales order (see Figure 12–1). At the moment this order includes three families, of which two, *Anaplasmataceae* and *Rickettsiaceae*, are significant to the discussion of Lyme disease co-infections. *Rickettsiales* bacteria are found in ticks, lice, fleas, mites, chiggers, and mammals.

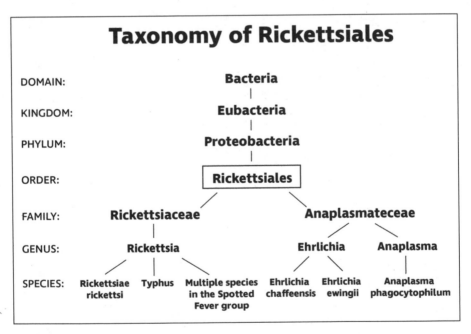

Taxonomy of Rickettsiales

DOMAIN:	**Bacteria**
KINGDOM:	**Eubacteria**
PHYLUM:	**Proteobacteria**
ORDER:	**Rickettsiales**
FAMILY:	**Rickettsiaceae** **Anaplasmateceae**
GENUS:	**Rickettsia** **Ehrlichia** **Anaplasma**
SPECIES:	**Rickettsiae rickettsi** **Typhus** **Multiple species in the Spotted Fever group** **Ehrlichia chaffeensis** **Ehrlichia ewingii** **Anaplasma phagocytophilum**

Figure 12–1

The family *Anaplasmataceae* consists of the genus *Ehrlichia*, with the species *Ehrlichia chaffensis* and *Ehrlichia ewingii*; and the genus *Anaplasma*, which includes *Anaplasma phagocytophilum*. The family *Rickettsiaceae* includes the genus

Rickettsia, which encompasses Rocky Mountain spotted fever, typhus, and the spotted fever group.

EHRLICHIA AND ANAPLASMA

There are two different species of *Ehrlichia* that infect humans: *E. chaffensis* and *E. ewingii*. The latter has only recently been discovered as a human pathogen,[1] and no tests to identify it are currently available in commercial labs. *E. ewingii* appears to cause an illness similar to infection with *E. chaffensis*, which will be the focus of this discussion.

Ehrlichia and *Anaplasma* both invade white blood cells, but each invades a different type. *Ehrlichia* invade monocytes; the resultant illness is human monocytic ehrlichiosis, referred to as HME. *Anaplasma* invade granulocytes and cause human granulocytic anaplasmosis (HGA), previously known as human granulocytic ehrlichiosis (HGE).

Ehrlichia was identified as the cause of a severe worldwide disease in cattle in 1910, but it wasn't until 1987 that this infection was first recognized in humans in the United States. The true incidence of this disease is unknown, since relatively few physicians are aware of it, and there is no system for reporting the illness.

Unlike the other Lyme co-infections, *Ehrlichia chaffensis* is mostly spread by the lone star tick, although it can also be transmitted by dog ticks and blacklegged ticks. Infection is most common in the south-central and southeastern United States, but there have also been cases reported in New England, the Mid-Atlantic States, the Midwest, and as far west as Texas.[2] In other words, it's spreading, and bacteria-laden ticks do not honor state boundaries.

Anaplasma was first described in 1990 in Wisconsin. It is spread by the bite of blacklegged ticks and is therefore a frequent co-infection of Lyme, although it can also occur by itself. The highest prevalence has been in the Upper Midwest, Connecticut, New York, and northern California, but, like HME, *Anaplasma* has expanded its range. A 2001 study at Yale University suggested that 20 percent of people with Lyme disease in Connecticut and Rhode Island were co-infected with HGA.[3] The authors suggested that anaplasmosis be considered in all patients diagnosed with Lyme disease in the northeastern United States. This seems like good advice for all patients with Lyme disease.

CLINICAL PRESENTATION OF HME AND HGA

The clinical presentation of HME and HGA are similar, and, to add to the confusion, both illnesses are often referred to as ehrlichiosis. These bacterial infections can be asymptomatic, but acute infection may cause a severe flu-like illness with fever, chills, fatigue, muscle aches, headaches, loss of appetite, nausea, vomiting, abdominal pain, diarrhea, sore throat, cough, and rashes. Headaches are often described as sharp or knifelike, often with pain behind the eyes.

Lymph nodes may be enlarged, reminiscent of infectious mononucleosis. On rare occasions, usually in immunosuppressed individuals, infection can be severe and cause respiratory failure, kidney malfunction, hepatitis, shock, and even death. Both *Ehrlichia* and *Anaplasma* may invade the nervous system, but HME is more likely to cause central nervous system symptoms such as confusion while HGA is more likely to result in symptoms of peripheral neuropathy and cranial neuropathy, including Bell's palsy.

Canine ehrlichiosis (*Ehrlichia canis*) is broadly recognized as causing chronic infection in dogs. Chronic infection of HME and HGA in humans, however, is not well documented in the medical literature. Yet upon testing, many patients with Lyme disease complex who are serologically positive for HME and HGA also have low white blood cell and platelet counts, consistent with active infection. Therefore it seems likely that HME and HGA do cause chronic human infections. Complaints usually include fatigue, headaches, and muscle aches. Dr. Joseph Burrascano described patients with these infections that he treated with long-term doxycycline, sometimes administered intravenously, who continued to be PCR positive, indicating persistent infection resistant to treatment.*

DIAGNOSIS OF HME AND HGA

It is impossible to distinguish these infections from Lyme on the basis of symptoms, but the laboratory can yield important clues. In the setting of a flu-like illness, particularly in the warmer months, routine blood tests showing low white blood cell and low platelet counts suggest HME or HGA. *Rickettsiae* can also cause these abnormal test results.

Antibody levels don't rise until two to three weeks after infection, so antibody tests performed too early may be negative. Antibody tests for HME and HGA need to be requested separately. PCR tests are currently available and are more specific, but have a high percentage of false negatives. Blood smears may reveal classic morulae—microcolonies of the invading bacteria inside the white blood cells—but this is also a low-yield finding. Elevated liver enzymes and anemia are common in acute illness, and occasionally there will be a low sodium level. Infection in the lungs can result in abnormal chest X-rays. As with the other tick-borne infections, laboratory tests are not the final word, particularly those obtained at a commercial laboratory rather than labs which specialize in detecting tick-borne infections.

---

*   Personal communication.

Meredith was twelve years old and living in northeastern Massachusetts when she came home one summer afternoon with a rash on her abdomen. It looked like a large red circle about the size of a grapefruit, with a small dot in the center. Her parents thought it was some kind of allergic reaction to an insect bite, until five days later when she developed a high fever, lethargy, and aching throughout her body.

Meredith's parents took her to the local emergency room, where she was diagnosed with the bacterial infection cellulitis. The doctors considered this to be the result of an insect bite that had become infected; they prescribed oral antibiotics and sent her home. Meredith continued to run a high fever, so her parents brought her back to the emergency room. She was admitted to the hospital for intravenous antibiotics. At this point the rash was starting to clear in the center, giving it a ring-like appearance.

Inexplicably, Meredith's doctors did not order blood tests for Lyme. When Meredith's routine admission blood tests returned showing depression of both her white blood cell and platelet counts, the doctors still did not order additional testing, but continued treatment for staph cellulitis. Meredith's mother called and asked me what I thought; the diagnosis was clear—Lyme disease and anaplasmosis. The diagnosis of HGA is more likely than HME, since the former is mainly in blacklegged ticks and the latter is mainly in lone star ticks.

TREATMENT OF HME AND HGA

The treatment of choice for these infections is one of the tetracycline drugs. This is one of the reasons why doxycycline is widely prescribed for Lyme disease—it will also treat HME and HGA. Response to treatment is usually rapid, although coexisting infections render treatment more difficult. Adding rifampin to the antimicrobial regimen has improved outcomes in difficult-to-treat cases.[4] In addition, the Byron White formula A-Bio is often helpful.

Meredith's story provides another important point: many patients who present at urgent care centers or emergency rooms with an EM rash are diagnosed with cellulitis. Cellulitis is an infection of the skin, usually caused by staph, and is potentially dangerous if it spreads to the blood. However, cellulitis is painful and quite tender, unlike an EM rash. Unfortunately, the antibiotics generally prescribed for cellulitis are often not appropriate for treating Lyme, HME, or HGA.

RICKETTSIA

In a further bit of nomenclature confusion, the order Rickettsiales contains the family *Rickettsiacae* and the genus *Rickettsia*. The best known species in this genus is *Rickettsiae rickettsi,* Rocky Mountain spotted fever (RMSF), which is only one of a dozen spotted fever illnesses. RMSF is transmitted by wood ticks and dog ticks, and therefore is not a Lyme co-infection. Its name is derived from the place where the first description of the disease occurred (in Idaho), but this is misleading, as infection is most prevalent on the East Coast and south-central United States. Typhus is also in the *Rickettsia* genus, but, like RMSF, is not a Lyme co-infection and is not discussed here.

In addition to RMSF, this genus contains the lesser-known spotted fever group. These include a number of infections, some of which can be transmitted by black-legged ticks and therefore may be Lyme co-infections. It has been well documented that spotted fever group infections can be transmitted within ten minutes of tick attachment.[5] They often leave a scab or eschar within days of the bite, followed by fever, headaches, muscle aches, and rashes. Nausea and vomiting are not uncommon. The spotted fever group infections are similar to RMSF early on in the illness, but symptoms tend to be considerably less severe and more reminiscent of a Lyme-like illness.

Reports of chronic symptoms following infection of RMSF describe significant neurological issues. It seems likely that the spotted fever group infections also have the capacity to cause chronic illness.

DIAGNOSIS OF *RICKETTSIA*

Routine laboratories offer IgM and IgG antibody testing for RMSF by immunofluorescence (IFA) and enzyme linked assays (ELISA). Specialized laboratories also offer PCR testing for RMSF. However, antibodies to RMSF may cross-react with the more benign spotted fever group infections.[6] Patients with positive RMSF serology but no history suggesting acute RMSF should be given the presumptive diagnosis of a spotted fever group infection. There is often a decrease in white blood cell and platelet counts, similar to infections with *Ehrlichia* and *Anaplasma.*

Josh grew up in upstate New York and had a history of several tick attachments. At age seven he exhibited difficulty with reading and math, but was otherwise asymptomatic until age eleven, when he began having mood issues. Josh became anxious and washed his hands compulsively. His parents said that his worst symptom was irritability; he would fly off the handle at the slightest provocation, and his attitude became quite defiant.

I first saw Josh when he was twelve years old. By then he also reported the following symptoms: poor short-term memory, light-headedness, sharp chest pains, hand tremors, occasional headaches, and tinnitus. On physical examination Josh had some skin mottling, and his reflexes were hyperactive. Otherwise his exam was unremarkable.

Laboratory tests were significant for the following:

Test	Result	Normal Range
Mycoplasma IgM	2259 U/ml	<770
Mycoplasma IgG	2926 U/ml	<100
RMSF IgM	1.08	<0.90
RMSF IgG	Negative	Negative

And this was his Lyme Western blot:

Band	IgM	IgG
18 kDa	-	-
23–25 kDa	-	-
28 kDa	-	-
30 kDa	-	-
31 kDa	+	-
34 kDa	+/-	-
39 kDa	-	-
41 kDa	+	++
45 kDa	-	-
58 kDa	++	+
66 kDa	-	-
83–93 kDa		-

Josh's potential for exposure to tick-borne infections was high since he had known tick attachments in upstate New York. The Western blot suggested infection with Bb; although not performed at the time, we could have done an IgM 31 epitope assay to see if the positive 31 band was indeed from Bb. The indeterminate IgM 34 band was consistent with active Lyme disease. The high antibody level to Mycoplasma IgM and IgG was a slam-dunk for active Mycoplasma infection. The positive IgM to RMSF suggested active infection with the spotted fever group, although IgM to any microbe in the absence of IgG reactivity can be a false positive when other infections are active. Bartonella titers were negative, but the severe neuropsychological symptoms made me suspicious of this infection.

I started Josh on amoxicillin. While this antibiotic will hit Bartonella in the extracellular spaces, it is much more active against Bb. Josh reacted favorably. He felt better in general, and was happier, though still irritable. Chest pains were less common, and headaches remitted. I interpreted this response as consistent with active Lyme disease.

Josh then started on A-Bart, and his mood immediately worsened; he was more grumpy, oppositional, and anxious, consistent with Bartonella *infection. He went on Nutramedix Burbur-Pinella to assist detoxification, and it helped a lot. He stopped the A-Bart and began SMZ-TMP to treat* Bartonella. *This was well tolerated, and symptoms again improved a notch.*

I then recommended A-RMS/4B, the Byron White fomula that treats rickettsial infections, and at three drops Josh's irritability and anxiety again spiked. It seemed more likely than not that Josh was also suffering from chronic infection with the spotted fever group.

Josh's symptoms improved a lot, but he continued to have angry outbursts. I prescribed LA Bicillin, 1.2 million units intramuscularly once weekly. This low dose has been effective in treating pediatric acute-onset neuropsychiatric syndrome (PANS),[7] an autoimmune disorder that can be triggered by microbial infections (including Mycoplasma[8], Bartonella[9], *and perhaps* Bb[10]*), resulting in mood and behavioral issues. (PANS is described in more detail in Chapter 17.) After a Herx, Josh's angry outbursts subsided.*

Consideration was also given to treating Josh with doxycycline for all of the above-mentioned infections, including Mycoplasma *and* Rickettsiae, *but was not initiated, as the treatment he was on appeared to be working well.*

TREATMENT OF *RICKETTSIA*

The treatment of choice for spotted fever infections is the tetracycline group, usually doxycycline. Rifampin and chloramphenicol have been used in patients who do not tolerated doxy. In addition, the Byron White formula A-RMS/4B is useful as an adjunct to treatment.

TAKE-HOME POINTS

1. *Ehrlichia chaffensis, Anaplasma phagocytophilum,* and *Rickettsia* (spotted fever) infections may all result in low white blood cell and platelet counts.

2. While *Ehrlichia chaffensis* is occasionally a resident of the black-legged tick, it is most often transmitted by the lone star tick, and therefore may be associated with other infections transmitted by the lone star tick: STARI and Q fever (see Chapter 13).

3. A scab at the site of the tick attachment suggests *Rickettsia* infection.
4. Chronic infection with bacteria in the Rickettsiales order is not well documented in the medical literature; however, clinical experience suggests otherwise.
5. The treatment of choice for all infections caused by bacteria in the Rickettsiales order is any of the tetracycline group of antibiotics. Doxycycline is the one most commonly prescribed.

Chapter 13

The Other *Borrelias*

N ot all spirochetes are created equal. Until recently the most famous bacterial spirochete was syphilis, a sexually transmitted disease caused by *Treponema pallidum*. The Spirochaetales order includes a number of less-known bacteria, but *Trepenoma* and *Borrelia* remain the largest and best known genuses of the group, each containing multiple species. Worldwide there are over three hundred species in the *Borrelia* genus, and over one hundred in the United States. Luckily, many of these bacteria are benign—they colonize our mouths and gastrointestinal tracts but do not cause problems.

Lyme disease is often portrayed as an illness caused by one particular bacterium, but in reality it can be caused by a handful of different *Borrelia* species. *B. burgdorferi* is the primary causative agent of Lyme in the United States, while *B. afzelii* is its European counterpart, and *B. garini* is the Asian culprit. There are a host of other *Borrelia* species that cause a Lyme-like illness in other parts of the world: *B. californiensis*, *B. mayonii*, *B. spielmanii*, and *B. valaisana*. The terminology biologists use when referring to all the *Borrelia* species that cause a Lyme-like illness is *Borrelia burgdorferi sensuo lato*. When referring to *B. burgdorferi* specifically, the term is *Borrelia burgdorferi sensuo stricto*.

SOUTHERN TICK-ASSOCIATED RASH ILLNESS

Southern tick-associated rash illness (STARI) is believed to be caused by *B. lonestari*. The CDC continues to describe STARI as an acute illness characterized by a rash, which may not even require antibiotic treatment.[1] Recognition of STARI as causing systemic and/or chronic illness is controversial, although research indicates that it can cause the disseminated features of Lyme disease.[2]

We owe the discovery of STARI to Dr. Edwin Masters, a family physician in Missouri who was no ordinary doc. He began documenting a Lyme-like illness in his Missouri patients in 1995. The patients had tick bites followed by EM rashes, and, when untreated, went on to develop disseminated infections such as carditis and arthritis. Some of them had positive Lyme ELISA tests.[3] In other words, they had the same clinical presentation as Lyme disease, and in fact fulfilled strict CDC surveillance criteria for Lyme, but the CDC refused to affirm that Masters's patients had Lyme disease.

The controversy was because of the tick vector. The tick in Masters's patients was not the blacklegged tick, but rather the lone star tick (*Amblyomma americanum*), easily distinguishable by the white star or dot on its back. Masters claimed that his patients were suffering from an illness caused by a *Borrelia* spirochete on the Lyme spectrum, while the CDC maintained (and continues to maintain) that this is not the case. Although biopsies of skin rashes in some of these patients demonstrated spirochetes, *Bb* colonies could not be cultured from the samples. Additionally, the spirochetes found in lone star ticks were not *Bb*.

At present, the consensus is that STARI, a.k.a. Masters's disease, is caused by *Borrelia lonestari,* but there are no commercially available assays to test for this bacteria. (I recommend interested readers check out Pam Weintraub's four-part article on Dr. Masters, a colorful, brilliant, and tenacious physician "who did hand-to-hand combat with the Centers for Disease Control and Prevention over the existence of Lyme disease in southern United States."[4])

Many lone star ticks also carry *Ehrlichia chaffensis*, and this infection can coexist with STARI. Lone star ticks may also carry *Coxiella burnetii*, the causative agent of Q fever. (Q fever does not cause a Lyme-like illness, nor is it a Lyme co-infection.*)

The name STARI is unfortunate. It suggests that this infection is limited to the Southern states, when in fact the lone star tick, with its incumbent pathogens, has wide distribution both to the west and north.[5] The name STARI also implies that this illness only results in a rash, when in fact systemic symptoms are common.

The CDC initially maintained that the EM rash in STARI was different than the rash with Lyme, but in fact there is no evidence of a significant difference. The presentation of STARI is therefore a Lyme-like illness following a lone star tick attachment; the Lyme Western blot test will be negative. There is a lack of data on treatment of STARI, but Dr. Masters's reports suggest that this infection should be treated aggressively, in a manner parallel to that of infection with *Bb.*

TICK-BORNE RELAPSING FEVER

The other *Borrelia* infections not included with *Borrelia burgdorferi sensuo lato* are the tick-borne relapsing fever (TBRF) group. The medical literature describes a

---

*   Q Fever is not discussed here, but interested readers can find more information at www. columbialyme.org/patients/tbd_qfever.html.

classic presentation of TBRF: approximately one week following a tick attachment, patients experience recurrent cycles of high fevers lasting several days, alternating with non-feverish periods that last seven days. The fevers are preceded by chills, and can be as high as 106 degrees. During this "crisis phase," patients can become delirious, agitated, and suffer palpitations and shortness of breath. The fever rapidly drops after thirty minutes or less, and patients then experience the "flush phase," with drenching sweats and, occasionally, hypotensive episodes.

TBRF is caused by a long list of *Borrelia* species worldwide, but in the United States the causative organisms are *B. hermsii*, *B. parkeri*, *B. turicatae*, and *B. miyamotoi*. Lice as well as ticks can transmit these infections. The first three species noted above are transmitted by soft ticks (*Ornithodoros*), which are found on small mammals, including mice, prairie dogs, squirrels, and chipmunks, as well as burrowing owls. People are most often exposed when sleeping in cabins or rustic buildings.

B. hermsii is perhaps the most common of this group, especially in the Western United States. Antibodies to this microbe are often positive at commercial labs, but the assay lacks specificity, so the presence of antibodies on this test may actually be reflective of infection or colonization with another *Borrelia* species.

The last species on the list above, *B. miyamotoi,* is a recently discovered microbe in the TBRF class. It inhabits the blacklegged tick, and is often overlooked as a Lyme co-infection. *B. miyamotoi* was initially isolated in Japan in 2005, and human infection first described in Russia in 2011. The first case in the United States was not reported until 2013, but *B. miyamotoi* is no stranger here. Up to 10 percent of ticks in California are colonized by this microbe,[6] and in 2013 Krause and colleagues documented *B. miyamotoi* infection in 21 percent of patients in southern New York who were being evaluated at a Lyme disease clinic for a "viral-like illness."[7]

Recent studies suggest that most patients with *B. miyamotoi* do not recall having high fevers. Rather, infection with *B. miyamotoi* may present just like *B. burgdorferi*, although without EM rashes despite early reports.[8] In other words, *B. miyamotoi* may be categorized as a TBRF on the basis of genetics without actually causing relapsing fevers; rather, *B. miyamotoi* causes a Lyme-like illness. According to Dr. Jyotsna Shah, CEO and science director of IGeneX, other *Borrelia* species in the relapsing fever category can also cause a Lyme-like illness rather than high fevers.[†]

Fatigue, headaches, and muscle aches are the norm. Other symptoms often include joint pains, neck pain, eye pain with conjunctivitis, light sensitivity, rashes, cough, abdominal pain, diarrhea, nausea, and vomiting. Bleeding into the skin can

---

†   Personal communication.

cause petechiae (tiny flat red, purple, or brown dots) and ecchymoses (bruises). Neurological issues may include meningitis, cranial neuropathies, neuropsychiatric symptoms, cognitive difficulties, and seizures, although these are more common in louse-borne than in tick-borne relapsing fever. Myocarditis, cardiac arrhythmias, hepatitis, disseminated intravascular coagulation (DIC), and respiratory failure are rare complications that have been reported.

It has been demonstrated that *B. miyamotoi* can be transferred transovarially. Rather than tick offspring acquiring the bacteria by taking a blood meal from a previously infected animal, adult ticks colonized with the bacteria can transmit the microbes directly to their newly hatched larvae.[9] Although yet to be proven, this discovery raises the question of whether other *Borrelia* species have the capacity for transovarial transmission.

Laboratory diagnosis of *B. miyamotoi* infection can sometimes be confirmed by examination of blood smears during the acute phase of illness. Traditional tests for *Bb,* including the ELISA and Western blot antibody tests, will not detect *B. miyamotoi* or other infections in the TBRF category, but PCR analysis as well as antibody testing for *B. miyamotoi* is available. IGeneX offers antibody testing via Western blot as well as immunoblot to detect infection with TBRF. The latter utilizes recombinant proteins and is more sensitive than the Western blot, but is not specific to one species—it covers *B. americana, B. miyamotoi, B. coriaceae, B. parkeri, B. hermsii, B. turicatae, B. turcica,* and *Candidatus Borrelia texasensis.*

Treatment of TBRF parallels that of *Bb.* Mild and moderate cases can be treated with the same oral antibiotics and herbs that are used in the treatment of Lyme disease. Severe cases, particularly those with heart, pulmonary, central nervous system, and hematologic complications, should be treated aggressively with IV antibiotics.

TAKE-HOME POINTS

1. Lone star ticks are not confined to the southern states, and neither is STARI.
2. Consider STARI in patients with a Lyme-like illness following a lone star tick attachment.
3. STARI is not limited to a rash; it can result in disseminated infection. Patients with STARI deserve antibiotic treatment.
4. Lone star ticks can also transmit *Ehrlichia chaffensis* and *Coxiella burnetii,* the causative agents of ehrlichiosis and Q fever.

5. *B. miyamotoi* is transmitted by blacklegged ticks, and is likely a frequent Lyme co-infection.

6. *B. miyamotoi* does not typically result in relapsing fevers; clinically it is similar to Lyme disease.

7. Consider infection with *B. miyamotoi* in patients who have a Lyme-like illness but test negative for *Bb*.

Chapter 14

Powassan Virus

I
t is unlikely that all the microbes contained in the blacklegged tick menagerie have been identified to date; in fact, the list of known diseases spread by ticks keeps expanding. In addition to bacteria and protozoa, one of the infections now being tracked is Powassan virus (POWV).

As with other tick-borne infections, there is a wide spectrum of illness associated with POWV, although most patients are only minimally symptomatic,[1] In general only patients with severe neurological complications are tested for POWV, which may explain why only about one hundred cases were reported to the CDC over the five-year period from 2012 to 2017. The incidence of infection with POWV is therefore presumed to be far greater than the CDC's statistics suggest.

In 2017, researchers in Wisconsin tested ninety-five patients with suspected tick-borne infections for both *Bb* and POWV, and compared their results with fifty "control" patients undergoing routine medical evaluation. Sixty-three (66.5 percent) patients in the former group had evidence of current or prior infection with *Bb* and nine (9.5 percent) had antibodies to POWV, while in the latter group four (8 percent) had antibodies to *Bb* and two (4.0 percent) to POWV.[2] These results are similar to another report in which 10.4 percent of 106 patients with recent tick exposure suspected of having acute tick-borne disease were serologically positive for POWV.[3]

DIAGNOSIS OF POWV

Blacklegged ticks can transmit POWV within fifteen minutes of attachment.[4] Symptoms typically occur in one week, but can be delayed for up to a month. The onset of POWV can mimic other tick-borne infections, with symptoms of fever, headaches, muscle aches, and weakness. POWV can also cause meningitis, with nausea, vomiting, stiff neck, and confusion, as well as encephalitis (infection of the brain). These patients may experience respiratory distress, gait imbalance, coordination difficulties, seizures, speech difficulties, blurry vision, double vision, paralysis, and coma; 10 percent of neuroinvasive POWV infections are fatal. For those who survive, 50 percent have long-term neurological deficits that can mimic chronic neuroborreliosis.[5]

The first diagnostic step in a patient with the sudden onset of neurological symptoms is a CT scan or MRI to rule out conditions such as a tumor or an intracranial bleed. POWV can occasionally cause cerebral hemorrhage, but the majority of scans demonstrate only nonspecific abnormalities. A lumbar puncture will consistently yield abnormal findings in the cerebrospinal fluid (CSF) in patients with POWV. Pleocytosis (elevated white blood cells) is common—predominantly due to high levels of lymphocytes rather than neutrophils; neutrophils suggest bacterial infection while lymphocytes are more consistent with viral invasion. The protein levels in the CSF will be elevated, and sometimes the glucose will be as well. The CSF should be checked for POWV antibodies, although it is more likely that serum testing will reveal positive serologies. Powassan testing is most often done in state laboratories and then confirmed by the CDC.

TREATMENT OF POWV

Sadly, there are no medications to treat POWV. Patients with evidence of severe encephalomyelitis should be hospitalized and treated with supportive therapy. It is possible that many patients with Lyme disease complex are also suffering from the long-term consequences of undiagnosed POWV.

TAKE-HOME POINTS

1. POWV is a common co-infection of Lyme disease, but most patients have minimal symptoms.
2. A small subset of patients with POWV experience severe neurological deficits and death. Anyone with evidence of meningoencephatitis should be admitted to the hospital for a complete neurological evaluation and support.
3. There is no treatment for POWV.

Section Three
IT'S ALL CONNECTED

Western doctors like to compartmentalize. Each specialty has its own organization, its own credentialing system, its own journals, and its own conferences. That way physicians can specialize in a specific organ system and practice their specialty as if it is only remotely connected to the rest of the body. But the very idea that we are not an interconnected whole is misguided.

The endocrine system discharges hormones that regulate specific cellular functions. The immune system releases cytokines that talk to immune cells and engineer inflammation. And the nervous system dispatches neuropeptides that talk to other nerve cells. But all these systems are in continuous dialogue. There are receptors for each of the neuropeptides on every cell in our bodies. Cytokines talk to nerve cells and endocrine glands. Neuropeptides talk to immune cells. Hormones regulate all of the above.

It doesn't stop there. Stress and emotions also talk to all of the above. Robert Ader and Nicholas Cohen introduced the term psychoneuroimmunology (PNI) in 1975, after demonstrating that behavioral stimuli could impact immune function.[1] In other words, what we feel impacts cellular function. Later, PNI was lengthened to psychoneuroendocrineimmunology, in recognition of the role that hormones play in this dynamic. But it is not a stretch to consider expanding this to psycho-neuroendocrine-gastrointestinal-immunology, since the GI tract makes its own hormones that not only regulate digestion but also talk to the brain, giving a whole new meaning to the phrase "gut emotions."

In fact, the GI tract not only makes hormones, it also has more nerve cells than the spinal cord and more immune cells than the rest of the body combined. Meanwhile, other organs like the heart also send out messenger molecules. You get the point. The fact is—we are a vast informational network in which our cells are in continuous dialogue. And the reductionist attitude we have used to understand human function has limited our appreciation of the human condition.

That said, while I will be discussing the impact of tick-borne infections on specific organ systems, it is important to keep in mind that none of these function in isolation. When a microbe triggers an inflammatory response, the impact is felt throughout our entire bodies.

Chapter 15

Endocrine Dysfunction

The endocrine system is comprised of the body's glands, which produce and secrete hormones that regulate the function of cells throughout the body. The endocrine system is foundational, since nothing works correctly when hormones are out of balance. One of the great things about hormones is that they are quantifiable—their levels can be measured, and thereby glandular function can be assessed. This chapter will discuss some of the more common endocrine imbalances that occur in patients with chronic tick-borne infections.

First, though, it helps to have a big-picture understanding of the endocrine system and how it operates. The "central switchboard" of the endocrine system is the hypothalamus, located in the undersurface of the brain. (See Figure 15-1 below.)

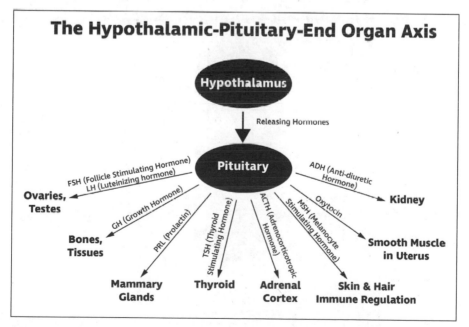

The Hypothalamic-Pituitary-End Organ Axis

Hypothalamus

Releasing Hormones

Pituitary

FSH (Follicle Stimulating Hormone)
LH (Luteinizing hormone)

ADH (Anti-diuretic Hormone)

Ovaries, Testes

Kidney

GH (Growth Hormone)

ACTH (Adrenocorticotropic Hormone)

MSH (Melanocyte Stimulating Hormone)

Oxytocin

Bones, Tissues

PRL (Prolactin)

TSH (Thyroid Stimulating Hormone)

Smooth Muscle in Uterus

Mammary Glands

Thyroid

Adrenal Cortex

Skin & Hair Immune Regulation

Figure 15-1

The hypothalamus coordinates endocrine function by secreting hormones down the pituitary stalk to the adjacent pituitary gland, which sits directly under the brain. The pituitary gland in turn releases other hormones that regulate a myriad of cellular functions as well as regulating other hormone-producing glands. (In addition to its role in regulating the endocrine system, the hypothalamus also oversees the autonomic nervous system, which will be discussed in Chapter 16.)

ADRENAL DYSREGULATION

The two adrenal glands, which sit on top of the kidneys, are each about the size and shape of a walnut. They secrete a symphony of hormones that enable cells throughout the body to deal with the ups and downs of everyday life. One example is their role in reacting to a sudden stress, such as a car accident. The autonomic nervous system, which is also centrally controlled by the hypothalamus, signals the adrenal medulla in the center of the adrenal gland to release catecholamines—epinephrine and norepinephrine, better known as adrenaline and noradrenaline—into the bloodstream. These hormones generate the aptly named fight-or-flight response.

Acute stress also stimulates the release of cortisol and DHEA from another part of the adrenal glands, the adrenal cortex. Release of these hormones is under the direct control of the hypothalamus, as depicted in Figure 15–2. The hypothalamus secretes corticotrophin releasing hormone (CRH) down the pituitary stalk,

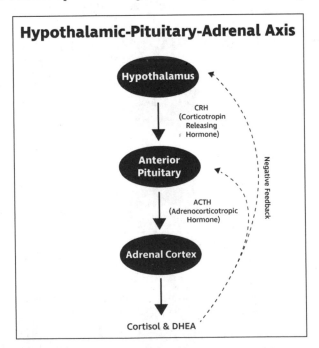

Figure 15–2

which triggers the release of adrenocorticotropic hormone (ACTH). ACTH travels through the blood stream to the adrenal cortex, where it stimulates the production and release of cortisol and DHEA.

This process works well as a necessary response to acute stress; the release of catecholamines is short-lived. However, chronic stress takes a toll on proper adrenal function. At first the adrenal cortex continues to increase production of cortisol and DHEA, helping the body adapt to the rise in metabolic demands. At this stage, the adrenal glands actually become enlarged; but over time they often get tired and lose their reserve, leading to low adrenal function.

Think of a long horse race where a jockey keeps whipping his steed. The horse works harder with each lash, but at some point runs out of energy and can't go one step farther. When people are sick for a long time, at first their adrenal glands work overtime, but they subsequently get tired and slow down—entering a state called adrenal insufficiency. Hans Selye first described the stages of adrenal fatigue in 1936, which he termed the General Adaptation Response.[1]

- Stage 1. The Alarm Stage
  o Elevated catecholamines—flight or fight
  o Elevated cortisol and DHEA
  o Decreased resistance to stress
- Stage 2. Resistance
  o Elevated cortisol and DHEA
  o Increased resistance to stress
- Stage 3. Exhaustion
  o Low cortisol and low DHEA
  o Decreased resistance to stress

Cortisol is important for more than helping deal with stress. Think of cortisol as WD-40 for most cellular functions: without it, metabolism slows and gets rusty. Cortisol helps control blood sugar, reduces inflammation, affects salt and water balance, modulates blood pressure, and assists with memory. And—this is really important—*low cortisol levels undermine immune function.*[2]

DHEA is similarly important for many metabolic functions. It is a precursor for the male and female hormones testosterone and estrogen. DHEA is also vital for energy production, immune function, bone growth, neurotransmitter activity, blood sugar regulation, and control of inflammation.

All people with chronic illness should ideally undergo adrenal evaluation. The symptoms of adrenal insufficiency start with fatigue, especially poor stamina and post-exertional malaise. Additional symptoms are listed in Table 15–1.

SYMPTOMS OF ADRENAL INSUFFICIENCY
Fatigue—mental and physical
Weakness, poor stamina, post-exertional exhaustion
Listlessness, depression
Low blood pressure, postural light-headedness
Anorexia, weight loss
Salt cravings

Table 15–1.

LABORATORY EVALUATION OF ADRENAL FUNCTION

The adrenocortical hormones are derived from cholesterol. Despite the common misperception that all cholesterol is diet-related, most circulating cholesterol is manufactured in the liver. The adrenal cortex converts cholesterol into pregnenolone, which is a precursor molecule for both cortisol and DHEA. Therefore, evaluation of pregnenolone levels, as well as levels of DHEA and cortisol, are recommended. How and when they are obtained can influence the results. The first step in the lab workup is to measure these in the blood:

- Serum pregnenolone
- Serum DHEA-S
    - Most circulating DHEA is in its sulfated version, DHEA-S
- Serum cortisol
    - Drawn from 7:00–9:00 a.m., when serum levels peak

Cortisol has a diurnal rhythm. Levels peak by 9:00 a.m., then decrease during the day, and should be low by bedtime. Levels start rising again around 4:00 a.m to start the new day. Keep in mind that a single morning blood test only gives an indication of cortisol production at one point in time, so multiple blood draws or an alternate method of analysis must be used to track cortisol levels over time.

Most endocrinologists evaluate adrenal insufficiency with an ACTH (Cosyntropin) stimulation test. This entails drawing blood for a baseline cortisol level, then injecting ACTH, which should stimulate the adrenals to produce more cortisol. Blood levels are then retested thirty and sixty minutes after injection. Dr. William Jeffries wrote a book, *Safe Uses of Cortisone*, that changed medicine's way of evaluating adrenal function.[3] He suggested that a serum cortisol drawn in the morning should be at least 15 mcg/dl, and that the level should at least double after an injection of ACTH.

The ACTH stimulation test is an artificial laboratory situation, and injecting very high levels of ACTH may not accurately indicate adrenal reserve. It doesn't provide an accurate picture of what is happening at home and work on a day-to-day basis. Therefore, in clinical practice, a more useful addition to a morning serum cortisol level is salivary cortisol testing, from a saliva sample collected at four different times during the day. Salivary levels closely mirror that of serum levels.[4] This test gives a more accurate picture of what is happening during a twenty-four-hour period. There are a handful of other tests available, such as twenty-four-hour urine collections, but it is preferable to have a chart of levels over the course of the day, as these results will impact treatment recommendations.

Below is a sample of salivary test results from three different chronically ill people, illustrating how the cortisol levels correspond with symptoms:

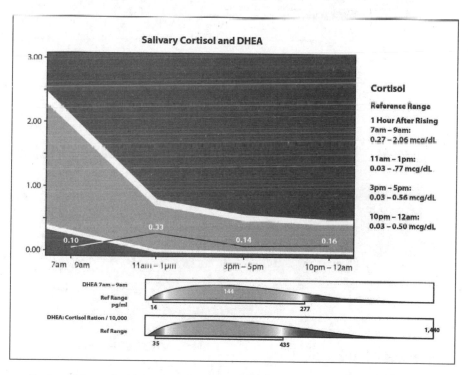

Patient A has a hard time getting up in the morning, but energy is okay the rest of the day.

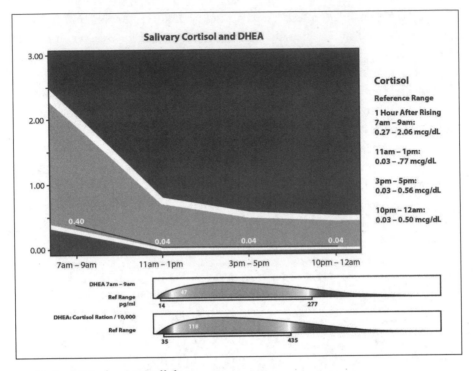

Patient B is dragging all day.

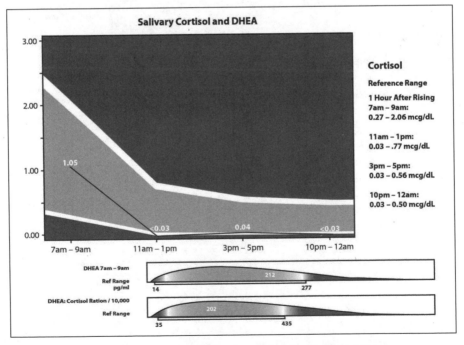

Patient C has energy in the morning, but is finished by lunchtime.

TREATMENT OF ADRENAL INSUFFICIENCY

Hydrocortisone is the bioidentical equivalent of cortisol. Prior to the 1980s it was only prescribed in high doses to quell inflammation in patients with conditions such as multiple sclerosis, lupus, asthma, and colitis. While effective and sometimes lifesaving, high doses of hydrocortisone can cause serious side effects, limiting its utility. High-dose cortisone will inevitably suppress both immune and adrenal function—and should therefore be avoided whenever possible in people with Lyme disease complex, as it will often result in a flare of the infections.

There are exceptions to this recommendation, since high doses of cortisone can be lifesaving in some situations; if their use is indicated, patients should be covered with aggressive antibiotic dosing. (By contrast, hydrocortisone cream, available over the counter to treat itchy rashes, is not absorbed and is not a problem. However, fluorinated cortisone creams, available by prescription, will be absorbed, and can pose a potential problem over the long run.)

When William Jeffries published *Safe Uses of Cortisone* in 1981, he introduced the idea of treating people with low doses of hydrocortisone.[5] Jeffries claimed that the baby was thrown out with the bathwater when the use of cortisone was limited to high doses. He demonstrated that using low doses of hydrocortisone to normalize cortisol levels in individuals with adrenal insufficiency actually improved their adrenal function and boosted immune competence. Patients often witnessed immediate improvement in energy and well-being.

The adrenal glands of a healthy non-stressed individual manufacture an average of 40 mg of cortisol daily. Under acute stress, a healthy person augments that production. However, under chronic stress, the ability to produce even normal levels of cortisol may decline. Low-dose hydrocortisone replacement aims to supplement levels into a normal range of circulating cortisol.

The patients with the lab results above all gained benefit from this approach. Patient A's output of cortisol in the morning was low but his remaining cortisol levels were normal; he benefited from taking hydrocortisone 10 mg upon awakening. Patient B was prescribed hydrocortisone 5 mg three times daily—at 7:00 to 8:00 a.m., 11:00 to 12:00 noon, and at 3:00 to 4:00 p.m.—based on salivary levels. Patient C was prescribed hydrocortisone 5 mg to take three times daily, but at different intervals—at 11:00 a.m., 3:00 p.m., and 6:00 p.m. All three patients noticed an immediate improvement in energy, wakefulness, and a decrease in post-exertional fatigue. They were also all advised to increase their dosage if they found themselves in a situation, such as an acute infection, which produced additional stress.

In addition to low doses of hydrocortisone, there are numerous combinations of herbs and glandulars that can benefit adrenal function. These typically contain eleuthero, panax ginseng, rhodiola, licorice, and/or desiccated bovine adrenal gland. These products can normalize adrenal function on their own in patients with mild adrenal fatigue, as well as providing benefit when used in conjunction with hydrocortisone replacement in those with more severe adrenal insufficiency.

> *Sally was eighteen years old at her first visit to my office. She had been experiencing multiple symptoms consistent with chronic infection for several years, but her worst symptom was fatigue. Sally was so exhausted that she typically didn't get out of bed until 2:00 p.m., and remained lethargic all day. However, Sally's energy would improve around 10:00 p.m., and she would stay wide awake until collapsing around 5:00 a.m.*
>
> *Sally had previously seen an endocrinologist, who diagnosed adrenal insufficiency on the basis of a low morning cortisol (3.8 mcg/dl) and prescribed hydrocortisone 10 mg twice daily. However, her history provided clues that something else was going on. I suggested she get her serum cortisol level tested at 11:00 p.m. The result came back at 18 mcg/dl. This would have been normal at 8:00 a.m., but was significantly elevated for a nighttime result. Sally was suffering from a reversed cortisol pattern; this shift in the diurnal cortisol pattern is more typically seen in someone who works the night shift, is up all night and sleeps in the daytime. It was not normal for Sally.*

It is not uncommon for patients with Lyme disease complex to have elevated cortisol levels at bedtime, which can interfere with sleep. The supplements phosphatidylserine, ashwaganda, and *Magnolia officinalis* can decrease elevated cortisol levels.

In addition to normalizing cortisol levels, DHEA and pregnenolone should be supplemented if their serum levels are low. These are available in various forms: capsules, extracts, and transdermal creams by prescription. Average doses for DHEA are 10 mg daily for women and 25 mg daily for men. Pregnenolone dose averages 25 mg twice daily. Blood levels of these hormones should be monitored for those taking these supplements.

THYROID DYSFUNCTION

The adrenal gland is not the only endocrine organ affecting metabolism; the thyroid, also under control of the hypothalmus and pituitary, plays a large role. The hypothalamus secretes thyrotropin-releasing hormone (TRH) down the pituitary stalk, which informs the pituitary gland to secrete thyroid-stimulating hormone (TSH). TSH enters the bloodstream and stimulates the thyroid gland to produce and release thyroxine (T4) and triiodothyronine (T3). T4 and T3 then signal back to

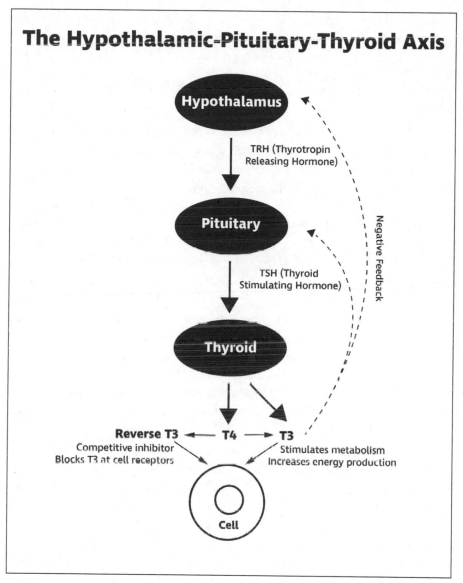

Figure 15–3

the hypothalamus and pituitary in a classic feedback loop. This is illustrated above in Figure 15–3.

Thyroid hormones attach to receptors on cells throughout the body, sending a message to boost the metabolic rate, i.e. increase energy production. Think of them as a foot pressing the accelerator pedal; without them, the car sits still. Low thyroid levels classically result in fatigue, weight gain, cold intolerance, hair loss, dry skin, constipation, and slow mentation. High levels tend to cause agitation, weight loss, sweating, palpitations, heat intolerance, tremors, and insomnia. In any given individual, the symptoms can be mixed—a person with thyroid dysfunction may show some but not all the symptoms of either category, and in some cases a patient may exhibit some symptoms of both categories.

REVERSE T3

Although the thyroid gland primarily makes the hormone T4 (thyroxine), it is T3 (triiodothyronine) that does most of the work. It turns out that T4 is converted to T3 in tissues throughout the body. T3 is not as bound to protein and therefore is more available to attach to specific receptors on cell membranes.

The story does not end there. T4 is converted not only to T3, but it can also be metabolized to reverse T3 (rT3). Think of rT3 as T3's evil twin brother: it binds with the same receptor sites as T3, but blocks its action. Technically, rT3 is a competitive inhibitor of T3. The more rT3 in circulation, the more it blocks the action of thyroid hormones, even if circulating levels of both T4 and T3 are normal. (Refer to Figure 15–3.)

The rate of conversion of T4 to rT3 can be great enough that serum levels of T3 fall. Endocrinologists refer to this as euthyroid-sick syndrome (ESS), because the thyroid gland itself is functioning normally even though circulating T3 levels are below the normal range. (Euthyroid means a normally functioning gland.) Many endocrinologists believe that no treatment is indicated, but this remains controversial. In the case of patients with chronic illness, withholding treatment appears shortsighted.

Under normal conditions, roughly 40 percent of T4 is converted to T3, and about 20 percent into rT3 daily. However, as much as 50 percent of T4 converts to rT3 when a person is under stress or if his or her body needs to conserve energy. Excessive amounts of rT3 will block T3's ability to provide energy, and thus will reduce metabolic function on a cellular level.

This appears counterproductive—if people are sick, they tend to make more rT3, blocking T3 action and resulting in even less energy production. It may be that this provided an evolutionary advantage, because it forced people who were ill to rest. Perhaps there is even a lesson in this—to honor the body's need to rest when stressed. But for those who are chronically ill, the overproduction of rT3 can be a major contributor to fatigue.

The key to determining a healthy balance in thyroid function using lab results is to calculate the ratio of T3 to rT3. T3 levels can be reported two ways, either as Free T3 or Total T3. If measuring Free T3, the ratio, ideally, is greater than 20:1; if measuring Total T3, it should be equal or greater than 7:1. There is a website that allows easy calculation, since the units reported by the laboratory are often different: stopthethyroidmadness.com/rt3-ratio. Most patients with low T3:rT3 ratios feel better and have more energy when prescribed additional T3. However, as with all laboratory tests, it is important to treat the patient and not just a lab abnormality; some people feel better when blood tests are not within specified ranges. Always perform follow-up thyroid testing after changing a patient's dose.

TYPES OF LOW THYROID CONDITIONS

A significant number of Lyme patients are hypothyroid. Many have classic hypothyroidism—their thyroid glands are simply low functioning. Some are depleted in iodine, an element necessary for production of thyroid hormones; some have a multinodular goiter (enlargement of the thyroid gland). Then there are Lyme patients who have Hashimoto's thyroiditis, also known as autoimmune thyroiditis, a condition in which the thyroid gland is under attack by their own immune system. In the initial phases the inflammation associated with Hashimoto's can mobilize excessive release of T4 and T3, and result in symptoms of hyperthyroidism. Over time, however, the thyroid gland often burns out, resulting in hypothyroidism.

All these conditions are fairly common in the general population, and it is unclear if they are more common in people with Lyme disease complex, although their presence contributes to the overall symptom picture. Overactive or hyperthyroid conditions including Graves' disease are uncommon in Lyme patients, and are not discussed here.

LABORATORY EVALUATION OF THYROID FUNCTION

Every patient with Lyme disease complex should have comprehensive thyroid testing performed, which includes the following:

- TSH
- Free T4
- Free T3
- Reverse T3

Figure 15–3 illustrates how production of thyroid hormone is regulated; if the thyroid gland is not making enough T4 and T3, the feedback will inform the pituitary gland to release more TSH. In other words, TSH levels move inversely to levels of T4 and T3. Increased TSH is, in fact, the earliest sign of a failing thyroid gland. However, the TSH level needs to be interpreted with caution. Many doctors use only the TSH as a screening tool for thyroid dysfunction, but this test alone is not adequate in evaluating thyroid function in the chronically ill patient. The TSH level needs to be interpreted in the context of the person's clinical condition, as well as levels of T4 and T3.

Many clinical laboratories state that the "normal range" of TSH is 0.450–4.500 uIU/ml, but the upper limit of normal has declined over the past decade. The National Academy of Clinical Biochemistry has suggested that the TSH reference range be lowered to 2.5 uIU/ml.[6] Even this new interpretation of normal range doesn't account for individual differences; there is a lot of variability of "normal" on the basis of genetic and environmental factors.[7]

Thyroid autoantibodies, including anti-thyroglobulin and thyroperoxidase (TPO) antibodies, are elevated in Hashimoto's thyroiditis. As previously stated, thyroid levels are often normal or even high early on in this condition, but elevated antibodies indicate a need to monitor thyroid function on a regular basis, since most patients become hypothyroid over time.

Endocrinologists refer to people with elevated TSH but normal T4 and T3 levels as having "subclinical hypothyroidism," suggesting that they do not require treatment. However, these patients have been found to have an increased risk of heart disease and other conditions, so while they may not be overtly hypothyroid, they are not metabolically healthy, either.[8]

It is important to note that while TSH levels usually coordinate with serum levels of thyroid hormones, TSH does not correlate with tissue thyroid levels.[9] Clinical experience has shown that most people feel better when TSH is less than 2.0 uIU/ml—keeping in mind that it is important to treat the person and not the number, a philosophy that holds for all lab testing. However, if the TSH is elevated and the T4 and T3 are low, the patient is clearly hypothyroid and should be treated with a combination of T4 and T3 (see below).

Many chronically ill patients have absolutely normal TSH, T4, and T3 levels but elevated rT3 as determined by a low T3:rT3 ratio. There are supplements, particularly selenium, that may improve conversion of T4 to T3 and increase the ratio, but most with this condition require additional T3 to normalize the ratio, generally leading to a noticable improvement in energy.

If TSH is normal, T4 is normal, and T3 is low, the so-called euthyroid-sick syndrome, rT3 will probably be elevated, with a decrease in the T3:rT3 ratio. These patients also feel better when T3 is added.

The pituitary gland should increase TSH production when T4 and T3 levels fall, prompting the thyroid to produce more hormone. However, some chronically ill patients have a normal TSH but low or low-normal T4 and T3. These lab results indicate that the pituitary gland is not responding appropriately to low thyroid function. These patients typically feel better when taking thyroid replacement. Repeat blood tests will show T4 and T3 in the normal range but low TSH, because there is no longer a stimulus to the pituitary gland to boost TSH output. This is confirmation that the pituitary is low functioning, and the TSH level should no longer be considered a parameter of thyroid function. As described later in this chapter, low pituitary function is often associated with mold toxins.

TREATMENT OF THYROID DYSFUNCTION

Most endocrinologists recommend treatment of hypothyroidism with only T4. They base this on the assumption that the body will convert what it needs to the more biologically active T3. However, numerous studies have demonstrated that T4-only preparations do not provide adequate T3 levels to most tissues.[10,11] Additional studies have confirmed improvement in clinical outcome when T3 is added to T4.[12,13]

In clinical experience, many patients with hypothyroidism on T4 replacement alone improve when T3 is added. Combination T4/T3 preparations such as NP Thyroid and Armour thyroid can be used to treat routine hypothyroidism, with dosage adjusted on the basis of repeat thyroid tests as well as clinical response. Supplemental T3 (liothyronine) can be added if the T3:rT3 ratio is still low. Although the half-life of T3 is about twenty-four hours, levels of T3 peak approximately four hours after ingestion.[14] Therefore, patients using the immediate release form of T3 can benefit by splitting the dose, taking it first thing in the morning and again after lunch. More sustained levels can be obtained by using extended release T3, which can be compounded in a specialty pharmacy. Again, the dose should be adjusted based on repeat blood tests and clinical response.

Some patients experience difficulty keeping both the T4 and T3 in optimal ranges when using a combination T4/T3 medication. These patients do best taking T4 (levothyroxine) and T3 (liothyronine) separately. T4 has a long half-life of five days, and therefore only needs to be taken once daily.

It is important to recognize that some patients don't tolerate prescription thyroid preparations at all, and some tolerate only certain products. Some don't do well on Armour thyroid but do respond to NP Thyroid, perhaps owing to the fillers in Armour. Some people do not tolerate either, perhaps because of a pork allergy. There are patients who do not respond to thyroxine, but who do well on the brand-name preparations Synthroid or Tirosint. Similarly, some don't feel well on generic liothyronine but feel good on brand-name Cytomel. Those patients who don't tolerate either often do well with USP thyroid from compounding pharmacies, perhaps because they are reacting to the fillers in the usual prescription medications.

Anyone taking thyroid replacement should be aware of the symptoms of taking too high a dose, which are similar to those of ingesting too much caffeine—edginess, anxiety, palpitations, tremors, and/or sleep problems. It is important to monitor blood pressure and pulse when initiating treatment. It takes three and a half weeks for TSH to normalize after adjusting doses, so repeat blood tests can be checked four weeks after a change in dose.[15]

DIABETES INSIPIDUS

The pituitary is an amazing gland. It is tiny—only about the size of a pea—but secretes nine different hormones, each regulated by its own stimulation and feedback mechanisms. While its multitude of functions is awe-inspiring, there are a lot of opportunities for things to go wrong.

Most patients with pituitary dysfunction and Lyme disease complex have been exposed to mold toxins. Mycotoxins can cause multiple endocrine problems, as discussed in more detail in Chapter 19. This chapter will be limited to a discussion of low ADH.

ADH is antidiuretic hormone, also known as arginine vasopressin or just vasopressin. ADH is actually made in the hypothalamus but is stored in the pituitary gland. Under normal conditions, the pituitary secretes ADH when a person is dehydrated. The ADH circulates in the blood and gives a message to the kidneys, telling them to conserve fluid by concentrating the urine. Conversely, low levels of ADH will cause increased urination. This occurs whether or not the person is adequately hydrated. When someone has chronically low levels of ADH, his body acts as if he is taking a diuretic; this condition is called diabetes insipidus (DI).*

DI should not be confused with diabetes mellitus, a totally distinct condition associated with high blood sugar. What the two conditions have in common is excessive urination. When people with DI are asked if they pee a lot, they often answer, "Yes, but I drink a lot." The truth is the other way around: they drink a lot because they pee a lot.

Patients with DI continue to urinate regardless of hydration status, usually totalling over three liters daily. This then causes them to get thirsty and drink a lot—but they can never really catch up, and are always dehydrated. These symptoms of excessive urination and thirst are termed polyuria and polydipsia. Symptoms can be exacerbated by both caffeine and alcohol, which inhibit secretion of ADH, making them bad choices for anyone trying to stay hydrated, but particularly poor choices for the person with DI.

The simplest way to make the diagnosis of DI is to measure the ADH level after a twelve-hour fast of both food and fluids. Normally people secrete ADH when dehydrated, prompting their kidneys to concentrate urine and conserve water. Therefore extremely low or undetectable levels of ADH on a blood test performed when a person is dehydrated is consistent with the diagnosis of DI.

---

*   Diabetes insipidus caused by pituitary dysfunction is termed central diabetes insipidus. In addition, there are other origins of diabetes insipidus.

Treatment for DI can start with a pituitary glandular supplement. Several companies make these; many people with DI have particular success using Pituitrophin by Standard Process. The majority of patients who take this supplement report that they no longer are continually on the lookout for the next bathroom, and they can sleep through the night without waking multiple times to urinate.

Prescription desmopressin, a synthetic form of vasopressin, can be used if a pituitary glandular supplement is not successful in alleviating symptoms. Desmopressin is available in multiple forms: oral tablets, nasal spray, and as a subcutaneous injection. Patients taking this medication will need to have their electrolytes monitored. Unfortunately, about 20 percent of my patients who are prescribed desmopressin don't tolerate it; the most common side effects are headaches and fluid retention.

Surgical trauma, head injury, toxins, and inflammation can cause DI. People with Lyme disease complex have plenty of inflammation, and it is not unlikely that cytokines—signaling molecules released by the immune system that may cause inflammation—can interfere with pituitary function. But in my clinical experience 90 percent of patients with Lyme disease complex and DI have mold toxins. The pituitary gland appears particularly vulnerable to these toxins, so much so that if a patient presents with DI, exposure to mold toxins should be high on the list of suspected issues.

TESTOSTERONE DEFICIENCY

Low libido is a common complaint in people with Lyme disease complex. Many times this is simply related to being tired and depressed, but it may also be due to low testosterone, so the level of this hormone should always be checked.

Testosterone is famous as a sex hormone; low testosterone is associated with decreased sex drive in both males and females, and with impaired erectile function in men. Testosterone is also necessary for muscle size and strength, exercise tolerance, bone density, fat distribution, and red blood cell production.

In addition, testosterone is required for the activation of dopamine and norepinephrine as well as for opioid receptor binding, which is particularly relevant for people with Lyme disease complex, since alterations in neurotransmitter function will affect mood, energy, and pain tolerance. Consequently, low testosterone may result in increased pain, depression, and fatigue.[16] Testosterone also has immune modulating properties, and may protect against inflammation.[17,18] Some have postulated that this may be why women, who naturally have much lower levels of testosterone, suffer more than men from inflammatory conditions such as autoimmune illnesses and allergies.

Testosterone has different origins in men and women. In women, testosterone is produced in the adrenal glands and ovaries. In men, the hypothalamus sends gonadotrophin-releasing hormone (GnRH) down the pituitary stalk, signaling the pituitary to release follicular stimulating hormone (FSH) and luteinizing hormone (LH). These travel through the blood and stimulate the Leydig cells in the testicles to produce testosterone, which feeds back to the hypothalamus and pituitary. (See Figure 15–4.)

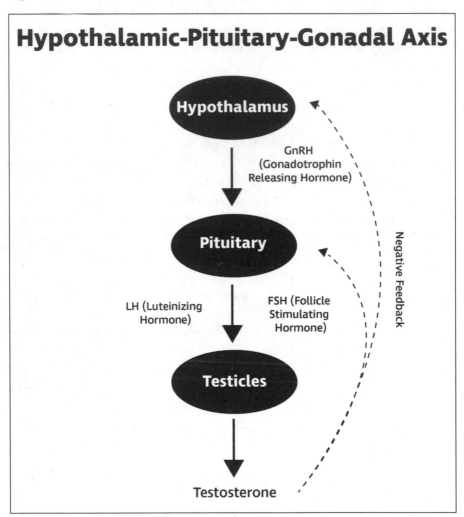

Hypothalamic-Pituitary-Gonadal Axis

Figure 15–4

Most circulating testosterone is bound to a protein called sex hormone binding globulin (SHBG). Some testosterone is converted to estrogen in both men and women via the aromatase enzyme. The remainder of the free (unbound) testosterone is bioavailable; when testing, it is important to measure free testosterone, the biologically active component.

Like cortisol, testosterone has a diurnal rhythm, and levels peak in the early morning. (Perhaps that's when we are biologically programmed to be making love!) Therefore, blood should be drawn before 9:00 a.m.

Once results are obtained, particularly if a man has low testosterone, it is important to determine the source of the problem prior to initiating treatment. Low testosterone can be a result of hypothalamic, pituitary, or testicular issues. If exogenous (literally "from outside the body") testosterone is prescribed to a man who has a hypothalamic or pituitary issue, it will further suppress those structures and may exacerbate, rather than treat, the problem. The first step in the evaluation process is to check out the hypothalamus with a clomiphene stimulation test.

Clomiphene is a fertility drug that blocks estrogen at the hypothalamus. Its use prompts the hypothalamus to release more GnRH, which in turn stimulates the pituitary to discharge FSH and LH, which in men informs the Leydig cells in the testicles to produce testosterone. During a stimulation test, clomiphene 50 mg is prescribed at twice daily for seven days, then the testosterone level is tested on the morning of day eight. If this results in a doubling of the testosterone as compared to the baseline level, the problem is in the hypothalamus.

In this instance, treatment with daily clomiphene will maintain normal testosterone levels. Regular monitoring with blood tests is necessary to appropriately adjust the dose.[10] It is important to also monitor estradiol, because the aromatase enzyme conversion of testosterone to estrogen can result in levels that exceed normal ranges for men. If this occurs, an aromatase inhibitor such as di-indole meth ane (DIM), chrysin, or anastrazole by prescription can be added.[†]

If, however, there is no response to clomiphene stimulation, the next step is a human chorionic gonadotrophin (hCG) stimulation test. hCG is an LH analogue and directly stimulates the Leydig cells in the testes to produce testosterone. If testosterone does not respond to clomiphene, but doubles in response to hCG, the problem is in the pituitary.

An hCG stimulation test is performed by administering hCG 1000 units by subcutaneous injection on Monday, Wednesday, and Friday for two weeks, then repeating the testosterone level test on the second Saturday. The test is considered positive if the hCG is successful in doubling the testosterone level; treatment is with hCG injections two to three times weekly, while monitoring both testosterone and estradiol levels.[‡] As described above, an aromatase inhibitor can be added to increase levels of testosterone and maintain normal estradiol levels.[20,21]

---

†   This testing and treatment protocol is based on a seminar by Dr. Eugene Shippen presented in Reading, Pennsylvania in April 2002.

‡   Ibid.

If testosterone does not respond to either clomiphene or hCG, then treatment with testosterone, either transdermal or by injection, is indicated.

The majority of male patients with low testosterone levels with Lyme disease complex have pituitary dysfunction; fewer have hypothalamic issues, and in general the more elderly have testicular dysfunction. Patients with Lyme disease complex have plenty of inflammation, and pro-inflammatory cytokines suppress testosterone.[22] Opiates can also suppress the pituitary and hypothalamus, resulting in low testosterone.[23] Heavy metals and mold toxins can have a similar effect.[24]

Women with low testosterone are usually postmenopausal, but premenopausal women with Lyme disease complex may also have low levels. This is probably related to the downstream effects of chronic inflammation on both ovarian and adrenal function. Females with low testosterone should have their DHEA levels checked; if DHEA is low, it should be supplemented, but DHEA by itself does not usually normalize a low level of testosterone.

Testosterone replacement in women can be administered transdermally, via sublingual extracts and lozenges, by subcutaneous injection, or by pellet implants. Aromatase inhibitors may also raise testosterone levels. Too much testosterone can cause excess hair growth and deeper voice, but the earliest sign of intolerance is usually irritability, a signal to lower the dose. Appropriate dosing often leads to an improvement in general well-being, energy, mood, and pain control, as well as libido.

INSULIN RESISTANCE

Under normal conditions, eating leads to a rise in blood sugar, which triggers the pancreas to release insulin. The insulin attaches to specific receptors on cell membranes. This relays a message to the cells that they should open the door and let the sugar into the cell. The result is that the sugar level in the blood returns to baseline, and so does the insulin level.

However, if the receptors on the cell membranes do not respond appropriately, the pancreas will release more and more insulin, in effect knocking harder and harder until the doors open and allow in the blood sugar. This is insulin resistance, a prediabetic condition. (See Figure 15–5.) At some point the higher levels of insulin can no longer do the job, and blood sugar starts rising, resulting in Type 2 or adult onset diabetes mellitus (AODM).

Just a few decades ago it was unusual to see a patient under the age of forty with AODM. Now children are being diagnosed with it. What has changed?

Sugar intake has increased dramatically in the past three centuries. In 1700, the average American intake of sugar was estimated at five grams daily; in 1800, it

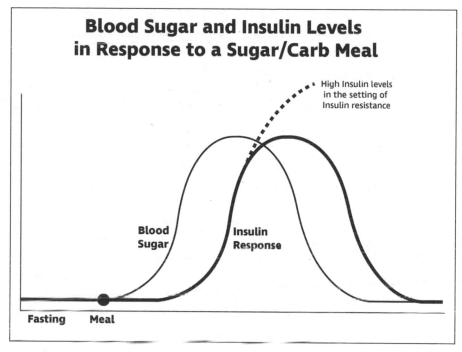

Figure 15–5

was 22 grams daily; in 1900, 112 grams daily; and in 2009 it was 227 grams a day.[25] Sugar intake has increased a whopping 30 percent in adults in the United States in the past thirty years.[26] For reference, one twelve-ounce can of Dr Pepper contains forty grams of sugar.

In the 1960s, the Harvard School of Public Health declared that saturated fats were the cause of heart disease, and food manufacturers began promoting low-fat foods while substituting lots of sugar to give them taste. This was in spite of Dr. John Yudkin's research dating back to the 1950s suggesting that sugar was a major miscreant in the genesis of heart disease, the number one killer in the United States both then and now.[27,28] But Harvard maintained that Yudkin's data were flawed and instead indicted fat, leading the US government to make wholesale recommendations to drastically reduce Americans' fat intake.[§29]

It turns out that the sugar industry secretly paid for the favorable Harvard research[30]—that's right, the Harvard folks took gobs of money to influence Americans' diets to increase sugar (and carbohydrates) while lowering fats, and generate an epidemic of obesity, insulin resistance, and diabetes.[**] Nearly 40 percent

---

§   Those recommendations included the substitution of partially hydrogenated fats, a.k.a. trans fats, for butter. Trans fats are now known as major contributors to heart disease (and perhaps cancer). They are banned in New York, and the FDA has proposed a national ban.

of adults and 19 percent of children in the United States are obese, a staggering increase since 1999.[31] The incidence of diabetes increased 90 percent from 1995–1997 to 2005–2007.[32]

Elevated insulin directs the metabolism to channel calories into fat, thus increasing weight, which in turn increases insulin resistance. It's a downward spiral, and it's easy to see why there are so many more overweight people today than there were just two generations ago. But even before diabetes sets in, high insulin levels can lead to high blood pressure, elevated cholesterol and triglycerides, and an increased risk of heart disease. This cluster of conditions is called metabolic syndrome.

Elevated insulin may also result in fatigue and drowsiness. People who get tired after eating lots of carbohydrates are often insulin resistant, although food sensitivities can also result in sleepiness after eating. And here is the direct link to Lyme disease complex: Inflammation from the infection results in insulin resistance, which in turn leads to more inflammation. The pro-inflammatory cytokine TNF-α is able to induce insulin resistance, and fat is a site for the production of inflammatory cytokines including TNF-α, Interleukin-6, and others.[33]

Blood tests to diagnosis insulin resistance start with a fasting insulin level. It is wise to also test for fasting blood sugar, fasting triglycerides, and a hemoglobin A1c, which indicates blood sugar averages over the previous four months. A fasting insulin level greater than 5 uIU/ml suggests a possible problem.

Treatment starts with a low-glycemic diet—avoiding foods that stimulate high insulin release. The worst offenders are glutinous grains, rice, corn, white potatoes, and, of course, sugar. Most weight loss diets are based on this idea—avoid sugar and carbohydrates and emphasize protein. Not only can these Paleolithic-type menus often control AODM even without medication, they also decrease inflammation and lead to weight loss. Many patients with Lyme disease complex feel better avoiding sugar and carbohydrates.

Nutritional supplements that can enhance insulin sensitivity include chromium, alpha lipoic acid, omega-3 essential fatty acids, magnesium, and zinc. The most common medication to treat insulin resistance and early diabetes is metformin.

IT'S ALL CONNECTED

Endocrine function is foundational to health and well-being. Hormones regulate every cell in the body, and are in continuous communication wth the nervous and

---

** In his book *The Case Against Sugar*, Gary Taubes tells the sordid story of how the food industry paid off the Harvard School of Public Health and managed to suppress the evidence of sugar's negative impact on our nation's health. (Random House, ©2016)

immune systems. Chronic illness often results in endocrine dysregulation. This chapter has outlined hormones of the endocrine system; the gastrointestinal system manufactures its own set of hormones, and is described in the next chapter.

TAKE-HOME POINTS

1. Adrenal insufficiency results in fatigue, immune suppression, and other problems. Everyone who has Lyme disease complex should have their adrenal function evaluated.
2. People with Lyme disease complex should have thyroid testing. Proper evaluation of thyroid function includes measuring reverse T3.
3. Low pituitary function is prevalent, particularly in patients with mold toxins. Diabetes insipidus is the most common problem associated with low pituitary function.
4. Low testosterone can result in fatigue, weakness, depression, and increased pain as well as low libido. Low levels deserve a careful evaluation and treatment.
5. Insulin resistance increases weight, may lead to diabetes, increases risk of heart disease, increases inflammation, and causes fatigue. Paleo or low-glycemic diets can be anti-inflammatory.
6. It's all connected: the endocrine system impacts every cell in the body.

Chapter 16

Gastrointestinal Issues

The gut is finally getting the respect it deserves. From an evolutionary perspective, the alimentary canal is the brain of our unicellular predecessors like amoebae and paramecia. In some ways it is still a "brain": in addition to digestion and absorption, the gut contains more nerve cells than the spinal cord, produces the majority of neurotransmitters (including 90 percent of serotonin), encompasses more immune cells than the rest of the body combined, and produces its own hormones that communicate with all other cells in the body. Recent research has demonstrated the profound impact of the gut microbiome on metabolism. Good health requires a healthy GI tract.

People with recurrent abdominal pain, gas, bloating, constipation, and/or diarrhea are likely to be referred to a gastroenterologist. More often than not the doctor will look up and down, but not find any abnormalities—no ulcers, no tumors, nothing visibly wrong. Hence, the default diagnosis of irritable bowel syndrome (IBS). IBS is the most common diagnosis made in a gastroenterologist's office.

It is estimated that the prevalence of IBS in the United States is 10 to 15 percent—that's over thirty million Americans.[1] It's not clear who is more irritated—the patients or the doctors—probably both, and often from lack of answers. But a careful functional evaluation often reveals underlying conditions, many of which occur in patients with Lyme disease complex. These include food sensitivities, yeast overgrowth, parasites, small intestine bacterial overgrowth, gastroparesis, malabsorption syndromes and leaky gut syndrome. These issues complicate and compound the clinical picture, making overall treatment more difficult.

FOOD SENSITIVITIES

There are two categories of food sensitivities. Type 1 allergy reactions are fairly obvious; they typically result in hives, eczema, congestion, asthma, swelling, and, in the worst case scenario, anaphylaxis. Type 1 reactions are mediated via the IgE antibody, and are usually immediate in onset. Type 2 reactions are often delayed, and symptoms may not be classically "allergic"; e.g. fatigue, sleepiness, joint pains, headaches, brain fog, hyperactivity, and nonspecific GI complaints. Type 2 reactions may have more than one mechanism, but the IgG4 antibody is often implicated. Table 16–1 lists the clinical spectrum of Type 2 food reactions.

The Clinical Spectrum of Food Sensitivities			
Respiratory	Congestion	**Gastrointestinal**	Abdominal pain
	Sinus pain		Indigestion
	Cough		Diarrhea
	Wheezing/asthma		Constipation
	Recurrent otitis, Recurrent sinusitis, bronchitis, and pharyngitis		Bloating
			Post-cholecystectomy syndrome
Neurological	Headaches		Biliary colic
	Migraine headaches		Inflammatory bowel disease
	Cognitive dysfunction		
	Mood swings	**Genitourinary**	Canker sores
	Irritability		Urinary frequency
	Anxiety		Enuresis (bed-wetting)
	Depression		
	Seizure disorders		Nephrosis
	Hyperactivity		Premenstrual syndrome
	Attention deficit disorder	**Systemic**	Recurrent vaginitis
Musculo-skeletal	Muscle aches		Edema
	Joint pains		Fatigue
	Rashes	**Cardiac**	Palpitations
	Rheumatoid arthritis		

Table 16–1.

The possibility of food sensitivities should be considered in all patients with chronic GI complaints; studies have confirmed the association of IBS with food intolerances.[2] This is particularly true if the person reports a childhood history of recurrent ear infections, sore throats, sinusitis, chronic congestion, constipation, diarrhea, abdominal pain, headaches, fatigue, or attention deficit hyperactivity disorder (ADHD), since these conditions are often associated with food sensitivities.

Interestingly, people with delayed food reactions often crave the food that causes the reaction. This is referred to as the allergy-addiction syndrome.[3] For example, if Johnny is chronically congested, gets frequent colds and ear infections, suffers chronic constipation, and drinks four glasses of milk daily—and gets cranky if he doesn't get it—dairy is likely a problem. People who crave bread and starchy food are usually sensitive to wheat, gluten, and/or yeast. Yeast is almost always a problem in the person who craves sugar as well as carbs (candidiasis sensitivity syndrome is discussed below). People often go through withdrawal for a few days when they stop eating the food that is causing an allergy-addiction syndrome; common withdrawal symptoms are irritability, headaches, and fatigue.

Tony was twenty-seven years old at his first visit. He told me that he had been fatigued as long as he could remember. As a child he had suffered from frequent colds, recurrent sinusitis, and strep throats. Then at age thirteen he developed chronic indigestion, flatulence, and fluctuating diarrhea and constipation. By his twenties he also had frequent headaches and joint pains.

When Tony was twenty-five years old he decided to eliminate all gluten from his diet. His GI symptoms and headaches totally remitted, his energy improved, and his joint pains diminished.

Prior to the 1960s, only a half dozen foods accounted for 95 percent of Type 2 food reactions; wheat, dairy, eggs, corn, citrus, and sugar/yeast were by far the most common. Second-tier foods included beef, pork, soy, and gluten. Back then it was rare to find someone who reacted to rice, lamb, or avocado. But things have changed over the past two generations, and now people react to almost anything.*

The most common food sensitivities I have witnessed among patients with Lyme disease complex are gluten, dairy, and eggs. Many patients with both Lyme and food sensitivities report that they developed the reactivity after becoming infected, suggesting that chronic infections can alter immunity and result in heightened reactivity. In fact, alpha-gal syndrome is a recently identified type of food allergy to red meat that often begins after a bite by a lone star tick.

Type 1 IgE mediated food allergies are relatively easy to diagnose, whether by history or with blood and skin tests. Type 2 food sensitivities are more difficult to

---

* I suspect there are multiple factors that account for the increase in reactions to foods: the wholesale change in diet over the past century with a huge increase in sugar and decrease in whole grains; mineral depletion in the soil; exposure to hundreds of thousands of chemicals such as pesticides and herbicides; changes in the intestinal bioflora; GMO foods; leaky gut syndrome; epigenetic issues; and chronic infections like Lyme that alter immune function—to name a few.

nail down. Symptoms such as sleepiness or headaches may or may not suggest an allergic issue. In addition, reactions are often delayed, occurring hours to days after ingesting the offending food. And reactivity can also vary depending on how often the food is ingested. Further complicating this scenario is that many people with Type 2 food sensitivities are reacting to more than one food, and they are usually eating the offending foods daily.

Skin testing for Type 2 food reactions is not accurate. Many laboratories offer blood tests to pinpoint offending foods, usually measuring IgG4 antibodies to one hundred or more foods. Although results are not totally reliable, with both false positives and false negatives, they do provide the opportunity to test a lot of foods with a simple blood draw.

The Elimination-Challenge Diet

The gold standard of diagnosis is an elimination-challenge diet. The overall strategy is quite simple: remove suspected foods from the diet for a period of time, then reintroduce them one at a time, watching carefully for any reactions.

Alternatively, an elimination-challenge can be performed on a single food item. The problem with this approach is that many people with food sensitivities are reacting to multiple foods. If only one of them is removed from the diet while the person continues to eat the other offenders, the results of eliminating a single irritating food may be unclear.

The most common elimination diet involves removing milk, wheat, corn, eggs, citrus, tomatoes, coffee, caffeine, chocolate, artificial additives (including preservatives and coloring), sugar (including natural sweeteners like honey, syrup, molasses, etc.), soy, gluten (barley, rye, oats, wheat, and spelt), and yeast (which includes all breads unless specifically stated "no yeast," pastries, alcohol, vinegar, peanuts, peanut butter, cheese, mushrooms, dried fruit [including raisins], smoked or processed meats, fermented foods [sauerkraut, pickles, olives], fruit juices, melons, berries, grapes, and all sweets).

Labels should be read carefully, as soy and corn oil are in a lot of processed food (the latter particularly in "vegetable oils"). To achieve the most accurate results, any food eaten more than once weekly should also be removed.

If you go on an elimination diet, it needs to be 100 percent, because any cheating will confuse the results. Children typically stay on the basic elimination diet for five to seven days before "challenging" by reintroducing foods one at a time, but adults often need to stay on the diet two weeks before challenging. This is because withdrawal symptoms (think caffeine cessation) such as fatigue, headaches, irritability, and aching clear more quickly in children than adults. Food cravings may be strong during this period, since chances are that the foods being craved are the ones causing problems.†

The following foods are allowed during the elimination diet: limited starches such as quinoa, millet, rice, sweet potatoes, legumes other than peanuts, and amaranth; meats, fish, chicken, and turkey; salad, squash, and greens in general—although any salad dressing should not contain soy oil or vinegar; olive oil with basil and garlic is recommended. Fruit is limited to one serving of fresh fruit daily, excluding citrus, melons, berries, and grapes. Drinks are limited to spring water (no tap water) and herbal teas. Sample menus include a breakfast of rice, buckwheat, or gluten-free oatmeal with cinnamon and unsweetened almond milk. Lunch can be salad, tuna, or chicken (without mayo) and rice cakes. Dinner can be meat, fish, or chicken, with vegetables, potatoes, or rice. Acceptable snacks include vegetables, rice cakes with almond butter, hummus, or tahini. All fruit and vegetables should be organic.

When it is time to begin the challenge, one food per day is introduced, and always as a pure food. For example, if the food being challenged is milk, other dairy products such as ice cream or cheese are not appropriate. Instead, you should drink milk in moderate quantity at least three times during the day; e.g., three glasses of milk total. If the reaction is clear, the challenge for milk is stopped. In this case, the milk is again eliminated, and the next food challenged on the next day. It is best to keep the challenges pure; for example, don't use bread to challenge wheat, because it has many other ingredients, including yeast. Wheatena cereal made with water, or whole wheat crackers without additives, are better options. Yeast can be challenged using brewer's yeast tablets, five or six per meal.

If the symptoms of a reaction are not clear, the food is continued for another day or two before moving on. Alternately, if there is a severe reaction to a food challenge and the symptoms are carrying over to the next day, the baseline elimination diet is resumed for at least one day beyond the resolution of symptoms before the next challenge is performed.

The foods listed above have been chosen because they are the ones to which most people react. Of course people can be sensitive to any number of foods in addition to these. If any other foods are suspect, and in particular any foods eaten frequently, they should be added to the list.

The proper interpretation of the results depends on keeping a careful diary of symptoms during both the elimination and challenge period. Some find it helpful to make a table that lists symptoms, then grade these at several different times of the "challenge" day, with a new page for every day of the trial.

---

†   I highly recommend *An Alternative Approach to Allergies* by Theron Randolph and Ralph Moss (New York: Harper and Row, 1980). The authors give an excellent description of the stimulation-withdrawal syndrome associated with these sensitivity syndromes.

Treatment of Food Sensitivities

Once an offending food is identified, it should be completely eliminated from the diet until all symptoms of food sensitivity have resolved, at which point the food can be reintroduced on a rotation basis—i.e. it can be eaten every four days, assuming it is tolerated. Anyone with multiple food sensitivities should also be evaluated for leaky gut syndrome and maldigestion, which are discussed later in this chapter.

Supplements like quercitin (a bioflavanoid that stabilizes mast cells—immune cells that release histamine during a process called degranulation) and diamine oxidase (which breaks down histamine), taken thirty to forty-five minutes before eating, can help block food reactions. The prescription medications cromolyn sodium (Gastrocrom) and ketotifen also inhibit mast cell degranulation; they are also taken about thirty to forty-five minutes before meals.

Gluten deserves special mention. Celiac disease is only one type of gluten sensitivity; it can be diagnosed by antibody tests and small bowel biopsy. But gluten sensitivity without celiac is not uncommon. It can result in similar GI issues as well as headaches, joint pain, brain fog, and fatigue.

CANDIDIASIS SENSITIVITY SYNDROME

When conditions allow for overgrowth of yeast in the gut, some people develop sensitivity to yeast, a.k.a. candidiasis sensitivity syndrome (CSS). Yeast sensitivity merits particular attention, because a reaction to yeast can result in many symptoms that overlap with those of Lyme disease complex. Risk factors that increase the likelihood of developing CSS include frequent or prolonged use of antibiotics, corticosteroids, or oral contraceptives; mold allergy and/or mold exposure; multiple food sensitivities; multiple pregnancies; and high intake of sugar, carbohydrates, and alcohol.

CSS is more common in women, since female hormones encourage yeast growth. Almost all people with CSS have GI complaints, particularly gas and bloating, and they usually crave sugar and carbohydrates. Symptoms are worse with sugar and carbohydrate intake as well as premenstrually, when sugar cravings typically spike. Many women describe recurrent or chronic yeast vaginitis as well as oral thrush and skin mycoses (fungi on the skin).

A typical scenario occurs when children with food sensitivities, especially to dairy products, suffer chronic congestion and frequent ear infections. They are prescribed recurrent courses of antibiotics, leading to yeast overgrowth in the gut and subsequent sensitization to yeast. That's when the sugar and carbohydrate cravings kick in—in essence, they are feeding their yeast. Patients with Lyme disease complex need to be particularly aware of CSS, since the chronic antibiotics they take in the course of treatment can lead to yeast issues unless they are simultaneously taking anti-yeast agents and probiotics. When a patient with Lyme disease complex presents with CSS, it is advisable to initiate anti-yeast treatment before starting antibiotics.

Treatment of CSS is achieved with dietary changes, plus anti-yeast agents and probiotics. Everyone with CSS needs to avoid all sugar and alcohol, and most need to be off the yeast-containing foods listed in the description of the elimination/challenge diet. The more severely affected also need to stay on a very low carbohydrate diet.

Table 16–2 lists commonly used anti-yeast agents. Nystatin is a well-tolerated medication that is not absorbed systemically—it works only in the gut. Anyone taking long-term antibiotics should strongly consider simultaneous use of Nystatin to prevent yeast overgrowth. Fluconazole, on the other hand, is systemic in action; it is appropriate for patients with more severe yeast problems, with the dosing frequency ranging from daily to once weekly. Probiotics with 100+ billion colony forming units should be taken with food but away from antibiotics. Another probiotic, *Saccharomyces boulardii,* is a good addition. It is sometimes referred to as yeast against yeast, because it inhibits *Candida.* Anti-yeast agents may result in a Herxheimer reaction due to yeast die-off, so should be initiated slowly in patients with CSS.

COMMONLY USED ANTI-YEAST AGENTS		
Availability	**Agent**	**Considerations**
Prescription Agents	Nystatin	Not absorbed
	Fluconazole	Systemic
	Itraconazole	Systemic, active against a broad spectrum of fungi
	Voriconazole	Systemic, active against a broad spectrum of fungi
	Ketoconazole	High incidence of liver toxicity
	Amphotericin	IV medication that can be compounded to take as non-absorbable oral antifungal
Nonprescription agents	Caprylic acid	Coconut derived, well tolerated
	Grapefruit seed extract	Active against *Bb* spirochete and cyst form
	Undecylinic acid	Well tolerated
	Coptis (goldthread)	Antifungal in Traditional Chinese Medicine
	Biocidin	Gentian and other herbs Powerful broad-spectrum antifungal, antiparasitic, antibacterial

Table 16-2

DIGESTION ISSUES

Food entering the stomach is first exposed to the gastric secretion of hydrochloric acid. This digestive fluid performs a number of important functions. It initiates protein digestion, chelates minerals for absorption, eradicates bacteria and parasites, and stimulates the release of bile and pancreatic enzyme juices.

Too much acid gets all the attention as the cause of gastrointestinal complaints. It was long assumed that anyone with indigestion, heartburn, or peptic ulcer disease had too much acid—from stress, coffee, and/or alcohol. But in 2005 Dr. Barry Marshall of Australia won the Nobel Prize for his research demonstrating that gastric ulcers are actually caused by a bacterium, *H. pylori*.[‡4] What is often overlooked is the evidence that this bacterium thrives in a low acid environment, i.e. when there is a low output of hydrochloric acid. Most people with peptic disease have low gastric output of hydrochloric acid, a condition called hypochlorhydria,[5] not too much acid.

Nevertheless, the pharmaceutical industry developed a financial bonanza of agents that decrease stomach acid. Virtually everyone with indigestion, heartburn, or gastroesophageal reflux disorder (GERD) is prescribed a protein pump inhibitor (PPI) like omeprazole (Prilosec), or an H2 blocker like famotidine to cut acid production. These agents are only intended to be taken for short, six-week courses, but more often people end up taking them for years.

This is a problem for two reasons. First of all, low stomach acid is not good for you—the acid is there for important reasons. Secondly, PPIs actually decrease the tone of the gastroesophageal sphincter, thereby increasing the likelihood of reflux.[6] This reflux is less likely to cause heartburn because of its low acidity, but other problems now arise.

People with hypochlorhydria typically don't absorb minerals well and therefore are prone to iron deficiency and osteoporosis. They may also become deficient in amino acids because of the impairment in the breakdown of proteins. These people are prone to overgrowth of bacteria in the small intestine, which is described below.

PPIs are sometimes called Purple Meth because they are so difficult to discontinue. Try stopping the PPI and the heartburn is actually worse than before because the sphincter between the esophagus and the stomach has lost tone. Patients have to be weaned off slowly. Some people find that drinking calcium carbonate 250 mg powder in water at the end of meals makes the weaning process easier, as it increases the tone of the sphincter.

---

‡   Barry Marshall initially experienced stiff resistance from the medical establishment but eventually convinced them by swallowing some *H. pylori* and documenting that it gave him an ulcer. He eventually received the Nobel Prize for his discovery. The long lag time between his discovery and its acceptance in the medical community is not uncommon, as we have experienced with persistent infection with *Borrelia burgdorferi*.

Famotidine appears easier to discontinue, so some find it helpful to first transition from PPIs to this class of acid inhibitors. Additional suggestions include putting six-inch blocks under the head of the bed, and staying away from coffee, alcohol, and nonsteroidal anti-inflammatory drugs (NSAIDs). There are several natural agents that can settle the stomach including DGL (deglycyrrihiizinated licorice), aloe, slippery elm, and marshmallow extract.

Hypochlorhydria, low stomach acid, occurs in many people who are not on these medications. In fact, it may be more common than too much gastric acid. It is estimated that half of people over the age of sixty have hypochlorhydria, and 80 percent of people have low stomach acid by the age of eighty-five. Symptoms include bloating, constipation, belching, and early satiety. Low stomach acid may occur alone, but can also be associated with other problems. Hypochlorhydria is common in people with autoimmune conditions, multiple food allergies, and celiac disease.[7] Many people with gastroparesis (see below) have low stomach acid. People with pernicious anemia and inability to absorb vitamin B_{12} are achlorhydric: they make no stomach acid.

Treatment of hypochlorhydria focuses on replacing stomach acid. Many companies sell betaine hydrochloride with pepsin, usually in a 650 mg capsule. The best way to add this supplement is to start with one capsule at the onset of each meal, taken after one or two bites of food. The dose should be increased daily by one capsule per meal, except if this causes indigestion; then the dose is decreased by one capsule for that meal. Most people are good at finding their ideal dose, which may not be the same at every meal; they may need two capsules for breakfast, three with lunch and four with dinner.

The patient who is achlorhydric may require eight capsules for an average dinner. But ironically they may not tolerate even one capsule, because the stomach lining is not acclimated to even a small amount of acid. These folks should start with a half-teaspoon of vinegar to slowly accustom the stomach to acid. Alternatively, Standard Process makes a lower dose product with just under 300 mg of betaine hydrochloride per tablet.

The stomach is not the only organ of digestion, nor is hydrochloric acid the only chemical involved. As the partially digested food and gastric juices enter the small intestine, the pancreas releases enzymes that proceed with food digestion. In addition, the gall bladder squirts its bile contents through the common bile duct to assist in fat breakdown.

Pancreatic insufficiency, a deficiency in enzyme secretion, leads to maldigestion and malabsorption, particularly of fats. Common symptoms include diarrhea and flatulence, occasional bloating, and borborygmi (gurgling gut). Lab results via stool analysis reveal elevated fats and low chymotrypsin. Treatment is the replacement of pancreatic enzymes, taken at the end of a meal. These are available over the counter as well as by prescription.

People who have had their gall bladders removed can also experience difficulty digesting fatty foods, due to a reduction in bile. This will often improve if ox-bile supplements are taken after meals.

PARASITIC INFECTIONS

Most of us associate parasites with foreign travel. It's true that the risk of infestation increases in some parts of the world such as India and Africa, but you don't need a passport to get a parasite. They are actually quite common in the United States. It is estimated that 5–10 percent of Americans harbor *Blastocystis hominis*,[8] a single-celled parasite of the human gastrointestinal tract.

Parasitic intestinal infections with protozoa such as *Giardia* and with helminths (worms) can lead to serious illness. Although parasites are notorious for causing acute diarrheal illness, they can also hide asymptomatically in the GI tract for years. Ironically, chronic infestation often results in constipation.[9]

Parasites can have multiple impacts on the immune system. They can stimulate systemic inflammatory responses such as arthritis and may be a potent trigger of mast cell degranulation.[10] They can also result in immune suppression[11] and increase autoimmune reactivity.[12] It is highly likely that many people harbor these critters without problems, but if their immune system becomes dysregulated by chronic infection, the dormant parasites become a problem—not only resulting in GI complaints, but also contributing to systemic inflammation.

Patty was thirty-three years old and living in Ohio when she noticed a small red rash on her chest with a pale center. Over the next several years she developed progressive fatigue, arthritic and neurological complaints, as well as chronic indigestion and abdominal bloating. The GI symptoms decreased when she stopped eating gluten, but never totally resolved.

I initially saw Patty when she was fifty-eight years old. At that time she had chronic muscle and joint pains, multiple neuropathic symptoms, impaired cognition, and ongoing GI issues, including occasional abdominal pain, diarrhea, and excess flatulence. She also had drenching night sweats.

I treated Patty for Lyme disease, babesiosis, and bartonellosis with significant improvement. I also prescribed a high potency pancreatic enzyme replacement, which decreased her flatulence. Overall she felt about 80 percent improved.

Then she took Mimosa pudica seed. This herb is different from the Mimosa pudica used to treat Babesia—it is made from the seed rather than the stems and leaves. It does not appear to have antimalarial activity, but it is quite active against intestinal worms, a.k.a. helminths. Shortly after starting,

Patty reported that she evacuated multiple worms, including a five-inch tape-worm. She felt much better following treatment, with increased energy and improved general well-being. Since then, she has dramatically increased her activity and is now campaigning for office in her hometown.

Tests for parasites include direct testing, i.e. detection in a stool examination, as well as indirect testing—antibody detection in either blood, stools, or both. Blood tests may reveal an increase in eosinophils, a type of white blood cell that is also associated with allergy. However, definitive evidence of infection can be difficult to find, and the sensitivity of parasite testing is quite low.[13] Therefore, I often initiate treatment empirically, based on history and symptoms.

Mimosa pudica seeds expand in the gut to form a gelatinous mass that adheres to the parasites and facilitates their expulsion. There are no documented side effects, although some patients actually have Herxheimer reaction with GI distress and fatigue. Many patients have described worms in their stools after taking this herb.

More aggressive regimens are often necessary to treat helminths. Typically, multiple agents such as praziquantel, ivermectin, albendazole, and Alinia are prescribed on a rotational basis. So many of my patients have seen worms in their stools when taking these agents that I suspect a high percentage of us harbor these critters. But if otherwise healthy, we can live in harmony with them similar to our coexistence with the trillions of other microbes than inhabit our bodies. But when our immune systems get out of whack because of tick-borne infections, these colonizers become pathogenic and can cause inflammation both in the gut and systemically.

If patients experience ongoing inflammation despite adequate treatment for their tick-borne infections, consider a trial of anti-protozoal agents in order to eliminate any remaining intestinal parasites such as *Giardia* or *Blastocystis*. These agents include commercially sold extracts of multiple herbs such as Clarkia or Para A, as well as pharmaceuticals like tinidazole and nitazoxanide (Alinia). I am very cautious using metronidazole (Flagyl) because many of my patients have neurological side effects from this drug. Some of these medications also treat tick-borne pathogens; tinidazole attacks the cystic form of *Bb* (and Archaea—see SIBO discussion below), while Alinia is active against *Babesia*. As with many chronic infections, parasites can be resistant to treatment. Complete resolution may take long-term treatment and rotation of anti-parasitic agents.

SMALL INTESTINAL BACTERIAL OVERGROWTH

The small intestine is responsible for the majority of nutrient absorption. While the colon is teeming with trillions of bacteria, the small intestine harbors a relatively scant population of microbes. When the small bowel contains excess bacteria, or bacterial overgrowth, normal function is disrupted. Small intestinal bacterial overgrowth (SIBO) can result in malabsorption, nutrient deficiencies, and weight loss. Common symptoms include bloating, cramping, flatulence, diarrhea, constipation, and nausea. Symptoms are typically worse with carbohydrate intake.

Excess bacteria in the small intestine ferment sugar from carbohydrates, leading to the release of hydrogen. When additional organisms called methanogens, primitive bugs from the kingdom Archaea, are present, methane is released as well.[§] Hydrogen and methane are absorbed in the blood and sent to the lungs, where they are exhaled in the breath, which is why a breath test can detect SIBO (see below). If these microbes were limited to the colon, where fermentation normally occurs, it would not be a problem. However, their presence in the small intestine is another story.

SIBO with hydrogen production usually causes diarrhea, while methane-producing microbes are more likely to cause constipation. People who have alternating diarrhea and constipation may have colonization with both sets of microbes, as well as other GI conditions that cause maldigestion: vitamin B_{12} deficiency, fat malabsorption, food allergies, yeast overgrowth, leaky gut, gastroparesis, and parasites.

There are conditions that predispose a person to SIBO. A major risk factor is a diet high in alcohol, sugar, and carbs, which provides food for the errant microbes. Many patients with SIBO have hypochlorhydria. This makes sense, since stomach acid knocks out microbes before they get to the small intestine. The increase in numbers of people diagnosed with SIBO may very well be related to the flood of prescriptions for PPIs which suppress gastric acid production.

Another risk factor for SIBO is slow motility, which can be due to a number of conditions. Sluggish bowels allow more time for microbes to migrate from the colon to the small intestine. Bowel motility can be disrupted by celiac disease and other food sensitivities, Ehlers-Danlos syndrome (a congenital connective tissue disorder), parasites, some medications (particularly opioid drugs), and neuropathies associated with diabetes, as well as tick-borne infections. Structural bowel issues caused by surgery and diverticulosis can also lead to SIBO. People with SIBO have a higher incidence of autoimmune conditions, fibromyalgia, rosacea, and GERD than the general population.[14]

Many laboratories perform breath analyses for both hydrogen and methane, which can be used for diagnosis. Treatment of SIBO should then follow in a stepwise fashion:

- Identify and treat the underlying conditions that resulted in SIBO, such as hypochlorhydria.

[§]   Archaea constitute a domain of microorganisms without cell nuclei. Initially classified as bacteria, they now constitute a separate kingdom.

- Treat nutrient deficiencies, address issues of malabsorption, and repair the lining of the gut. Bone broth is highly recommended. (Additional recommendations are discussed in more detail under leaky gut syndrome, below.)
- Implement a Paleo-type, low-carbohydrate, low-fermentable-foods diet —the Simple Carbohydrate Diet, GAPS diet, and low FODMAPS diet are common variations.
- Consider beneficial probiotics. This is somewhat controversial in SIBO, but these bacteria are theorized to help maintain a neutral pH at the gut lining, and there are data that supports their use in SIBO.[15,16] On the other hand, some people with SIBO do not tolerate probiotics, and find they actually make symptoms worse.
- Employ antimicrobials to minimize the intestinal overgrowth.

It is possible that treating hypochlorhydria and implementing an appropriate diet will address the conditions for bacterial overgrowth, and SIBO will be alleviated. On the other hand, many people require antibiotics. If a breath test reveals only hydrogen, a long list of antibiotics may be effective, but the drug of choice is Xifaxan, which is non-absorbable and generally well tolerated (although some will experience die-off reactions). A typical regimen is 550 mg three times daily for two weeks; many people require repeated or prolonged courses.

If there is excess methane, effective antibiotics include neomycin, tinidazole, and metronidazole. It is recommended to simultaneously treat the hydrogen-producing offenders, since hydrogen feeds the Archaea organisms. Patients often do even better when adding anti-yeast agents, pancreatic enzymes, and biofilm busters. It is not uncommon for SIBO to coexist with parasitic and fungal overgrowth, and these also require treatment.

There are many non-pharmacologic antimicrobial options. Berberine and oregano oil are useful against hydrogen-producing bacteria. Effective herbs against methane producers include allicin, a garlic derivative, and Atrantil, a dietary supplement composed of quebracho, horse chestnut, and peppermint leaf extracts.[17]

One study found that herbals were as effective as pharmaceuticals,**[18] but as with tick-borne pathogens, people with SIBO respond variably to different antimicrobial regimens. And some people require prolonged and repeated cycles of treatment. Bacteria and Archaea organisms can adapt quickly, so rotating antimicrobials to avoid resistance is a good idea.

** Dysbiocide and FC Cidal (Biotics Research Laboratories, Rosenberg, Texas) or Candibactin-AR and Candibactin-BR (Metagenics, Inc., Aliso Viejo, California) for four consecutive weeks

GASTROPARESIS

In 2006, Dr. Virginia Sherr coined the term "Bell's Palsy of the Gut" to describe the severe constipation that occurs in some patients with Lyme disease complex.[19] Gastroparesis, also called delayed gastric emptying, is a condition in which the movement of food from the stomach to the small intestine is slowed or stopped.

Most often, however, there is decreased peristalsis of the entire intestinal tract, with severe constipation. There may be a sensation of fullness after eating, as if the food is just sitting in the stomach, which it is. Additional symptoms include nausea and vomiting, abdominal bloating, abdominal pain, and acid reflux.

Gastroparesis can occur for a number of reasons:

- Hypochlorhydria, or low stomach acid, as described above
- Dysbiosis—imbalanced gut microbiome, intestinal overgrowth conditions, parasites
- Dysfunction of the vagus—the tenth cranial nerve
- Dysautonomia, or disorders of the autonomic nervous system
- Neuropathies that can occur with diabetes as well as tick-borne infections
- Other nervous system disorders such as Parkinson's and multiple sclerosis
- Hypothyroidism
- Some connective tissue disorders such as scleroderma
- Ehlers-Danlos syndrome, a congenital hyperflexibility condition
- Medications, particularly narcotics
- Food sensitivities

Patients with Lyme disease complex may have several of these conditions concomitantly. An additional complication is the development of SIBO, as described above, and patients can develop malabsorption, become malnourished, and lose weight.

It is necessary to address the underlying condition, but poor gastrointestinal motility can be remarkably resistant to treatment. Multiple drug regimens often fail to alleviate this condition.[††] Magnesium can improve gastric motility, and some patients take very high doses that can result in diarrhea, which they have found preferable to chronic constipation; liquid magnesium oxide in capsules is often effective with doses as high as twenty capsules daily.

---

†† Plucalopride (Resolor) shows some promise in treating gastroparesis. It is currently available in Canada.

INFLAMMATORY BOWEL DISEASE

Inflammatory bowel disease (IBD) is an umbrella term used to describe disorders that involve chronic inflammation of the digestive tract. Crohn's disease and ulcerative colitis are the principal types of inflammatory bowel disease. IBD is distinct from irritable bowel syndrome in that inflammation with IBD can be demonstrated by biopsies, and complications can be serious.

Crohn's disease most commonly affects the small intestine, particularly the terminal ileum, but can cause inflammation everywhere from the mouth to the anus. It can cause severe abdominal pain, diarrhea, abscesses, fistulae formation, and blockage. Ulcerative colitis is a condition that causes inflammation with ulcerations in the colon and rectum, commonly resulting in abdominal pain and bloody diarrhea.

The underlying causes of IBD are probably numerous. Both Crohn's and ulcerativecolitis have been associated with food sensitivities, and strict avoidance of offending foods has resulted in remission in some patients[20,21]—yeast and dairy top the list.

In Chapter 10, I introduced Susan, who had been diagnosed with Crohn's disease but responded to treatment for *Bb*, *Babesia*, and *Bartonella* infections. Susan's experience is not unique. Martin Fried and colleagues studied children and adolescents diagnosed with acute Lyme disease with a history of EM rash and CDC positive Western blots who developed chronic abdominal pain, diarrhea, acid reflux, or blood in the stool following antibiotic treatment. Some were diagnosed with Crohn's or ulcerative colitis. Biopsies demonstrated evidence of colitis, gastritis, and duodenitis, and were also PCR positive for *Bb*, despite previous antibiotic treatment.[22,23] These studies not only demonstrated the capacity of *Bb* to cause IBD, but also the persistence of infection after antibiotic treatment for acute Lyme disease.

Fried and colleagues also found that *Bartonella* can cause IBD. They studied children and adolescents with a history of either tick attachment or cat scratch prior to the onset of chronic abdominal pain or heartburn. Serum *Bartonella* IgG was positive in all the subjects. Biopsies demonstrated gastritis and duodenitis, with PCR positivity for *B. henselae*. In addition, CT scans in many of the subjects demonstrated mesenteric adenitis, a condition characterized by inflammation and swelling of the lymph nodes inside the abdomen.[24] In that report Fried also described the skin changes often referred to as *Bartonella* striae.‡‡ In a follow-up study, Fried demonstrated positive PCRs for *Bb*, *Bartonella*, and *M. fermentans* as

---

‡‡ Other microbes have been implicated in Crohn's disease, notably atypical mycobacteria.

well as *H. pylori* associated with gastritis, duodenitis, or colitis at the site of the biopsy.[25]

Other investigators have described *Bartonella* as a cause of ileitis and colitis.[26,27] In addition, *Bartonella* can cause liver and spleen lesions that appear to be cysts by ultrasound, but which are demonstrated on biopsy to be inflammatory granulomas. These resolve with antibiotic treatment.[28]

LEAKY GUT SYNDROME

The intestines have a paradoxical function: to absorb essential nutrients and to deny entry to unwanted molecules such as undigested foods, toxic waste products, and bacteria. When the integrity of the mucosal lining is disturbed, it can result in disturbance of both these functions. Specifically, there is a degradation of the tight junctions between the cells of the intestinal lining. The technical designation of leaky gut syndrome (LGS) is intestinal hyperpermeability. The consequences are considerable:

- Maldigestion and malabsorption of critical nutrients
- Increased burden on hepatic detoxification systems
- Absorption of undigested food particles, leading to an increase in food reactions
- Increased susceptibility to toxic substances
- Inflammatory conditions and autoimmune issues

The more common conditions that lead to LGS include all the conditions discussed in this chapter and then some:

- Food sensitivities
- Celiac disease
- *Candida* overgrowth
- Parasitic infections
- Bacterial infections—including tick-borne disease
- SIBO
- Inflammatory bowel disease
- Nutritional deficiencies
- Drugs—alcohol, aspirin and other NSAIDs, corticosteroids, some antibiotics and chemotherapeutic agents

It is noteworthy that the causes and the results of leaky gut feed each other and lead to a downward spiral: e.g., food sensitivities lead to bowel inflammation and leaky gut issues, which then lead to more food sensitization; nutritional deficiencies undermine the integrity of the intestinal lining leading to malabsorption and more malnutrition; and chronic inflammatory issues from different causes result in intestinal inflammation leading to leaky gut and increased inflammation.

Testing for LGS is available through specialty labs. The person first provides a baseline urine sample, drinks a premeasured challenge drink containing lactulose and mannitol—two non-metabolized sugar molecules—and then collects urine for six hours. An elevation in the lactulose-to-mannitol ratio is consistent with a hyperpermeable gut lining. Alternatively, an elevated serum level of zonulin, a protein that modulates the permeability of tight junctions in the wall of the digestive tract (and which is upregulated when permeability is increased), indicates leaky gut.[29]

The treatment strategy is encompassed in the "4R" approach:

- Remove irritants, including allergenic foods, *Candida,* parasites, alcohol, and drugs that may be contributing to the problem. In other words, treat any underlying issues, including SIBO.
- Replace agents necessary for digestion: hydrochloric acid, pancreatic enzymes, and bile supplements.
- Re-inoculate with beneficial probiotics.
- Repair the intestinal lining. There is a long list of nutrients that can facilitate healing of the gut lining, and many companies combine them in a single capsule or powder. Among the most important nutrients are glutamine (the most prolific amino acid in the gut lining, also important for immune function), zinc, omega-3 essential fatty acids, gamma oryzanol, gamma-linolenic acid, N-acetyl-D-glucosamine, and lecithin.

The bottom line is that whenever there are gut issues, suspect that LGS may be a downstream issue that is aggravating the problem, and should be addressed.

TAKE-HOME POINTS

1. The GI tract is a complex organ system that is intimately involved with immune function, nervous system regulation, and endocrine balance as well as digestion and absorption.
2. It is essential to normalize GI function to keep the body healthy and optimize the ability to treat tick-borne infections.
3. Diagnosing problems in the GI tract takes a methodical investigation to uncover what may constitute several underlying issues.

4. The most common problem seen with antibiotic treatment is overgrowth of yeast and imbalance of intestinal flora. These issues can be prevented and addressed with anti-yeast agents and probiotics.

Chapter 17

Nervous System Disorders

A Lyme attack on the nervous system can impact the quality of life more than any other aspect of this disease. It's bad enough being tired and in pain, but feeling like you are losing your mind can be devastating. Constant anxiety and panic attacks make for more than a bad day. Depression can be so severe that several Lyme sufferers have committed suicide. The smallest task—like feeding the pets, watering the plants, folding the laundry, or making the bed—can seem overwhelming. Many Lyme patients describe having times where they are so confused that they can't complete a sentence, remember where they are driving, or even recall if they've already eaten. Addressing imbalances in the nervous system is important not only to improve quality of life, but also because it is crucial to proper immune and endocrine function.

A word of caution: severe mood disorders associated with central nervous system involvement are serious and may require psychiatric intervention and psychotropic medication as well as aggressive treatment of infections. Don't let them go untreated.

Infection with *Bb* results in a cytokine cascade leading to inflammation in the nervous system. This can cause meningitis, inflammatory neuropathies, myelitis (spinal cord inflammation), neurotransmitter imbalance, vasculitis with decreased bloodflow to the brain, transient ischemic attacks and strokes, neurodegeneration, and demyelination.[1,2,3] It's no wonder that people with Lyme have so many cognitive and mood disorders.

It is always important to consider co-infections in patients with severe neurological symptoms, particularly *Bartonella* and *Babesia*. Table 6–2 in Chapter 6 details a list of neurological issues associated with these infections. This chapter focuses on treatment, for both the more common and for the more severe nervous system issues. In addition to the treatments outlined here, remember that all the problems addressed in this chapter will improve when the infections are properly treated, in conjunction with the use of anti-inflammatory agents and detoxification support.

SLEEP DISORDERS

Insomnia is extremely common in patients with Lyme disease complex. Since sleep and the circadian rhythm exert major influence on immune function,[4] normalizing sleep patterns is essential to the healing process.

It has recently been discovered that the brain detoxifies while we sleep. The glymphatic system, essentially the waste clearance system of the central nervous system, removes neurotoxic waste products and is activated during sleep. Sleep disorders cause a build up of toxins in the brain that may lead to an increase in neuro-degenerative disorders and cognitive dysfunction.[5]

Sleep issues can be broken down into difficulty with sleep initiation, difficulty with staying asleep, and disturbances in sleep architecture, such as sleep apnea. Remedies for sleep problems, whether prescription or natural products, may address one sleep issue but not all. This often makes finding the right solution a matter of trial and error. Table 17-1 lists natural sleep aids, common dosages, and potential adverse effects: each are then described in more depth.

NATURAL AGENTS FOR SLEEP			
Name	Generic	Common bedtime doses	Most common side effects
Magnesium		250–1000 mg	Diarrhea
Melatonin		.5–3.0 mg orally or under tongue	Depression Daytime sleepiness
Valerian	*Valeriana officinalis*	300–500 mg	None known
Passionflower	*Passiflora incarnata*	5–10 mg	None known
5-HTP	5-Hydoxytryptophan	100–500 mg	Avoid if taking an SSRI
Tryptophan		500–2000 mg	Avoid if taking an SSRI
GABA	Gamma-aminobutyric acid	500–1000 mg	In excess can increase anxiety and cause tingling in the limbs

Table 17–1. Natural Agents for Sleep

- **Magnesium:** Magnesium is a muscle relaxant that also calms the nervous system. If sleep problems are not severe, taking magnesium at bedtime may do the trick. Some people take magnesium in the middle of the night when they wake up and can't fall back to sleep. Magnesium glycinate, malate, and citrate are well absorbed, while magnesium oxide is not. The dose can be increased until stools become soft—at some dose magnesium will give everyone diarrhea. ReMag is a highly concentrated liquid magnesium that appears to be extremely well absorbed.

- **Melatonin:** The body's biological clock is regulated by melatonin. This natural hormone is released by the pineal gland when the lights are turned off, so levels go down during the day and up at night. Melatonin is the body's signal to go into rest mode. Adequate levels shorten the time needed to fall asleep and reduce nighttime awakenings. Melatonin production naturally decreases as we get older.[6]

  Supplemental melatonin can be taken orally or sublingually, i.e. under the tongue, and liposomal varieties may be the best absorbed. Usual doses are one-half to three milligrams, although some people benefit from much higher doses. Melatonin is metabolized quickly in most people, so it is ideal for individuals whose issue is sleep initiation. But it also comes in a sustained-release oral preparation, which may help in staying asleep.

  Despite its quick metabolism, some people feel sleepy the next day, regardless of which type they take. There is also the occasional person who feels depressed on melatonin.

- **Herbs:** Valerian stimulates the central nervous system receptors that lead to sedation, but it does not cause morning hangovers. It is often combined with passionflower (*Passiflora*), which, despite its name, has relaxing and antianxiety effects. Other herbs that may be helpful and are often found in combination with both valerian and passionflower include lemon balm, wild lettuce, Jamaican dogwood, skullcap, hops, catnip, and chamomile.

- **5-HTP:** 5-hydroxy-tryptophan is a serotonin precursor that may help sleep as well as reduce pain. Typical doses are 100–300 mg at bedtime. The simultaneous ingestion of other protein should be avoided; it will compete with 5-HTP to cross the blood-brain barrier. This amino acid shouldn't be used by anyone taking an antidepressant in the SSRI class, as doing so could precipitate serotonin syndrome, which in severe cases can be fatal.

- **Tryptophan:** Like 5-HTP, this serotonin precursor is often effective for sleep disorders, especially if taken with 100 mg of vitamin B_6. Doses range from 500 to 2000 mg. The same precaution holds for those taking an antidepressant in the SSRI class.

- **GABA:** Gamma-aminobutyric acid is an inhibitory neuropeptide—it decreases the activity of other neurotransmitters that are firing too rapidly. GABA has a calming effect, and in some people it is also sedating. Typical doses range from 500 to 1000 mg.

- **Diphenhydramine:** The most effective over-the-counter drugs available for sleep contain some form of diphenhydramine, which is the active agent in Benadryl. Best known as an antihistamine, its sedative qualities have made it a popular sleep agent as well. As with many of these sleep-inducers, it can cause grogginess the next day. Diphenhydramine can result in cognitive dysfunction if taken on a long-term basis. Other antihistamines that are used for sleep include hydroxyzine and doxylamine.

- **THC**: Medical marijuana is increasingly available in states throughout the United States. Tetrahydrocannabinol is well known as the psychoactive agent in *Cannabis*, but there are *Cannabis indica* strains in which THC is sedating without the psychoactive component. People with difficulties falling asleep should consider smoking *Cannabis* using a pipe with a cooling chamber or taking a sublingual extract, both of which have a short onset of action. People who have difficulty staying asleep should try an edible form at bedtime; it takes sixty to ninety minutes to enter the bloodstream, and lasts an average of three to four hours. Edible THC comes in tablets, with an average dose of 10 mg at bedtime. If a patient has never tried marijuana, it is best to start at 2.5 mg.

  THC has an added advantage in that it increases the amount of time spent in stages three and four of the sleep cycle, thereby increasing the quality of sleep. It has been shown to decrease episodes of central sleep apnea, and also decreases REM sleep, which is when we dream.[7] Some patients formerly plagued by nightmares and night terrors have restful nights when they take THC at bedtime.

- **Progesterone**—Many women are low in this hormone, particularly if they are postmenopausal. Progesterone is both calming and sedating, and often improves sleep when taken at bedtime.[8]

  Men also require progesterone. It is produced in the adrenal glands and testes, and is necessary for adequate production of testosterone. Deficiencies in progesterone mimic testosterone deficiency: low libido, fatigue, depression, and erectile dysfunction. Progesterone in men can improve sleep, decrease episodes of central and sleep apnea, and enhance immune function.[9]

There is a long list of prescription sleep medications, each with highly variable individual responses. While finding the right sleep aid usually entails trial and error to see what works, there are some basic considerations they all have in common. All meds prescribed for sleep are potentially addictive, some more so than others. They can all make you groggy the next day. And they can all increase depression in susceptible people. It is not unusual for a medication to be effective without side effects, but to lose its effectiveness or cause side effects with extended use. These are not reasons to avoid sleep medications for anyone not getting adequate rest, but be forewarned of the possible complications associated with their long-term use.

Benzodiazepines like clonazepam (Klonopin) and lorazepam (Ativan) can both induce and maintain sleep. However, normal sleep architecture is often disrupted with their long-term use, so they are only recommended for short-term benefits. The same is true for zolpidem (Ambien); while not a benzodiazepine, it has similar characteristics and side effects.

Tricyclics have been replaced by SSRIs and SNRIs as antidepressants, but they are often recommended for sleep. Like THC, these medications have the benefit of increasing the time spent in stages three and four of the sleep cycle, thereby improving the quality of sleep.[10] Doxepin has the added advantage of antihistaminic action, and amitriptyline is often helpful in migraine prevention and treatment of neuropathic pain.

Trazadone is an antidepressant but not in the tricyclic or SSRI class that is rarely prescribed anymore for depression. But it is a good medication for people who wake early.

Some people appear to be getting adequate sleep, but wake feeling unrested. This is when a sleep study is indicated to rule out episodes of sleep apnea and low oxygen to the brain.

Proper sleep hygiene is critical. This includes avoiding workouts, caffeine, and nicotine near bedtime. Getting to bed at a regular time without using electronic devices an hour before bedtime is also important. While napping during the day is usually discouraged, it is often necessary for folks with Lyme disease complex.

ANXIETY

Anxiety can be incredibly distressful. My daughter Hannah, who has had Lyme, told me that she would rather have a migraine headache than suffer anxiety. I was considered a calm, even-keeled person before I had Lyme disease. The agitation and daily panic attacks that I experienced with *Bb*, *Babesia*, and *Bartonella* infections were overwhelming. I could barely talk or move, let alone function. In nontechnical terms, I was a nervous wreck.

Short-term stress, such as a car accident, can actually enhance immune function, but chronic anxiety can decrease immune competence and increase inflammation, so it is important to address this issue—not only because it causes distress, but also because it will adversely impact the ability to fight infection.[11]

There are some who claim that it is important to move through your darkest fears in order to find ultimate healing—the "no pain, no gain" theory. But anxiety caused by an organic illness is not a dark night of the soul, nor is it a productive time to deal with traumatic issues from childhood. Anyone with severe anxiety is strongly encouraged to take measures to decrease these awful symptoms. It's more the "no pain, no pain" philosophy. If anxiety is not severe, then some of the natural agents listed in Table 17–2 may do the trick.

NATURAL AGENTS FOR ANXIETY			
Name	Generic	Common doses	Most common side effects
Magnesium		250 mg 1–3x/day	Diarrhea
Calcium		250–500 mg, 1–3x/day	None
Vitamin B complex		B-50 complex contains 50 mg of each B vitamin 1–3x/day	Insomnia Agitation
Kava	*Piper methysticum*	100 mg, 1–3x/day	Liver irritation
Theanine		100–200 mg, 1–3x/day	None
GABA	Gamma-aminobutyric acid	250–500 mg 1–3x/day (500–1000 mg at night for sleep, higher doses to stimulate growth hormone)	In excess it can increase anxiety and cause tingling in the limbs

Table 17–2. Natural Agents for Anxiety

- **Magnesium**: Magnesium can be a powerful relaxer. Some people take it at bedtime to help them sleep. [12] The faster it is absorbed, the better it works. Natural CALM, which is an effervescent form of magnesium citrate, gets into the bloodstream quickly. Magnesium glycinate and malate are also well absorbed. As noted above, ReMag is a highly concentrated liquid that appears to be extremely well absorbed.
- **Calcium**: This is another mineral that can have calming effects. [13] Calcium citrate is inexpensive and well absorbed.
- **Kava**: This herb is well known for its relaxing and soothing properties. [14] It can also be sedating, relieve pain, and protect the nervous system. However, some people describe an uncomfortable, spacey feeling from kava, and it can irritate the liver. Liver tests should be performed regularly if taken long term.
- **Theanine**: This amino acid is a relaxant that increases alpha waves, promoting both mental and physical relaxation without causing sleepiness. [15] Typical doses are 200 mg three times daily.
- **GABA**: Gamma-aminobutyric acid is an amino acid that can slow brain activity, and it has been useful in treating anxiety as well as sleep issues. [16]
- **Psy-Stabil**: A homeopathic remedy made by Pekana. Many patients have reported relief of anxiety taking fifteen to thirty drops three times daily.

- **Vitamin B complex**: This can be an effective treatment for anxiety in some people, but in others it can make it worse. The most effective are methylated B vitamins, which are discussed in detail in Chapter 19.[17]
- **CBD**: This extract derived from hemp oil decreases neuroinflammation and can decrease anxiety and pain. CBD is discussed in more detail under medical marijuana in the pain section below.
- **Rescue Remedy**: Manufactured by Nelsons, contains five flower essences: rockrose to alleviate terror and panic, impatiens to mollify irritation and impatience, clematis to combat inattentiveness, star-of-Bethlehem to ease shock, and cherry plum to calm irrational thoughts. It is available in liquid drops, spray, and pastilles.
- *Pulsatilla* **tincture**: Used at five to ten drops directly in the mouth can help to allay a panic attack. Note that this is the plant tincture of root or tuber, and not the homeopathic preparation.

Anxiolytics is a fancy name for drugs that decrease anxiety. By far the most commonly prescribed drugs in this category are in the benzodiazepine class, and include Valium, Xanax, Ativan, and Klonopin. They all tend to cause sleepiness and have been useful in treating sleep disorders as well as anxiety. For those having frequent panic attacks, they are more effective in preventing the episodes when they are taken regularly. Some of them, like Klonopin and Ativan, can be chewed and dissolved under the tongue for quick relief of an anxiety attack.

These drugs can be habit forming, with significant withdrawal symptoms such as a spike in agitation and even seizures when they are discontinued. And, as noted above, over the long term they can interfere with normal sleep architecture, impair cognition, and cause depression. This won't happen if their use is limited to an as-needed basis. There are a handful of other prescription medications that can help anxiety, including some antidepressants, buspirone, and gabapentin.

Alcohol, sugar, and caffeine can all increase anxiety, and, of course, should be avoided. Adequate sleep is a must. Emotional Freedom Technique, a practice in which tapping on selected acupressure points relieves emotional distress, is often highly effective at resolving panic and anxiety. There are many sites on YouTube that walk through the process.

DEPRESSION

There is no easy formula to distinguish between mood disturbances with a psychological origin from those caused by an organic illness. It is not unusual for someone with a chronic disease to feel down, but if depression is severe, it is possible that that neuroinflammation is resulting in "brain on fire." The depression associated with neuropsychiatric Lyme can be extremely virulent, filling people with blackness and despair and continual thoughts of ending it all. These thoughts can overwhelm everything else that is happening, and have even been seen in children with Lyme disease complex.

This condition is serious. At the very least, it drains many patients of energy, as if someone has pulled the plug. But it can also crush their spirit and destroy their will to live. Depression is often compounded by sleep disturbances and anxiety. Recent studies have documented the association between inflammation and depression.[18] Depression is associated with a decline in immune function generally and in natural killer (NK) cell activity in particular.[19] NK cells play a role in killing both tumor cells and virus-infected cells; in short, depression makes it more difficult for the body to heal.

NATURAL AGENTS FOR DEPRESSION			
Name	Generic	Common doses	Most common side effects
St. John's wort	*Hypericum perforatum*	300 mg 1x/day–3x/day	Light sensitivity Interaction with drugs
SAMe	S-adenosyl methionine	400 mg 1–4/day	None known
DHEA	Dehydro-epiandrosterone	2.5–25 mg (F) 5.0–50 mg (M)	Fluid retention Insomnia Virilization
Magnesium		250 mg 2x/day	Diarrhea
Tyrosine		500 mg 2x/day 2000 mg 3x/day	Diarrhea Nausea/vomiting
DLPA	D,L-Phenylalanine	100 mg 1x/day- 500 mg 3x/day	Nausea Heartburn Headache
5-HTP	5-Hydroxytryptophan	50–100 mg 3x/day	Avoid if taking an SSRI
Tryptophan		500–1000 mg 2x/day	Avoid if taking an SSRI
Vitamin B complex		B-50 complex contains 50 mg of each B vitamin, 1–3x/day	Insomnia Racy
Vitamin B$_{12}$	Cobalamin	500–2000 mcg orally or sublingually or nasally; 1000–25,000 mcg IM daily to once weekly	High doses may be overstimulating in fragile people and those with certain genetic variants

Table 17–3. Natural Agents for Depression

Natural supplements have been helpful in reducing mild to moderate depression, and recent studies have demonstrated their effectiveness in more severe cases as well. Although side effects are less common than with prescription drugs, they are not totally benign. For anyone suffering from depression, they are definitely worth trying. Table 17–3 contains a list of natural antidepressants, along with their side effects. Each is then described in more detail below.

- **St. John's Wort**: This is one of the best known of the natural antidepressants. It is widely used in Europe and has received a lot of attention in the United States as well. In early studies, St. John's wort demonstrated benefits in relieving symptoms of depression including a decrease in sadness, hopelessness, and feelings of low self-worth.[20] However, subsequent studies have not confirmed that it is any better than placebo,[21] and further studies are clearly indicated.

   St. John's wort can bind with a variety of neurotransmitters and on rare occasions has caused mania. It can also interfere with the metabolism of other drugs by initially inhibiting but then stimulating the cytochrome enzyme system, thereby impacting blood levels of other medications such as blood thinners, hormonal contraceptives, and atovaquone.[22] St. John's wort should not be combined with other antidepressants. It is important that anyone who wants to try St John's wort first lets his or her doctor know.

- **SAMe** (pronounced "sammy"): S-adenosyl methionine, as it is officially known, is produced naturally in our bodies. It is important in metabolism because it is a methyl donor that helps other molecules, such as neurotransmitters and DNA, change into their active states. SAMe production is impaired in people who are depressed. Taking SAMe supplements can increase the level of many neurotransmitters and is often helpful in alleviating depression.[23] It has also been beneficial in treating osteoarthritis because of its ability to promote the manufacture of cartilage.

- **DHEA**: Chronic stress, including chronic infection, often leads to low levels of DHEA. Replacing this adrenal hormone can improve mood,[24] as well as immune function and energy level. (See Chapter 15.)

- **Magnesium:** This mineral has been effective in the treatment of depression as well as anxiety and sleep disorders.[25]

Replacement of specific amino acids can also increase neurotransmitter synthesis and improve mood. These amino acids need to be taken without other protein in order for them to get into the brain at effective levels. They include:

- **Tyrosine:** This is converted into epinephrine, norepinephrine, and L-dopa, all of which are important in the function of the nervous system. Taking supplements of tyrosine may help mood and energy.[26]
- **Phenylalanine:** Supplements of this amino acid have been effective in reducing both depression and pain.[27]
- **5-HTP:** This amino acid, 5-hydroxytryptophan, is converted into serotonin. Supplements can improve both mood and sleep.[28] It is also an appetite suppressant when taken a half hour before meals. Anyone on an SSRI antidepressant should not take 5-HTP.
- **Tryptophan:** For some people this amino acid has been a highly effective treatment for depression and sleep disorders.[29] Like 5-HTP, it is converted into serotonin, and should be avoided when taking SSRI antidepressants.

Additional supplements that may decrease depression include the following:

- **Fish oil:** Americans suffer from a widespread deficiency of omega-3 essential fatty acids,[30] which has been linked to a variety of issues including coronary artery disease and mood disorders. Of note, high doses of omega-3 essential fatty acids have been shown to help depression, and to stabilize patients with bipolar disorder (formerly known as manic depression).[31] Vitamin E (200 IU—400 IU of mixed tocopherols daily) should also be taken when supplementing with fish oils; this prevents them from oxidizing, i.e. going rancid, in the body.
- **Vitamin B complex:** The challenges of a chronic illness put extra demands on nutritional requirements for the B vitamins. One study found that 53 percent of middle-class psychiatric patients with no clinical signs of malnutrition had laboratory-proven deficiencies of at least one B vitamin.[32] The entire complex of B vitamins is important in all aspects of neurological function.
- **Vitamin B$_{12}$:** This B vitamin deserves special attention. Mood as well as energy are often improved with supplements of B$_{12}$. This is independent of treating a vitamin deficiency, and is beneficial even in some patients with high B$_{12}$ levels. Some of this benefit is probably related to the impact of B$_{12}$ in facilitating methylation (see Chapter 19). Intranasal preparations, available at compounding pharmacies, probably get into the central nervous system better than oral preparations, and intramuscular B$_{12}$ is particularly effective. It is not clear that taking it under the tongue is any more effective than when swallowed.

    There are several forms of B$_{12}$. Methylcobolamin has unique properties that help repair nerve tissue.[33] I have been prescribing very high doses, ranging from 1 milligram (1000 micrograms) to 25 milligrams (25,000 micrograms) injected into muscle as often as once daily, and many patients describe improvements in energy, mood, cognition, and neuropathic symptoms such as pain and tingling sensations. Higher doses are only available at compounding pharmacies. It is impossible to overdose on B_{12}, even when given these high pharmacologic doses, but more fragile patients may find it too stimulating.[34]

Not everyone's ability to metabolize B vitamins is the same. In particular, there are people who have genetic mutations in the methylation pathway that can inhibit conversion of B vitamins to a usable form. In these cases, methylcobalamin may be therapeutic, but it is not always tolerated; these people should try hydroxycobolamin. (See Chapter 19 for a complete discussion of methylation.)

- **Folate**: A component of the B complex, folate is derived from foliage, hence its name. Studies have demonstrated its capacity to increase the effectiveness of antidepressants.[35] This effect is probably related to the impact of folate on methylation. Methylation is a complex metabolic cycle that takes place in most all the cells in our bodies, and is particularly important for detoxification, neurotransmitter metabolism, and DNA repair and activation. People with MTHFR mutations don't efficiently convert folate to its active metabolite, 5-methyltetrahydrofolate, 5-MTHF. This slows methylation and is associated with an increased risk of depression and other problems. These people need to be supplementing with the active form of folate, 5-MTHF. (See Chapter 19 for a detailed description of methylation.)

There is a theory that B vitamins are contraindicated in Lyme patients because they feed the bacteria. There is no evidence for this theory, and my experience has been just the opposite. Everyone with a chronic illness should consider taking B complex. But those with a sensitivity to yeast should make sure that their vitamins are not yeast-derived.

Pharmaceutical antidepressants can be effective in patients with Lyme disease complex who suffer from depression. Unfortunately these medications won't transform the chronically ill person from a couch potato to the poster child for the power of positive thinking. But if they improve mental outlook, they will make life more bearable, and facilitate healing. People with Lyme often react differently to these drugs, especially if there are methylation issues, so anyone with a serious mood disorder should consult with a psychiatrist or psychopharmacologist who has experience treating people with Lyme disease, if at all possible.

In addition to these considerations, there are many adjuncts that can be useful when addressing depression. Normalizing sex hormone levels, estrogen, progesterone, and testosterone, is important. Low doses of T3 (thyroid hormone) can be beneficial.[36] Exercise, yoga, light therapy, bodywork, acupuncture, and EFT (Emotional Freedom Technique) have all been helpful in people with depression. Going outdoors and getting sunlight in addition to appropriate exercise is essential. And, of course, a support network of friends and/or family is paramount to recovery.

IRRITABILITY

One of the more common symptoms of Lyme is irritability, and sometimes rage. One couple I was treating, both of whom had Lyme, said that they had been married fifteen years with barely an argument. After they became ill, they have been having blowouts every day.

Parents describe their formerly easygoing children as oppositional, cranky, defiant, aggressive, and sometimes combative. Spouses describe their partners as grouches. In Lyme support groups, this syndrome is often referred to as "Lyme rage." Patients (and their families) need to realize that this is a symptom of the infection caused by inflammation of the nervous system, and they need to be patient, compassionate, and prepared to apologize. Some of the natural agents used to treat anxiety may help mellow out irritability, but if it is severe, medication may be appropriate. Depakote, Zyprexa, and Risperidal have all been useful in reducing Lyme rage.

There are some excellent practitioners using homeopathics, including essential oils and flower essences, to treat all types of mood disorders. Administering effective treatments requires some expertise. Consider seeing a well-trained practitioner, and don't hesitate to reach out to others who have traveled this road.

COGNITIVE PROBLEMS

Most people with Lyme disease complex have problems with short-term memory. I experienced this myself; prior to Lyme I had particularly good retention of numbers—they would make arithmetic patterns in my head that I found easy to recall. But when my Lyme was bad, people would have to repeat their phone numbers at least three times while I was writing it down because I couldn't keep more than one number in my head long enough to put it on paper. I left my keys at the post office on three separate occasions—luckily, I couldn't get too far without them. I would lose my train of thought in the middle of a sentence and be unable to find the simplest of words. Stories abound of people who got lost driving in their hometowns, had no idea where they parked the car, repeatedly left the oven on, and couldn't find anything once they had put it down.

Dr. Dale Breseden has done primary research on dementia and has authored a book entitled *The End of Alzheimer's*[37] in which he describes dementia as a multifactorial process: toxins, inflammation, and nutritional and hormonal imbalances. This applies to patients with Lyme disease complex as well. The ability to focus, concentrate, and maintain attention can all go down the drain. Treating the infections, inflammation, and concurrent imbalances are the first line in addressing impaired cognition. Patients with impaired cognition need to be assessed for detoxification issues (such as impaired methylation), mold toxins, and heavy metals. (These issues are discussed in detail in Chapter 19.)

Kris Kristofferson has gone public with his diagnosis of Lyme disease after being misdiagnosed with fibromyalgia then Alzheimer's dementia. Reportedly, he has had a complete recovery after being treated for Lyme.[38]

In addition to treating the infections and detoxification issues, there are some supplements as well as some pharmaceutical products that can assist with memory. Natural agents to enhance memory are listed in Table 17–4, and discussed individually below.

NATURAL AGENTS TO HELP COGNITION		
Name	**Common doses**	**Most common side effects**
Ginkgo biloba	120–160 mg 2–3x/day	None known
Phosphatidylserine	100 mg 3x/day	None known
Phosphatidylcholine	420 mg 2x/day	None known
Acetyl-L-carnitine	500 mg 3x/day	None known
Theanine	100–200 mg 3x/day	None known
Vitamin B complex	B-50 complex contains 50 mg of each B vitamin, 1–3x/day	Insomnia Agitation

Table 17–4. Natural Agents to Help Cognition

- *Ginkgo biloba*: This potent antioxidant is the best known natural treatment for memory loss. It can improve circulation by regulating the tone and elasticity of blood vessels, and it can reduce damage to nerve cells.[39] It would appear well suited to help alleviate some of the cognitive symptoms associated with Lyme disease. While ginkgo has shown promise in animal studies, research studies in humans have shown mixed results. It may be that ginkgo improves memory in people whose brains have more neuroplasticity than those with Alzheimer's.
- **Phosphatidylserine**: High concentrations of this compound are normally found in the brain. Taking supplements of phosphatidylserine can

improve memory, even in people with Alzheimer's disease. It can also help relieve depression.[40]

- **Phosphatidylcholine:** Phosphatidylcholine is the major lipid, or fat, of cell membranes and blood proteins. Phosphatidylcholine serves as the body's main source of choline, an essential nutrient and precursor to the neurotransmitter acetylcholine. It can improve memory in some people.[41]

- **Acetyl-L-carnitine:** This nutrient helps transport fats into mitochondria to be utilized for energy production. It is also important in clearing toxic accumulations of fatty acids and enhancing neurotransmitter activity. Supplements can be helpful with mental function, memory loss, and depression.[42]

There are a few prescription medications that may help memory problems in patients with dementia. These can also be effective in patients with Lyme disease complex, although there may be cardiac and gastrointestinal side effects. In my clinical experience, patients have benefited from memantine in particular.

There are several drugs that are used to help people with difficulties in staying focused. These medications are mostly in the amphetamine class, or are related to amphetamines, and they have gained widespread use in the treatment of ADD. Some Lyme patients on Adderall report that it has changed their lives because they are more able to focus and be functional. Doses need to be individualized, as these drugs can result in agitation and anxiety, and blood pressure and pulse need to be monitored.

Modafinil and armodafinil can improve wakefulness, cognition, concentration, memory, and motivation. Unlike the other stimulants, these usually have a calming effect in adults.[43] A few of the drugs used for Parkinson's can also improve alertness, attentiveness, and thought clarity, but they have little effect on wakefulness.[44] These include Eldepryl, Symmetrel, and Parlodel.

Some of the antidepressants may also help with concentration. They are not as strong as the other medications used for cognition and concentration, but they may be better tolerated. They may also be used in combination with the medications described above.

Table 17-5 lists prescription medications that may help with cognition, attention, and alertness.

PRESCRIPTION MEDICATIONS TO HELP COGNITION AND WAKEFULNESS		
Class	**Brand name**	**Generic name**
Acetylcholine-esterase inhibitors	Aricept	Donezepilhydrochloride
	Reminyl	Galantamine hydrobromide
	Exelon	Rivastigmine tartrate
NMDA receptor blockade	Namenda	Memantine
Stimulants	Ritalin Metadate CD Concerta	Methyphenidate hydrochloride
	Dexedrine spansules	Dextroamphetamine sulfate
	Adderall and AdderallXR	Dextroamphetamine Amphetamine
	Ionamin	Phentiramine
	Cylert	Pemoline
Anti-Parkinson drugs	Eldepryl	Selegiline hydrochloride
	Symmetrel	Amantadine hydrochloride
	Parlodel	Bromocriptine mesylate
Antidepressants	Wellbutrin	Bupropion
	Effexor	Venlafaxine
	Zoloft	Sertraline
	Norpramine	Desipramine hydrochloride

Table 17–5. Prescription Medications to Help Cognition and Wakefulness

DYSAUTONOMIA

The autonomic nervous system (ANS) can be thought of as the automatic nervous system. It controls those body functions that occur without conscious thought, such as heart rate, breathing, and directing blood flow to different organs and muscles. The ANS has two branches, sympathetic and parasympathetic, both regulated by the hypothalamus. Activation of the sympathetic branch is mainly stimulating; it can trigger the flight-or-fight reaction with a release of catecholamines from the adrenals. The parasympathetic arm is calming, although it does stimulate gastrointestinal function. The interplay of the two ANS branches is designed to maintain homeostasis, or balance, in the body.

However, in patients with dysautonomia, the ANS is in chaos. Most people with dysautonomia experience light-headedness, especially when going from lying or sitting to standing. Their heart may race and pound as if it had a mind of its own, and blood pressure may run high, low, or both—sometimes to the point of passing out. Patients can feel hot then cold, with chills and sweats; anxiety and even panic attacks may occur without explanation. A host of other symptoms, such as blurry vision, diarrhea, frequent urination, and fatigue, can also be attributed to dysautonomia. (See Table 17–7.)

SYMPTOMS ASSOCIATED WITH DYSAUTONOMIA
Excessive fatigue, post-exertional malaise
Light-headedness, or dizziness
POTS: Postural orthostatic tachycardia syndrome
Heart rate increase greater than 30 beats per minute for 5–30 minutes upon moving from sitting or lying to standing
NMH: Neurally Mediated Hypotension
Blood pressure drops upon moving from sitting or lying to standing
Sinus tachycardia (racing heart) and sinus bradycardia (abnormally slow pulse)
Blood pressure fluctuations
Shortness of breath
Flushing/mottling/livedo reticularis/erythromelalgia
Motion sickness
Gastrointestinal symptoms
Abdominal distention, constipation, gastroparesis
Nausea, reflux, vomiting
Mydriasis, blurry vision
Neurogenic bladder
Urinary incontinence
Hypotonicity—failure to empty
Excessive sweating or lack of sweating
Heat and cold intolerance, Raynaud's phenomenon
Sexual problems
Erectile dysfunction
Women: vaginal dryness and orgasmic difficulties
Anxiety, panic attacks

Table 17–6. Symptoms Associated with Dysautonomia

Two common syndromes come under the heading of dysautonomia: postural orthostatic tachycardia syndrome (POTS) and neurally mediated hypotension (NMH). In the former, heart racing occurs when standing up, but blood pressure remains fairly stable. In the latter, blood pressure drops when standing up, sometimes to the point of passing out. Many people with dysautonomia have components of both. Checking vital signs while the person is lying, then sitting, and then standing is an easy way to evaluate for this. A tilt table test, in which the patient is strapped to a table and vital signs are checked as it goes from horizontal to vertical, is an expensive way of essentially doing the same thing, but at times this method can pick up more subtle autonomic issues.

The mechanism for dysregulation is probably related to the effects of the inflammatory messengers (cytokines) on the ANS. Treatment needs to address inflammation as well as the infections that are the underlying cause of the inflammation. In my clinical experience, *Babesia* causes the worst dysautonomic symptoms. Most people experience more energy when their dysautonomia is stabilized. There are several interventions that can help alleviate this problem:

- If blood pressure is low, lots of water with added sea salt (¼ teaspoon per glass) or an electrolyte mixture is recommended.
- Licorice in the form of tea, capsules, or extract can also help the person with low blood pressure retain fluid and electrolytes.
- Fludrocortisone is a prescription medication that has a similar effect to licorice in raising blood pressure, but is stronger—it is also a mild corticosteroid, but not strong enough to suppress adrenal or immune function.
- Beta-blockers are medications that can slow the pulse in people with POTS; they may also lower blood pressure, so should be used with caution in people with NMH.
- Midodrine effectively lowers the pulse in people with POTS. It may also raise blood pressure, which then needs to be monitored.
- Dysautonomic episodes can result in mast cell degranulation and the release of histamine. The result is that symptons associated with inflammation and histamine often occur in conjunction with episodes of dysautonomia, and anti-inflammatory and antihistamine agents may lessen reactions. (See Chapter 18.) Most people experience more energy when their dysautonomia is stabilized.

NEUROPATHIC SYMPTOMS

Many people with tick-borne infections suffer with symptoms caused by irritation of the nerves. These symptoms include all types of pain syndromes— burning, shooting, stinging, electric shocks—as well as itching, creepy-crawly sensations, tingling, vibration sensation, pins and needles, and numbness. These are the result of inflammation hitting the nerves or the nerve-roots, which is where the nerves come off the spinal cord. Symptoms can range from mild to disabling.

Neurologists evaluate neuropathy with electromyography (EMG), nerve conduction velocity (NCV), and punch biopsy of the skin, which can demonstrate small nerve pathology. The diagnosis of chronic inflammatory demyelinating polyneuropathy (CIDP) can be made by EMG and punch biopsy. CIDP may occur with Lyme disease complex, and continue even after infections are no longer active, presumably via autoimmune mechanisms. The treatment is with intravenous gamma-globulin (IVIg), which is discussed in Chapter 18. Of note is that most insurance carriers at present only accept inflammatory changes in the nerves documented by EMG to cover this treatment, which is quite expensive.

There are some natural agents that are worth trying for neuropathy:

- **Phenylalanine**: This was discussed under depression. It can also help with mild to moderate pain in some people.
- **B complex vitamins, calcium, and magnesium:** These can all relax nerve endings and sometimes mitigate symptoms. In particular, high-dose vitamin B_{12} injections can be effective, especially methylcobolamin, as described above under depression.
- **Capsaicin:** This extract derived from the chili pepper plant can modulate neurotransmitters that transmit pain signals. When applied topically as a cream or impregnated in a pad and placed on an inflamed area, capsaicin produces heat and alleviates local pain.[45] It has been helpful in neuropathies such as shingles as well as Lyme disease complex. It is also beneficial for muscle and joint pain. Capsaicin is not recommended for those who don't like heat.
- **Alpha lipoic acid:** ALA is a powerful antioxidant and has been demonstrated to not only be neuroprotective, but also facilitate healing of damaged nerves. Intravenous ALA has been particularly effective in treating neuropathic pain.[46]
- **Melatonin:** While the standard use of this hormone is to initiate sleep, there is evidence that it is neuroprotective,[47] and it may actually assist in the healing of damaged nerves.

Topical lidocaine patches may give temporary relief from neuropathic symptoms. These are available by prescription at 5 percent, but also over the counter at 4 percent. Other OTC pads contain methylsalicylate, an aspirin analogue, combined with menthol or capsaicin; these topical pads have benefited many patients.

Some people have found relief from neuropathic symptoms with acupuncture, but the response has been inconsistent.

Nonsteroidal antiinflammatory drugs (NSAIDs) like ibuprofen (Motrin; Advil) can also decrease pain. The biggest problem is that they can also cause gastric irritation, so they should always be taken with food. Acetaminophen (Tylenol) does not have the same GI toxicity, but it can result in major liver problems with chronic use, especially if alcoholic beverages are consumed at the same time. The good news is that taking 500 mg of N-acetylcysteine (NAC) with each dose of acetaminophen will counteract the liver toxicity—but alcohol should still be avoided.

Stronger pain medications abound. Some patients respond to anti-seizure agents like gabapentin, SNRI antidepressants such as duloxetine, and tricyclic antidepressants such as amitriptyline. Sometimes combinations of medications such as gabapentin and duloxetine are even more effective. These agents all act at the level of the central nervous system so they can be useful for any pain, including headaches. But they can also cause side effects such as sleepiness, dizziness, cognitive difficulties, coordination problems, and depression.

Narcotic pain relievers also act centrally, broadly addressing any pain, but they have a similar spectrum of side effects, with the added complication of being habit forming. Tramadol is not as strong as other narcotics such as hydrocodone or oxycodone, while still activating opiate receptors and modulating neurotransmitters. It is usually well tolerated, and stronger than the NSAIDs, so should be considered prior to other narcotics. Overall, however, narcotic drugs are addictive, and stopping them suddenly can result in serious withdrawal issues. With the current

MEDICATIONS AND NATURAL AGENTS USED IN TOPICAL PREPARATIONS FOR NEUROPATHIC PAIN	
Class	**Agent**
Anti-inflammatory	Ketoprofen Piroxicam Emu oil
Block pain receptors	Gabapetin Ketamine Dextramethorphan Amitryptiline Carbamazepine Cyclobenzaprine
Local anesthetics	Lidocaine Piruvacaine
Dilate blood vessels	Isosorbide dinitrate Nifedipine
Transporting agent	DMSO

Table 17–7. Medications and Natural Agents Used in Topical Preparations for Neuropathic Pain

opioid crisis in America, careful consideration should be given before starting this course of treatment, especially where effective alternatives exist.

Pharmacists with compounding skills can make topical preparations containing various agents that block pain receptors and reduce inflammation. Table 17–6 lists some of the medications that can be compounded together and applied as creams or gels. Because these preparations act locally with limited systemic absorption, they can have profound effects on local pain with little or no side effects. They are available only by prescription, and most compounding pharmacists are happy to consult with providers to determine which preparations would be of most benefit.

Cannabis products also come in balms (which often contain essential oils) and gels, and are useful in alleviating local pain. Cannabis is described in more detail later in this chapter.

MUSCLE TWITCHING AND CRAMPING

Twitching, spontaneous muscle jerks, and muscle cramps all fall under the umbrella of neuromuscular irritability, but muscle cramps can be particularly severe and deserve to be addressed as a discrete symptom. The first line of treatment is magnesium; magnesium glycinate, citrate, and malate are easily assimilated. A highly concentrated and highly absorbable liquid magnesium called ReMag is particularly effective at alleviating symptoms of neuromuscular irritability. ReMag has 60,000 ppm pico-sized particles of magnesium—pico is one thousand times smaller than nano.

Magnesium absorption is first dependent on adequate gastric acid, but once it accesses the blood, it then needs to traverse each cell's membrane against a concentration gradient, since magnesium is concentrated within cells. It appears that ReMag is a good vehicle for increasing intracellular magnesium.

Topical magnesium can also be helpful, although these highly concentrated preparations can irritate or even burn the skin; MagneSul by Xymogen is a topical product that has been well tolerated by patients in my practice.

There are other supplements that may help neuromuscular irritability. Potassium and calcium are sometimes effective. Quinine, which has been used to treat both malaria and babesiosis, has been recommended for leg cramps. Scientific documentation of its efficacy is lacking, but anecdotal reports suggest it helps. Unfortunately, benefits occur at higher doses—much greater than in tonic water—which are potentially toxic to the liver and kidneys. Electrolyte balance is important to deter muscle cramps. There are homeopathic remedies that are sometimes effective.

One interesting connection I have noted is that muscle cramps are particularly common in patients with babesiosis, and quinine has been employed to treat this infection. Quinine is produced from the medicinal plant *Cinchona officinalis*; the herbal extract of this plant (sold by Nutramedix as Quina) often helps patients with babesiosis—which in turn can help resolve muscle cramps.

A note of caution. If twitching (a.k.a. fasciculations) is accompanied by weakness and in particular if it involves the tongue, an evaluation for amyotrophic lateral sclerosis (ALS) should be performed.

MEDICAL MARIJUANA

Now is a good time to talk about medical marijuana (MMJ). MMJ has been legalized in the majority of states and in the District of Columbia, although states vary in the types of medical conditions approved for its use. Marijuana has 483 phytocannabanoids, which are naturally occurring compounds that can affect many body processes such as appetite, mood, and sleep. Most people have heard of one of them—THC, or tetrahydrocannabinol, the psychoactive component of marijuana. It has been clearly established that THC is quite beneficial for pain, sleep, nausea, appetite, and PTSD, so there are numerous medically valid reasons for its use.[48] Most of the remaining phytocannabanoids are cannabadiols (CBDs).

There are two strains of cannabis: indica and sativa. The difference between the two strains are terpenes, which modulate the activity of THC and CBD. For example, indica is effective for pain but can be sedating, so it is best used evening and nighttime. Sativa is also pain-relieving, but is activating and may increase energy, so it is better suited for daytime use. There are now a profusion of hybrid strains available that essentially cross categories.

CBDs were once considered physiologically inactive unless paired with THC, but it turns out that is not the case. There is a compelling amount of scientific research documenting their independent activity, and increasingly there is extensive clinical experience as well.

It turns out that we make our own CBDs. All vertebrates going back 600 million years on the evolutionary tree have an endocannabanoid system which modulates immune and nervous system function. CBDs are potent anti-inflammatory agents, they regulate neurotransmitters, and they may enhance immune competence. CBDs decrease neuroinflammation and are neuroprotective. They can significantly reduce pain and anxiety.[49,50,51]

CBDs can be extracted without THC, particularly when obtained from hemp, which is a strain of *Cannabis sativa* but is not a controlled substance—it is legal everywhere and can be purchased on the Internet. If the problem is pain, consider CBDs in the form of hemp oil in the daytime. It has less than 0.3 percent THC, so there is no psychoactive or sedating effect. My patients have had excellent responses to both oral capsules and a liposomal sublingual extract (taken under the tongue), and it is activating, sometimes increasing energy. Conversely, CBD helps sleep in some people, probably secondary to its impact on reducing anxiety. In some patients it helps cognition.

In the evening, a marijuana extract with equal parts THC and CBD will have additive pain-relieving effects. There are a number of delivery systems available, including smoking, vaping, edibles, and sublingual extracts. I recommend the extracts since the onset is reasonably quick, usually less than thirty minutes, and the dose can be easily titrated by the number of drops under the tongue.

Both hemp-derived CBD and marijuana are available as salves that can be applied topically to relieve pain. Whether taken systemically or applied locally, many patients are able to decrease the need for pain medication.

It is notable that states that have legalized medical marijuana have experienced a 25 percent decrease in opiate overdose deaths.[52,53] This makes perfect sense: the vast majority of addicts developed their habit from prescription painkillers, then ended up either purchasing the drugs on the street or started heroin after prescriptions were no longer available. MMJ has had a major impact as an alternative to narcotics for those seeking pain relief.

Two additional pain considerations: Testosterone can help pain tolerance in men who are low in testosterone.[54] If testosterone is low, a patient deserves a full workup as described in Chapter 15. In addition, low-dose amphetamines can potentiate the effect of opioid medications.[55]

MULTIPLE SCLEROSIS

Lyme can look a lot like multiple sclerosis (MS). The definition of MS is "neurological lesions disseminated in time and space." This means that neurological abnormalities in the brain and spinal cord occur in different places and at different times. There are no tests that definitively confirm this diagnosis, although almost all MS patients will have abnormal brain MRIs with signal flairs, abnormal cerebrospinal fluid with oligoclonal proteins (a type of immunoglobulin), and abnormal evoked potential tests, which evaluate nerve response to sensory stimulation.

Lyme can present with the same symptoms as MS, including optic neuritis. And Lyme can produce the same test abnormalities as MS, so everyone diagnosed with MS should be tested for Lyme. I have seen many patients who were diagnosed with MS but subsequently tested positive for Lyme, and responded to antibiotics with a resolution of their "MS" symptoms.

The reality is that these patients can have Lyme, or MS, or both. The biggest problem is when patients with Lyme are diagnosed with MS and then given high doses of steroids. People with Lyme usually experience a flare in symptoms rather than relief. I know one patient who was misdiagnosed with MS and went blind when treated with intravenous steroids. She subsequently recovered when treated for Lyme and babesiosis.

In addition to treating the underlying infection, always check out the role of food sensitivities.[56] Some patients with MS go into remission on elimination-challenge diets, and consistently relapse when they eat certain foods, particularly yeast. Heavy metal toxicity and vitamin B_{12} deficiency can each mimic MS and also need to be ruled out. Even without a deficiency state, high-dose vitamin B_{12} injections can often be helpful.

ALS (AMYOTROPHIC LATERAL SCLEROSIS, OR LOU GEHRIG'S DISEASE)

Dr. David Martz was an oncologist practicing in Colorado when he developed profound weakness and was eventually diagnosed with ALS. While he was still ambulatory, he decided take a last trip to Africa on a safari. He was prescribed Malarone for malaria prophylaxis, and did much better than expected on his trip. A smart colleague of his put two and two together, and diagnosed both Lyme and babesiosis. Dr. Martz experienced a full recovery from ALS.

Even doctors who don't believe in chronic *Bb* infection suggest that intravenous ceftriaxone may be of benefit in ALS patients owing to its impact on glutamate metabolism.[57] It is certainly appropriate to consider aggressive treatment of ALS patients with antibiotics if there is evidence of these infections, but it needs to be done carefully—a Herxheimer reaction could be lethal, and these patients often have mitochondrial dysfunction that antibiotics can worsen.

PARKINSON'S DISEASE

Lyme disease complex can manifest with Parkinsonian symptoms, particularly tremors and stiffness. As with MS and ALS, any underlying infection such as Lyme and its co-infections should be treated. In addition, patients should undergo aggressive detoxification as described in Chapter 19.

AUTOIMMUNE NEUROPSYCHIATRIC DISORDERS

Pediatric autoimmune neuropsychiatric disorders associated with streptococcal infections (PANDAS) occurs in some children when a strep infection triggers an immune response that results in brain inflammation. There is typically a sudden onset of symptoms, particularly anxiety, OCD (obsessive compulsive disorder), and eating disorders, as well as other personality, mood, and behavior disorders. These kids may also exhibit choreiform movements—random, involuntary movements that can affect the entire body.

Once it became clear that strep was not the only microbe that could trigger this syndrome, the name PANS, pediatric acute-onset neuropsychiatric syndrome, was added to the medical lexicon. Herpes simplex virus, influenza A virus, varicella zoster virus, Epstein-Barr virus (EBV), HIV, recurrent sinusitis, the common cold, *Mycoplasma pneumonia,* and *Bartonella henselae,* have all been identified as triggers.[58,59,60,61] My clinical suspicion is that *Bartonella* and *Mycoplasma* may be particularly problematic in their capacity to trigger autoimmune encephalitis.

There are many toxins in the environment that trigger autoimmune reactivity, and these may also be triggers for neuroinflammation with psychiatric illness; mold, asbestos, mercury, trichloroethylene (a common solvent), and bisphenol A (in plastics) are a handful of examples.[62,63]

The neuropsychological symptoms of PANS parallel the psychiatric symptoms of Lyme disease complex. Almost 50 percent of people who continue to be symptomatic after treatment of acute Lyme disease exhibit anti-neuronal antibody activity (found with inflammatory disorders of the nervous system).[64] There is a protein on the surface of *Bb* (outer-surface protein A) that has an amino acid sequence similar to a strep protein, so it makes sense that *Bb* can trigger a syndrome similar to PANDAS.[65] It is likely that *Bb* is yet another microbe that can trigger PANS, but that has not yet been documented.

Recall that these tick-borne infections make mischief by attacking software, not hardware—these awful psychiatric symptoms are caused by neuroinflammation. Frequently, symptoms related to the central nervous system improve even when the patient is taking an antibiotic that has poor penetration across the blood-brain barrier; this is consistent with the symptoms arising from an autoimmune response triggered by a microbial infection. Moleculera Labs offers a panel of specific anti-neuronal antibodies that are associated with PANS, and can be used to confirm the diagnosis of PANS.[66]

It is likely that genetics influences the tendency to develop autoimmune reactivity in response to microbes and toxins. Human leukocyte antigens (HLA) are protein markers that the immune system uses to recognize its own cells. Researchers have found that people with Lyme disease who have HLA-DR4 and HLA-DR2 alleles (alternative forms of the gene) have an increased likelihood of inflammatory responses to the infection.[67]

While children and adolescents with the acute onset of neuropsychiatric symptoms following a viral or bacterial infection fall under the designation of PANS, it has been my clinical experience that this syndrome also occurs in adults and it often is not sudden in onset. I believe we need to expand the nomenclature of PANS and start testing patients with severe neuropsychiatric symptoms for anti-neuronal antibodies regardless of age and speed of onset.

Antibiotics are important in the treatment of microbe-induced autoimmune neuropsychiatric disorders, and Long-Acting Bicillin administered by intramuscular injection has been surprisingly successful. Dr. Amiram Katz presented a series of more than two hundred cases of PANS associated with Lyme disease complex at a conference in 2018.[68] He found that a low dose of L-A Bicillin given intramuscularly was particularly effective in this population—his protocol was to administer 600,000 units once weekly if the child weighed less than one hundred pounds, and 1.2 million units once weekly if greater than one hundred pounds. The mechanism of action of this drug at these low doses is unclear, but according to Dr. Katz it has been consistently more effective than higher doses of L-A Billicin or intravenous antibiotics.

Since hearing of Dr. Katz's protocol, I have treated several adolescents with Lyme disease complex who suffered from poorly controlled anger with regular violent outbursts in addition to other mood issues. Most of them were infected with *Bartonella* as well as *Mycoplasma*. Some of the adolescents demonstrated antineuronal antibodies on the Cunningham Panel. Almost all of them have had positive responses to L-A Bicillin 1.2 million units IM once weekly.

Some patients recover on antibiotics alone, but others require intravenous gamma globulin (IVIg), which supports immune competence while providing substantial anti-inflammatory action.[69] Unfortunately, the majority of insurance carriers do not approve coverage for PANS, and IVIg is quite expensive. One exception is the state of Illinois, which has mandated that insurance carriers cover IVIg treatment for PANS. Hopefully other states will follow suit. (IVIg is discussed in more detail in Chapter 18.)

In the meantime, other anti-inflammatory agents, which are described more fully in Chapter 18, can be employed. Ibuprofen affords some relief in symptoms.[70] CBD has a solid record of decreasing neuroinflammation in general and autoimmune reactivity in particular.[71] Low-dose immunotherapy (LDI), discussed in Chapter 23, holds promise in the treatment of PANS; LDI treats the microbes as if they are an allergic trigger and signals the immune system not to react to these pathogens. Some practitioners have found low-dose naltrexone (LDN) helpful; this will also be discussed in Chapter 23.

Mast cell activation often contributes to the neuro-inflammatory response.[72] (Mast cell activation syndrome [MCAS] is discussed in detail in Chapter 18.) Some practitioners report that treatment with antihistamines and other agents that prevent mast cells from releasing histamine and other inflammatory mediators will mitigate symptoms.[73] Other immunomodulatory interventions include corticosteroid pulses, which must be done with caution in patients with Lyme disease complex. Responses are not usually sustained and I don't recommend it. Plasmapheresis is a process that filters the blood and removes harmful antibodies; responses to this treatment also are often not sustained.[74]

It is possible that psychiatric symptoms triggered by neuroinflammation and autoimmunity are a common cause of mental illness. A pilot study in which ten adolescents with severe anxiety and depression but no known organic illness were tested for auto-neuronal antibodies is described in more detail in Chapter 25; nine of the ten had high levels. This is an incredible statistic that provides much food for thought; further study is planned.

WHERE DO WE GO FROM HERE?

More often than not, the nervous system is the most severely impacted system in people with Lyme disease complex, and neurological symptoms cause the most misery. Treating sleep disturbances, pain syndromes, and mood disorders is important for healing as well as to relieve suffering. Stabilizing the nervous system enables the immune system to deal with infections, and vice versa—these "systems" are intimately interconnected. Our bodies operate as whole working units, and it is important to restore normal balance and function throughout to be successful at regaining health.

TAKE-HOME POINTS

1. Lyme disease complex can cause severe and disabling neurological symptoms.
2. It is imperative to aggressively address depression, anxiety, sleep disorders, impaired cognition, and pain syndromes.
3. Many neurological issues are linked to autoimmune inflammation linked to microbial triggers.
4. *Bartonella* and *Babesia* are particularly virulent in causing nervous system disorders.
5. Cannabis in the form of medical marijuana as well as hemp oil CBD modulates immune and nervous system function, and is often beneficial in the treatment of Lyme disease complex. The THC component of the indica strain is useful for pain and sleep disorders.
6. Nervous system issues are linked to disorders of inflammation, which are discussed in the next chapter.

Chapter 18

Inflammation

Chronic tick-borne infections do not act the same way as a typical microbial invasion. Wound infections or strep throats result in bacteria invading tissue, which stimulates a local immune response to contain the infection and repair the tissue damage. By contrast, the tick-borne pathogens are not found in one discrete place in a person's body; in essence, they attack software, not hardware. The result is that our metabolic functions regulated by the immune, endocrine, and nervous systems are in disarray, resulting in excessive inflammation and autoimmunity.

Autoimmunity occurs when someone's immune system attacks their own tissues. A classic example is rheumatic fever, which occurs when a person gets a strep throat, then antibodies to the strep bacteria cross-react with cells on their heart valves that have a cellular structure similar to the strep bacteria. It is a combination of infection and autoimmunity in a condition believed to be caused by molecular mimicry. That is, some human cells have a structure similar to some bacteria, and antibodies to the pathogens attack tissues in their own body. There is widespread acceptance that microbial factors are a primary cause of autoimmune conditions in rheumatic diseases.[1]

Lyme disease is associated with auto-antibodies that may be largely responsible for both arthritic and neurological issues.[2,3] Patients with multiple sclerosis have a high rate of antibodies to *Bb*.[4] Tick-borne infections have been shown to trigger the PANS syndrome as described in Chapter 17, in which adolescents develop anti-neuronal antibodies and neuropsychological illness following infection. In many patients with Lyme disease complex there is probably a genetic factor. For example, people with the HLA-DR4 and HLA-DR2 genetic alleles have a high incidence of Lyme arthritis.[5] Infection with *Bb* may precipitate Hashimoto's thyroiditis, another autoimmune illness, in genetically susceptible people.[6]

It has been my clinical experience that *Bartonella* and *Mycoplasma* may play a particularly significant role in the development of autoimmunity. Several researchers have demonstrated autoimmune-type illness in association with both microbes, including rheumatic, gastrointestinal, and neurological conditions as well as vasculitis.[7,8,9,10,11] In Chapter 10, I described a thirteen-year-old male patient in my practice who developed primary sclerosing cholangitis, an autoimmune condition of the biliary tract, following *Bartonella* colitis, which has responded to anti-*Bartonella* treatment.[12]

THE IMMUNE SYSTEM: BASICS

The immune system is enormously complicated. Even medical researchers don't fully understand how it works, but are learning more on a daily basis. Much of this chapter will talk about what happens when the immune system goes awry; first, though, it is helpful to review immune system fundamentals. From a functional perspective, the immune system's role can be summarized as boundary protection.

The immune system is in constant surveillance mode—imagine satellites circling the earth continually monitoring the planet's landscape. The most basic immune system function is discerning whether an object it encounters is self or nonself. Self is the body's tissues; nonself is viruses, bacteria, fungi, food, pollens, toxins, and so on. If the object is nonself, the next step is to distinguish whether nonself is a threat. If nonself is an invasive microbe, a toxin, or an errant malignant cell, for instance, it should be identified as a threat, while foods and pollens should not be identified as threatening. Finally, a healthy immune system should efficiently eliminate any nonself threat. Like a well-balanced individual, a healthy immune system is strong but calm. It does not feel a need to respond to nonthreatening elements, but it will target dangerous intruders and successfully dispose of them.

Cytokines are the messengers of the immune system. Some are pro-inflammatory (capable of causing inflammation), others are anti-inflammatory, and some trigger allergic responses. Cytokines not only allow communication between immune cells, they also send messages throughout the body by binding to receptors on other types of cells. There are receptors for cytokines on the endocrine glands, nerve cells, and likely on most of the cells of the body.

It is important not to castigate inflammation as a bad thing. Inflammation is required to deter microbes from invasion, to target malignant cells, and to eliminate toxins. A security system that keeps out invaders but lets in guests is ideal, but one which sounds the alarm all the time can result in chaos. The bottom line is that it is all about balance.

The following few pages contain a deeper dive into immune system function; those without a keen interest in physiology should feel free to skip them. However, this knowledge is helpful for understanding some of the testing and treatment options used when the immune system in disarray—as is often found with Lyme disease complex.

There are two main branches of the immune system: the innate and the adaptive arms. (See Figure 18–1.) The innate immune system is on 24/7 patrol, sending white blood cells, natural killer cells, and other combatants to attack invasive microbes at the first sign of invasion. But if the pathogens overwhelm those defenses, then the adaptive immune system is called into action. In general, the adaptive immune system is recruited by the innate immune system, but it can also spring into action independently if it detects a previously encountered specific threat; e.g., a previous strep infection.

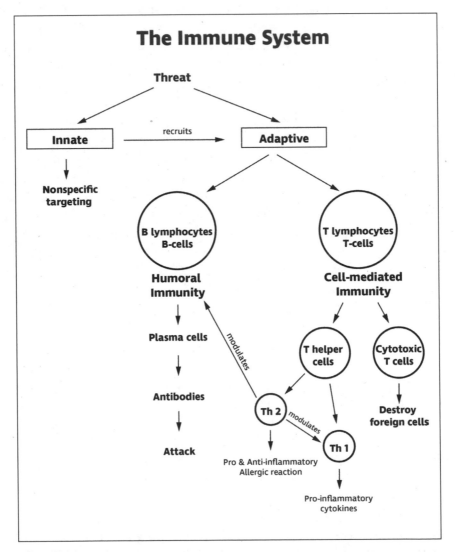

Figure 18–1

The adaptive immune system itself has two arms: humoral immunity and cell-mediated immunity. Humoral immunity involves B lymphocytes. These identify the outsider, then mature into plasma cells that secrete antibodies designed to target that particular invader. The antibodies attach to the microbe, then recruit other cells to assist in the destruction of the foreign agent. The B cells retain memory once the infection is halted—if there is ever reinfection with the same microbe, they can respond more quickly next time around.

Cell-mediated immunity is performed by T lymphocytes, which also respond to foreign antigens. T helper cells (a.k.a. CD4+) send messengers known as cytokines to other immune cells to support and coordinate an attack. Cytotoxic (literally "cell toxic") T cells (a.k.a. CD8+) directly kill the invaders. While B lymphocytes are designed to target hostile foreigners outside of cells, T cells are better at eliminating microbes within cells.

There are different classes of T helper cells. Th1 cells generate responses to intracellular microbes such as bacteria and viruses by manufacturing cytokines that promote an inflammatory response. Th2 cells release their own set of cytokines and generate antibodies to extracellular bacteria, toxins, and allergens. But Th2 cells also modulate the Th1 arm and B lymphocyte activity, and can be anti-inflammatory.

In summary, cytokines fall into two groups: pro-inflammatory and anti-inflammatory. The cytokines released by Th1 cells produce pro-inflammatory cytokines, particularly interferon gamma. Th2 lymphocytes release different cytokines, including several interleukins. Some of these are pro-inflammatory, and in particular can promote allergic responses, but others, like IL-10, will dampen the humoral arm and Th1 activity, and control excessive inflammation. The optimal scenario is a well-balanced Th1 and Th2 response, with both the Th1 and Th2 cells working together to maintain balance. During an acute infection, the Th1 arm becomes more active to eliminate the threat, but rapidly returns to its baseline of lower activity once the infection is resolved.

Problems occur when one side becomes overactive or dominant and suppresses the other side, resulting in excessive inflammation. The cytokine messengers that recruit other immune cells to target intracellular invaders can also lead to autoimmunity and uncontrolled inflammation. It appears that the presence of *Bb* and its cohorts upset the Th1-Th2 balance, promoting inflammation and autoimmunity while suppressing immune competence.

Th1 and Th2 are not the only classes of T cells; there are other T cell subsets, such as Th17, which releases interleukin-17. This highly inflammatory cytokine is thought to play a major role in the autoimmune response that triggers so much inflammation in patients with Lyme disease complex. It appears that at the earlier stages of chronic infection the Th1 arm remains dominant, but many patients progress to a severe hyperinflammatory autoimmune state related to activation of Th17 helper cells.[13]

This line is activated by extracellular pathogens, particularly those in hollow spaces such as the sinuses, lungs, GI tract, and bladder. While the role of the Th17 helper cells is to maintain a healthy mucosal barrier, too much stimulates autoimmunity. When Th17 is elevated, it suppresses Th1, leading to Th2 dominance.

Transfer factors, described in Chapters 8 and 20, can assist in restoring immune balance by stimulating Th1 activity. The herbs andrographis, echinacea, and berberine, and some supplements such as vitamin C, and beta-glucan, also boost Th1 activity. In addition, some peptides described in Chapter 23 can help restore Th1/Th2 balance.

LYME DISEASE COMPLEX IS THE BODY IN CHAOS

The bottom line is that *Bb* and its cohorts often disturb this well-balanced system, resulting in disorganized immune function. This manifests in both inflammation and immune suppression. Here is what happens: *Bb* and its co-conspirators confound the immune system, acting like a virus in the immune system's computer software. This leads to a hyper-inflammatory state. The confused immune cells begin targeting non-threats such as gluten and other foods, as well as the person's own tissues, resulting in more inflammation throughout the body. Inflammation in the intestines leads to a leaky gut; substances usually contained within the GI tract are absorbed, resulting in even more inflammation, food sensitivities, and increased toxic load. Exposures to molds that were previously not an issue now provoke additional reactions and more inflammation. Some people begin reacting to chemicals that are ubiquitous in our environment, and may develop multiple chemical sensitivity syndrome (MCS) as well as sensitivity to electromagnetic fields. With this increasing bedlam, immune function becomes less competent, and previously dormant viruses like Epstein-Barr (found in over 90 percent of the adult population) become active. Parasites that were asleep in the intestines are aroused. Detoxification pathways get overwhelmed. Since everything is connected, hormones are out of balance, the nervous system is in turmoil, and the body is in chaos. There are too many soldiers on the battlefield, but they are in disarray—and sometimes shooting their own compatriots instead of destroying the enemy.

Why not deal with this by just killing the bugs, since they were the initial trigger for immune disruption and inflammation? If it were only that simple. There is a misconception that there is a linear relationship between bumping off the microbes and clinical improvement: the more killing, the better we get. Although reducing the microbial load often leads to improved immune function, especially early in the disease process, it doesn't always work that way with these infections.

In addressing this conundrum, it is important to distinguish acute Lyme disease from the chronic multimicrobial infections found in patients with Lyme disease complex. A previously healthy individual who was recently infected typically does not experience the severe immune disruption that occurs in people who are chronically infected. The latter group have been under attack for a long time, and are much more prone to disorganization.

Remember the flat tire analogy? If you keep driving on it you not only destroy the tire and bend the rim, you risk bending a tie rod and breaking an axle. Fixing the tire does not fix the problem. With chronic infection, bringing the system into balance means dealing with all the issues that are in discord. That means optimizing hormone function, removing food culprits, eliminating mold, healing the gut, providing optimal nutrition, ensuring adequate sleep, calming the nerves, enhancing detoxification, and reducing pain—as well as treating the infections.

That is why Section 3 begins with a discussion on endocrine, gastrointestinal, and neurological function. In order to decrease inflammation, all these issues need to be addressed.

MAST CELL ACTIVATION SYNDROME

Mast cells are a type of white blood cell that act as the body's "first responder" to harmful stimuli. They are scattered throughout the body, and play an important role in fighting infection as well as repairing tissue. But they can also trigger inflammation and allergic responses. Mast cells contain more than two hundred pre-formed chemical mediators such as histamine, protease enzymes like tryptase, pro-inflammatory cytokines, and heparin. When triggered, mast cells release these mediators into surrounding tissues, then release a second wave of newly-synthesized mediators such as leukotrienes and interleukins. This process is called mast cell degranulation.

Mast cell activation syndrome (MCAS)* occurs when mast cells inappropriately and excessively degranulate. The chemical mediators released by mast cells can trigger local inflammation such as swelling and hives. They can also trigger systemic problems that range from mild to life-threatening, including anaphylaxis. Mast cells are in continuous dialogue with nerves: neurotransmitters activate the release of mediators from mast cells that, in turn, modulate nerve activity. The central nervous system communicates with mast cells directly through the tenth cranial nerve, the vagus.[14] This is also the nerve that has direct regulatory influence on the heart and the gastrointestinal system. What this means is that the communication route for control of essential body functions, the vagus nerve, can be flooded by inflammatory messengers—since everything is interconnected, mast cell degranulation can wreak systemic havoc. Table 18–1 lists symptoms that can be associated with MCAS.

---

* MCAS is one type of mast cell activation disorder. The other is systemic mastocytosis, a congenital condition in which there is an overabundance of mast cells.

SYMPTOMS CAUSED BY MCAS
Anaphylaxis
Flushing of the face, neck, and chest
Itching with or without rash
Hives, skin rashes
Angioedema (swelling)
Nasal itching and congestion
Wheezing and shortness of breath
Throat itching and swelling
Headache
Cognitive dysfunction
Anxiety, depression
Gastrointestinal symptoms: diarrhea, nausea, vomiting, abdominal pain, bloating, gastroesophageal reflux disease (GERD)
Bone/muscle pain
Dysautonomia: light-headedness, syncope/fainting, rapid heart rate, chest pain, low blood pressure, high blood pressure (at the start of a reaction), blood pressure instability
Uterine cramps or bleeding

Table 18–1. Symptoms caused by MCAS

There are a host of factors that can stimulate excessive mast cell degranulation. The more common include foods, medications, physical or emotional stress, direct pressure on the skin, cold or heat, and insect bites. (Table 18–2 lists triggers of mast cell degranulation.) Bacterial products and, no surprise, Lyme spirochetes, can also directly activate mast cells.[15]

TRIGGERS OF MAST CELL DEGRANULATION
Heat, cold, or sudden temperature changes
Stress: emotional, physical (including pain), or environmental (i.e., weather changes, pollution, pollen, pet dander, etc.)
Exercise
Fatigue
Food or beverages, including alcohol
Drugs (opioids, NSAIDs, antibiotics, and some local anesthetics) and contrast dyes
Natural odors, chemical odors, perfumes, and scents
Venoms (bee, wasp, mixed vespids, spiders, fire ants, jelly fish, snakes) Biting insects, such as flies, mosquitos, and fleas
Infections (viral, bacterial, and fungal)
Mechanical irritation, friction, vibration
Sun/sunlight

Table 18–2. Triggers of Mast Cell Degranulation

Histamine reactions can also be related to a decrease in the enzyme that metabolizes histamine, diamine oxidase (DAO).[16,17] In the healthy individual, the body rids itself of histamine as balance is restored. DAO deficiency leads to continued high histamine levels, even after the stimulus is gone. Many patients with Lyme disease complex have evidence of excessive histamine without demonstrating the full-blown syndrome of MCAS. Excessive mast cell degranulation often adds to the systemic inflammation in these patients and can play a role in autoimmunity.[18]

There are no definitive tests to diagnose MCAS. The lab test most commonly used is a serum tryptase level, preferably drawn within two hours of a reaction. Serum and urine histamine may be elevated. There are a host of other metabolites and messengers that can be measured, but none of them are a slam-dunk. The diagnosis is most often made on the basis of clinical presentation as well as response to treatment. Most patients with MCAS will have dermatographia, a condition that translates as skin writing: If the skin is lightly scratched, it will turn red, sometimes white, and may be raised. If a patient complains of many of the MCAS symptoms listed in Table 18-1, the diagnosis is likely.

It can take multiple interventions to treat MCAS. The most obvious is to avoid any known allergens, whether food, mold, cats, or medications. There are natural agents that stabilize mast cell membranes and increase the threshold for degranulation. Quercitin is a bioflavonoid that is naturally found in the rinds of citrus fruit. This supplement is strong enough that it can often block allergic reactions to foods. I recommend 250–500 mg taken a half hour before meals and at bedtime. There are non-citrus sources of quercitin for people allergic to citrus.

There are some drugs that also stabilize mast cell membranes and increase their threshold for degranulation. Patients may benefit from both cromolyn sodium (Gastrocrom)[†] and ketotifen. Both of these are often prescribed to block food reactions.

DAO (diamine oxidase), which metabolizes histamine, can also decrease reactions. I recommend 10,000–20,000 HDU, also taken a half hour before meals. Some people take this together with quercitin.

Antihistamines can reduce reactivity. Natural varieties include stinging nettles and bromelain, often combined with vitamin C. There are many pharmaceuticals available both over the counter and by prescription. Famotidine, which is often recommended for gastroesophageal reflux (GERD), is also a histamine (H2) blocker, and can be combined with the usual antihistamines, which are H1 blockers. However, famotidine will inhibit gastric acid secretion and its use for prolonged periods is therefore not recommended.

---

† Cromolyn sodium usually comes as a liquid and is quite expensive. However, it is also available in a powder at compounding pharmacies at a fraction of the cost.

Singulair (montelukast sodium), often prescribed for asthma, inhibits leukotrienes, which are a potent source of inflammation. Only available by prescription, it can be quite effective.

People with high reactivity may need to avoid foods containing histamine. The most common are listed in Table 18-3. In addition, some foods trigger histamine release—these are listed in Table 18-4—and some drinks that block activity of DAO are listed in Table 18-5.

FOODS CONTAINING HISTAMINE
Fermented alcoholic beverages, especially wine, champagne, and beer
Fermented foods: sauerkraut, vinegar, soy sauce, kefir, yogurt, kombucha
Vinegar-containing foods: pickles, mayonnaise, olives
Cured meats: bacon, salami, pepperoni, luncheon meats, and hot dogs
Soured foods: sour cream, sour milk, buttermilk, soured bread, etc.
Dried fruit: apricots, prunes, dates, figs, raisins
Most citrus fruits
Aged cheese including goat cheese
Nuts: walnuts, cashews, and peanuts
Vegetables: avocados, eggplant, spinach, and tomatoes
Smoked fish and certain species of fish: mackerel, mahi-mahi, tuna, anchovies, sardines

Table 18-3. Histamine Containing Foods

HISTAMINE-RELEASING FOODS
Alcohol
Bananas
Chocolate
Cow's milk
Nuts
Papaya
Pineapple
Shellfish
Strawberries
Tomatoes
Wheat germ
Many artificial preservatives and dyes

Table 18-4. Histamine Releasing Foods

DRINKS THAT BLOCK DAO
Alcohol
Caffeinated beverages
Energy drinks
Black tea
Maté tea
Green tea

Table 18–5. Drinks That Block DAO

Stabilizing mast cell activity can have a profound impact in quelling inflammation and bringing the body back into balance. For those patients suffering from excessive mast cell activation, removing the underlying triggers, including infection, allergens, and toxins, should always be considered.

ANTI-INFLAMMATORY AGENTS

CBDs and their role as anti-inflammatory, anxiolytic, and analgesic agents were discussed in Chapter 17. It is worth expanding the discussion here, as I have found CBDs so impactful in helping patients in their recovery process.

Humans make their own cannabinoids (known as endocannabinoids), and have built-in cannabinoid receptors. CBD stimulates the release of 2-Arachidonoylglycerol (2-AG), an endocannabinoid that activates both CB1 and CB2 receptors that are concentrated on immune cells as well as in the peripheral and central nervous system. CBDs modulate inflammation by a number of mechanisms, including suppression of some cytokines like tumor necrosis factor-alpha (TNF-α) and interleukin-6 (IL-6), stimulation of regulatory T cells, and inhibition of mast cell degranulation.[19,20]

CBDs moderate pain and the flow of neurotransmitters. They diminish nervous system inflammation, thereby improving cognition, memory, anxiety, control of appetite, vomiting, motor behavior, sensory, autonomic, and neuroendocrine responses. CBD has been recommended for patients with neurodegenerative disorders including Parkinson's and dementia, and has long been used to treat patients with multiple sclerosis.[21,22]

CBDs exert systemic anti-inflammatory effects, decrease autoimmune reactivity, and may also enhance immune competence.[23] CBDs derived from *Cannabis sativa* strains like hemp are activating, which means they can increase energy and wakefulness. Patients using these report more energy, less joint and muscle pain, decreased anxiety, and improved cognition. Most patients in my practice who use CBD take a liposomal sublingual extract twice daily, while some feel better on oral capsules, usually 25–50 mg twice daily. Either way, CBD needs to be taken for two to three weeks to feel the full effects.

There are a number of other natural anti-inflammatory agents. The following have been the most beneficial for people with Lyme disease complex:

- **Curcumin:** This is the active ingredient in turmeric, an Indian spice in the ginger family. It has been utilized by Ayurvedic healers in the treatment of multiple health issues for over four millennia.[24] Curcumin is well documented as an anti-inflammatory agent[25] as well as an antioxidant,[26] and has demonstrated benefits in conditions such as rheumatoid arthritis and ulcerative colitis.[27,28] It has been dubbed "natural Motrin" due to its ability to relieve joint and muscle pain. Curcumin is not well absorbed, so liposomal preparations may be more bioavailable.
- **Omega-3 EFAs:** These fish and flax oils are super-polyunsaturated, meaning they contain many double bonds in a long chain of carbon atoms. When these molecules are incorporated into cell membranes, they afford a fluidity that enhances the membrane's many functions. But multiple double bonds also means they are prone to oxidation, i.e. going rancid. That is why these EFAs are processed out of foods—they have a short shelf life. Most people who are not eating cold-water fish will be deficient in these fats.

  It has long been established that omega-3 EFAs have significant anti-inflammatory activity via multiple mechanisms, including suppressing anti-inflammatory cytokines.[29] They also enhance brain function by modulating neurotransmitters,[30] and have demonstrated benefit in the treatment of rheumatoid arthritis,[31] discogenic disease (degenerating discs in the spine),[32] and mental health conditions including ADHD, depression, and bipolar illness.[33] They also decrease the risk of cardiovascular disease, including heart attacks and strokes.

  Since people with Lyme disease complex have systemic inflammation, supplementation with EFAs is highly recommended. I suggest taking 1000 mg or more of EPA/DHA twice daily. Adding vitamin E in the form of natural tocopherols will protect these fats from oxidation once inside the body.

  Freshly ground flaxseeds are a rich source of alpha linolenic acid (ALA), which undergoes several enzymatic steps to be metabolized to EPA, eicosapentaenoic acid, the major anti-inflammatory prostaglandin in fish oil. Because many people have mutations that decrease this conversion, fish oil tends to have greater anti-inflammatory action than flaxseed oil. However, flaxseeds have other benefits such as improving bowel function and cardiovascular health.

Because flax oil is also super-polyunsaturated, it can go rancid easily. It is best to ingest flaxseeds freshly ground, and they should never be heated. Freshly ground flaxseed can be mixed into a protein shake, mixed in with yogurt, or sprinkled on salads.

- **Proteolytic enzymes**: These molecules break down protein and decrease inflammation by clearing inflammatory debris, dismantling circulating immune complexes, and enhancing macrophage activity.[34] Many of these enzymes, like trypsin and chymotrypsin, are produced within the digestive system and normally assist with protein digestion in the small intestine.

  People with chronic illness can enhance this pathway by taking supplemental, or exogenous, enzymes, which has been shown to be beneficial in decreasing inflammation. Bromelain comes from pineapple and papain from the papaya plant. Serrapeptase, synthesized by the silkworm, is both anti-inflammatory and fibrinolytic, meaning it can dissolve fibrous and scar tissue.[35] It is also effective as a biofilm buster.

  Combinations of enzymes can be found in preparations such as Wobenzym and Vitalzyme. It is important that these enzymes be taken away from food—that way they will be absorbed intact for their anti-inflammatory action, instead of assisting protein digestion in the gut.

- **Boswellia**: Extracts of *Boswellia serrata*, a plant that produces Indian frankincense, have been used for centuries to treat various chronic inflammatory diseases. It appears to decrease inflammation through a number of pathways including inhibition of cytokines like TNF-α and interleukin 1 beta, suppression of leukotriene B4 synthesis, and impeding the production of 5-lipooxygenase, a pro-inflammatory enzyme.[36] Studies have confirmed its benefits in osteoarthritis and rheumatoid arthritis.[37,38] It is often combined with curcumin and other anti-inflammatory agents.

- **Resveratrol**: Japanese knotweed, or *Polygonum cuspidatum*, contains trans-resveratrol, the active form of the compound, which has been shown to have significant anti-inflammatory, antioxidant, and DNA protective actions.[39] Clinically, it appears to have antimicrobial activity against *Bartonella*.

- **Nonsteroidal anti-inflammatory drugs (NSAIDs)**: like ibuprofen are the mainstay recommendations of Western physicians for patients with pain and inflammation. My experience with these medications in patients with Lyme disease complex is that they are often beneficial for pain, but less impactful at decreasing inflammation. They can cause gastritis, so they should to be taken with food. If taken on a chronic basis they can cause kidney damage.

Corticosteroids such as prednisone are often prescribed for inflammation. A long list of potential side effects is associated with these medications. People with Lyme need to be particularly wary of these medications because they suppress immune function and therefore allow the infections to flare. It is not uncommon for a patient to be given a Medrol dose-pack for poison ivy, for example, and then experience a Lyme relapse; this can occur even with a steroid injection into a joint. High-dose corticosteroids should be avoided unless it is a lifesaving situation, and those patients should simultaneously be on aggressive antibiotic treatment.

Decadron, a potent corticosteroid, is routinely administered intravenously to patients undergoing general anesthesia to control nausea and vomiting. I have seen patients relapse after surgery because of this. Anyone with Lyme who is undergoing surgery that requires general anesthesia should insist that they not be given any steroids.

It is important to distinguish high-dose from low-dose cortisone. Low doses seek to simply restore normal levels of circulating cortisol in patients with adrenal insufficiency. These low doses of hydrocortisone actually improve immune competence as well as adrenal function.[40] (See Chapter 15.)

A new generation of anti-inflammatory pharmaceuticals is biologicals. There has been a proliferation of commercials on TV that advertise the benefit of drugs like Humira for arthritis, psoriasis, and inflammatory bowel disease. Like corticosteroids, these medications suppress immune function, but their action is to inhibit cytokines such as TNF-α. The advertisements caution that people with infections should not take these medications, and I don't recommend them for people with chronic tick-borne infections.

INTRAVENOUS GAMMA GLOBULIN

Globulins are antibodies. There are four main classes of gamma globulin antibodies, but the most abundant is IgG. A deficiency of IgG can be genetic or acquired, and will result in difficulty fighting infection. Administration of intravenous gamma globulin, IVIg, stimulates immune function and, paradoxically, is also anti-inflammatory.

IVIg is concentrated antibodies, mainly IgG, derived from human donors. It is administered intravenously or subcutaneously. IVIg is extremely expensive, up to $10,000 per dose, and is typically administered every three weeks.

Since most people cannot afford to pay this cost out-of-pocket, those who need it rely on insurance coverage. It will come as no surprise that insurance carriers set a high bar for approval. In the case of people with Lyme, the criteria most likely to pass muster are low serum gamma-globulin levels (IgG) with either recurrent sinus or pulmonary infections, or evidence of inflammatory neuropathy (CIDP), documented by electromyography (EMG).

A blood chemistry profile that reveals low or low-normal total globulins should be followed up with a test for quantitative immunoglobulins and IgG subsets. Low numbers are diagnostic for hypogammaglobulinemia, a decreased capacity to make antibodies. The next step is a referral to an immunologist as well as a neurologist to determine if there is evidence of inflammatory neuropathy. While other recurrent or chronic infections will help meet insurance criteria for IVIg coverage, most carriers do not accept a diagnosis of chronic Lyme disease.

IVIg is not always well tolerated, and can cause flares in inflammation before there is noticeable improvement. However it is, as noted in Chapter 17, the agent of choice for patients with CIDP and PANS when antibiotics alone are not effective, and can markedly benefit selected patients with autoimmune conditions.

COAGULOPATHY

Hypercoagulability, the propensity of blood to inappropriately form clots, can be caused by both inherited and acquired conditions. People with predisposing genetic conditions can develop coagulation disorders when exposed to heavy metals, surgery, trauma, infections, and other stresses. Inflammation by itself can lead to abnormalities in blood clotting. In addition, inflammation can induce antiphospholipid antibodies, which can result in serious clotting abnormalities. Lyme disease is also associated with an increase in antiphospholipid antibodies.[41] Mutations in the MTHFR gene leading to elevated homocysteine levels are an added risk factor for abnormal clotting. (See Chapter 19.)

The abnormalities associated with chronic infection and inflammation typically result in low-level activation of the clotting system. Rather than causing blood clots, the blood becomes hyperviscous, decreasing blood flow through capillaries and thereby decreasing the delivery of nutrients and oxygen to cells. Recall that *Bb* thrives in low oxygen environments—so this tendency may actually be part of an overall *Bb* survival strategy. In addition, the excess fibrin associated with hypercoagulation can form a protective layer over the endothelial cells that line the inside of blood vessels and thereby protect germs from antibiotics.

Symptoms associated with these coagulopathies overlap with the symptoms of chronic infection such as fatigue and impaired cognition. Some patients notice that when their blood is drawn it comes out slowly. Laboratory evaluation is difficult since the standard tests for hemostatic abnormalities only reveal coagulation issues that result in actual blood clots. Dr. David Berg researched the reliability of using a panel of tests that includes fibrinogen, SFP (soluble fibrin monomer), F1+2 (prothrombin fragment 1+2), T/AT (thrombin/anti-thrombin complexes), and platelet activation by flow cytometry. He found that two or more abnormalities predicted the presence of low-level activation of the clotting system.[42] I suggest also testing homocysteine and antiphospholipid antibody levels.

Treatment is directed at thinning the blood. Low-dose subcutaneous heparin (5000 units twice daily) has been prescribed with excellent results in some patients.[43] Heparin has an additional benefit—it is anti-inflammatory.[44]

Alternatively, nattokinase is a nutraceutical that interferes with clotting by dissolving fibrin, and has been recommended to prevent cardiovascular disease.[45] Nattokinase can also break down biofilms. Dosages vary, but typically start around 2000 units twice daily on an empty stomach. Lumbrokinase is more powerful but is also expensive.

TAKE-HOME POINTS

1. Lyme and its co-infections trigger pandemonium in the immune system, resulting in excessive systemic inflammation and auto-immunity as well as immune suppression.

2. A multi-systemic approach is necessary to control inflammation: avoiding allergic triggers, healing the gut, balancing hormones, calming the nervous system, enhancing detoxification—as well as treating infections.

3. CBDs modulate immune function and nervous system activity. They have potent anti-inflammatory, analgesic, anxiolytic, and neuroprotective action.

4. Treatment of excessive mast cell degranulation can significantly reduce inflammation.

5. There are several natural anti-inflammatory agents that are well tolerated that can mitigate out-of-control inflammation.

6. High-dose corticosteroids should be avoided because they suppress the immune system and can lead to a flare in infections; ditto with biologicals.

7. Patients should be screened for hypogammaglobulinemia. Treatment with IVIg can boost immune function as well as decrease inflammation in selected patients.

8. Inflammation can facilitate "thick blood," which will decrease the delivery of nutrients, oxygen, and medications to cells. Patients who are not responding to treatment should be screened for a hyperviscosity syndrome.

9. A well-balanced immune system is dependent upon healthy detoxification pathways, which is the topic of the next chapter.

Chapter 19

Detoxification

Detoxification is the metabolic process that removes unwanted chemicals from the body. Detoxification ("detox") pathways eliminate the byproducts of normal metabolism and also contain a built-in reserve capacity for getting rid of additional undesired toxins. They are highly developed; most people's bodies are able to keep up with demands even when this system is stressed such as by taking medications or ingesting a moderate amount of alcohol.

At least that has been true historically. But these detox pathways are ill prepared to deal with the chemical onslaught from scientific "advances" of the past century including pesticides, industrial pollution, licit and illicit drugs, food additives, and food packaging materials, to name just a few. Add the stress of mold toxins, heavy metals, and chronic inflammation, and it becomes clear why our detox pathways are easily overwhelmed.

Imagine the wastebasket in your office filling with trash. You place it in the hall, where it is picked up along with a lot of other wastebaskets, then taken to a larger container by the back door of the building, and finally placed in the correct dumpsters outside, thereby being eliminated from the building. This is similar to how our cells release impurities into the circulatory system, which delivers these products to the liver, skin, and kidneys for removal. From there the final points of exit are sweat, stool, and urine. In addition to "direct delivery" from the cells to the blood, toxins from interstitial tissues are collected by the lymphatic system, a network of vessels that drain into the circulation.

Detoxification, however, is not simply about removal—it also entails neutralizing toxic substances so they can be carried through the body more safely. This process begins in the cells with a process called methylation.*

---

* Neil Nathan has authored an excellent text devoted to the topic of detoxification: Neil Nathan, *Toxic—Heal Your Body from Mold Toxicity, Lyme Disease, Multiple Chemical Sensitivities, and Chronic Environmetal Illness* (Las Vegas: Victory Belt Publishing, 2018).

METHYLATION

Methylation takes place in virtually all cells in the body. In addition to biotransforming metabolites for detoxification, methylation pathways encompass a series of about two hundred metabolic functions, processing neurotransmitters and sex hormones, producing energy, regulating glutathione activity, turning genes on and off, repairing DNA, and playing a number of other essential roles. This discussion will focus on methylation's role in detoxification, but it is important to note that, given its multiple functions, methylation is another example of how every system in the body is connected.

Figure 19–1 is a big picture of methylation, demonstrating the elegant complexity of the metabolic apparatus. Figure 19–2, which zeroes in on one portion of the methylation cycle, is less overwhelming. It starts with folate metabolism. Tetrahydrofolate (THF) comes from dietary folate, which is found in vegetables—i.e., foliage. THF needs to be converted to its active form, 5-methyltetrahydrofolate (5-MTHF), to perform its essential function within the body's cells. Enzymes are the catalysts used by the body in chemical conversion processes; the MTHF reductase enzyme (MTHFR) is the specific enzyme used to turn THF into 5-MTHF.

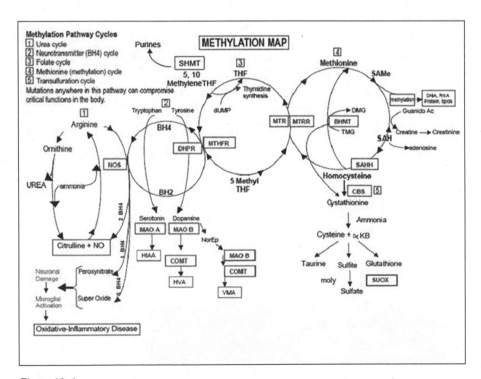

Figure 19–1

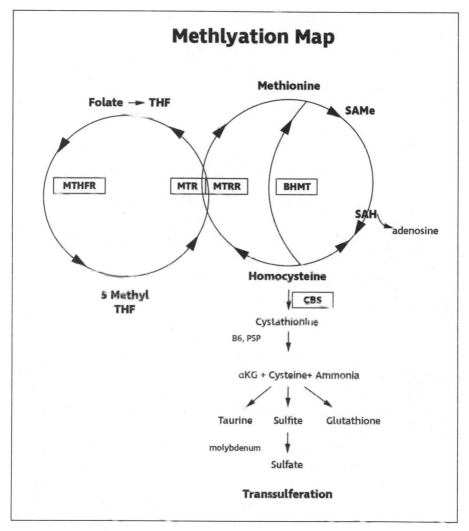

Figure 19–2

The MTHFR gene that encodes for production of the MTHFR enzyme can have mutations that will hamper the activity of the enzyme. When this happens, methylation cannot work efficiently; in our analogy, it's as if the wastebasket in each room is overflowing with THF and can't be emptied.

Mutational variations in these genes are termed alleles; note that there can be more than one variation (allele) of a particular gene. Alleles are formed when one building block of the DNA is different from that commonly found. This change is called a single nucleotide polymorphism (SNP), pronounced "snip." If the mutation comes from only one parent it is termed heterozygous; if from both parents it is a homozygous mutation. A heterozygous mutation (from just one parent) resulting in the C677T allele of the MTHFR gene will decrease conversion of folate to 5-MTHF by 35 percent; if the mutation is homozygous (from both parents), conversion drops to 70 percent.[1] But as you can see in Figure 19–2, if conversion of folate to its active form 5-MTHF is slowed, other conversions are also affected. In this case it will hamper the conversion of homocysteine to methionine; so people with an MTHFR mutation often have elevated serum homocysteine levels. If severe, levels may also be elevated in the urine, a condition termed homocystinuria.

The other major mutation in the MTHFR gene occurs in the A1298C allele. It is unclear if people heterozygous for this mutation run into difficulties, but homozygous A1298C mutations result in problems similar to C677T mutations. Similarly, people heterozygous for both the C677T and A1298C mutations (i.e., with a different faulty gene from each parent) are also markedly compromised.

MTHFR mutations are associated with an increased incidence of a long list of clinical problems. Elevated homocysteine is associated with a rise in cardiovascular disease, high blood pressure, migraine headaches, cancer, and dementia.[2] Since methylation impacts neurotransmitter activity as well as toxin elimination, people with these mutations have an increased incidence of depression, bipolar illness, and Parkinson's.[3] A large number of children with autism spectrum disorders have these mutations, and will see improvement when their methylation issues are addressed.[4] Autoimmune conditions such as inflammatory bowel disease are also more common in people with MTHFR mutations.[5] The good news is that MTHFR mutations can be bypassed by supplementing with 5-MTHF, the active form of folate.

Look closely at Figure 19–2. The MTHFR enzyme converts folate into its active form, 5-MTHF, which in turn facilitates the conversion of homocysteine to methionine via two other enzymes, methionine synthase reductase (MTRR) and 5-methyltetrahydrofolate-homocysteine methyltransferase (MTR). Reduced activity of these enzymes, which can occur due to different genetic SNP variations, will also lead to elevated homocysteine levels in the blood.

The MTRR enzyme converts vitamin B_{12} into its active form, methyl-B_{12}, using activated forms of vitamins B_2 and B_3 as cofactors. People with mutations in the MTRR gene don't perform this conversion properly, and therefore will need supplementation with methyl-B_{12}. The MTR enzyme itself requires the support of methyl-B_{12} and zinc. A mutation in the MTR gene actually depletes vitamin B_{12}. Low vitamin B_{12} can result in a potpourri of problems including fatigue, anemia, balance issues, neuropathies, cognitive dysfunction, and dementia. MTR activity is also inhibited by excess heavy metals such as lead and mercury.

There is a bypass pathway for homocysteine conversion to methionine that uses the enzyme betaine homocysteine methyl transferase (BHMT). This enzyme is dependent on zinc and betaine, a.k.a. trimethylglycine (TMG), which is synthesized from choline in the diet. Choline is converted into phosphatidylcholine as it supports the BHMT bypass pathway, and is then recycled back to choline. The BHMT bypass pathway can therefore be facilitated with supplements of phosphatidylcholine (a.k.a. lecithin), betaine, and zinc.

Phosphatidylcholine supplements are a good idea for a number of reasons. Phosphatidylcholine is the major phospholipid in cell membranes; it regulates enzyme activity, promotes mitochondrial energy production, defends against oxidative stress (described below), and protects neurons from damage. Phosphatidylcholine is also converted into acetylcholine, a major neurotransmitter, and can improve memory.[6] (Phosphatidylcholine is discussed in more detail later in this chapter.) An additional phospholipid, phosphatidylserine, can also facilitate the BHMT pathway, and is also beneficial for improving cognition and short-term memory.[7]

Meanwhile, if homocysteine is not properly metabolized, continued high levels will lead to a deficiency in methionine, since a "feedback loop" controls production. People with low methionine do not metabolize fat efficiently, which can lead to fatty liver. Additional problems include elevated histamine-mediated inflammation, a buildup of toxins, cardiovascular problems, and poor memory. And when methionine levels are low, there will be inadequate production of S-adenosyl methionine (SAMe).

SAMe is the major donor of methyl groups in the body. Methyl groups (CH_3—a carbon with three hydrogen atoms) facilitate the metabolism of proteins, lipids, and DNA. Methyl groups regulate the epigenetic activity of proteins that turn genes on and off. They are also essential in defense against microbial attacks and environmental toxins.

Under normal circumstances SAMe "gives up" its methyl group and is converted to S-adenosyl-homocysteine (SAH) and adenosine. SAH is converted into homocysteine, thereby completing the cycle. However, this last reaction can go the other way: homocysteine and adenosine can pair up to create SAH. This is what happens when there is an excess of homocysteine. SAH in turn inhibits SAMe production, limiting the body's access to methyl donors.

The presence of excess SAH may cause more vascular damage than homocysteine, and lowering the latter does not necessarily lower the former. This might explain why the risk of accelerated cardiovascular disease associated with elevated homocysteine does not change when homocysteine levels alone are normalized.[8]

As you can see from Figure 19–2, homocysteine can also be metabolized via the transsulfuration pathway. This pathway is particularly important for the synthesis of glutathione. In transsulfuration, homocysteine is first converted to cystathionine using the enzyme cystathionine beta synthase (CBS). The second step is conversion to cysteine, ammonia, and α-ketoglutarate using cystathione gamma-lyase (CTH). These steps are dependent on adequate levels of pyridoxal-5-phophate, the active form of vitamin B_6. Cysteine is then metabolized to glutathione, which is recycled to methionine, and the cycle repeats itself.

Glutathione is essential for removal of toxins from the body. It is also the body's most powerful antioxidant, protecting vulnerable tissues like the brain from oxidative stress. Oxidation occurs when oxygen molecules split into single atoms with unpaired electrons. Since electrons like to be in pairs, these "free radical" atoms scavenge the body looking for other electrons to form a pair. A chain reaction of electrons being pulled from molecules ensues, damaging cells in the process. Antioxidants keep free radicals in check, and glutatione is particularly good at doing so. Most glutathione production occurs in the liver.

When glutatione sacrifices an electron to quell a free radical, it changes from its reduced form to its oxidized state. In order for glutathione to continue to do its job, it needs to return to its reduced state. Selenium, vitamin C, and vitamin E assist in this transition. Other supplements that can augment glutathione synthesis include N-acetylcysteine (NAC) and glutamine. (See below for further discussion on glutathione.)

Transsulfuration is key to maintaining health. If CBS enzyme activity is deficient, homocysteine can accumulate and lead to the multiple issues listed above, particularly vascular disease. However, CBS mutations that accelerate enzymatic activity (C699T, A630A, N212N) can also lead to problems; this accelerated activity is referred to as up-regulation. CBS up-regulation results in increased production of ammonia, a toxin that will cause cognitive dysfunction. And the elevation in cysteine levels favors its conversion to taurine rather than glutathione. Therefore, CBS up-regulation leads to decreased glutathione synthesis.

In addition, since CBS up-regulation diverts homocysteine down the transsulfuration pathway, homocysteine is not properly converted into methionine and then SAMe, and there is a loss of methyl donors. The combination of low glutathione and lack of methyl donors leads to a dangerous detoxification profile with a potential for elevated ammonia, sulfates, and hydrogen sulfide. People with this profile often cannot tolerate sulfur in their food or supplements.

In summary, elevated homocysteine is clearly a serious issue, and it can be related to any one issue or combination of issues:

- MTHFR mutations, which decrease the conversion of folate to 5-MTHF
- MTR mutations, which decrease the conversion of homocysteine to methionine
- MTRR mutations, which decrease conversion of homocysteine to methionine
- CBS deficiency, which decreases the conversion of homocysteine to cysteine

People with elevated homocysteine levels should consider the following supplements:

- 5-MTHF, the active form of folate. They should not take folic acid.
- Methylcobalamin, the active form of vitamin B_{12}
- Trimethylglycine, a.k.a. betaine
- Riboflavin 5'-phosphate, the active form of vitamin B_2
- Niacin (vitamin B_3)
- Pyridoxal 5'-phosphate, the active form of vitamin B_6
- Phosphatidylcholine (lecithin)
- Phosphatidylserine

Many patients do well on combinations of these supplements that are available through many manufacturers. For example, Thorne makes Methyl Guard, which contains 5-MTHF and the active forms of vitamins B_2, B_3, and B_{12} as well as trimethyglycine; Integrative Theraputics has an Active B-Complex with active forms of these vitamins, as does Xymogen Methyl Protect.

However, supplementation is not always enough. Think back to the office garbage scenario—if you empty several overflowing wastebaskets and dump them in the hallway all at once, the hallway gets clogged with garbage. If a person's methylation is seriously compromised, then rapidly accelerating it with these supplements will lead to toxins being released quickly into the bloodstream, often at a faster rate than the liver and kidneys can process them. The result will be more inflammation, which will feel like a Herxheimer reaction.

It is imperative to introduce these supplements slowly, particularly if a patient has an elevated homocysteine level and is quite ill. I suggest starting with low doses of vitamins B_2, B_3, and B_6 as described above, then phosphatidylcholine and phosphatidylserine, reserving methylcobalamin for next to last, and finally adding 5-MTHF. Start each at a low dose, and gradually increase them while monitoring serum homocysteine levels.

Low homocysteine levels are consistent with CBS up-regulation. Furthermore, normal homocysteine levels in the setting of a homozygous MTHFR mutation also suggests CBS up-regulation; the MTHFR mutation will increase homocysteine and the CBS one will decrease it, so they cancel each other out. Either way, the person is at risk of having ammonia toxicity, low glutathione, low methionine, and low SAMe. It is uncommon to find elevated serum ammonia levels unless someone has chronic liver disease, but sometimes a patient with a healthy liver will report smelling or tasting ammonia.

Anyone at risk for ammonia toxicity should be given glutathione, discussed in greater detail in the following section on mold. Glutathione should be started slowly and only increased as tolerated. Patients with sulfur intolerance should also supplement with molybdenum, 500–1000 mcg twice daily. Additionally, yucca is an excellent binder for ammonia. Low-sulfur diets, which omit cruciferous vegetables and decrease protein intake, are often recommended; however, I have not seen these dietary restrictions providing noticeable benefit.

It is important to put these and other genetic mutations in context. In most cases there is no one-to-one association between a gene and a disease (exceptions are conditions such as sickle cell anemia, cystic fibrosis, and Huntington's chorea). There are multiple genes with multiple mutations as well as a host of environmental and lifestyle factors that contribute to the pathogenesis of most chronic illnesses. That said, mutations in the methylation pathway can constitute a major hurdle when treating chronic infections.

Most people do not need to be tested for all these mutations. The MTHFR mutation is the most common, so I order it along with a homocysteine level on all patients. Consider getting the other SNPs tested by ordering a genetic analysis at www.23andme.com, then submitting the results via www.geneticgenie.org to obtain a full methylation and detoxification profile for the patient who is particularly fragile. In addition, the different metabolic intermediaries can be measured in the blood; Health Diagnostics and Research Institute in South Amboy, New Jersey, offers a comprehensive profile.

MOLD

Dr. Joe Brewer specializes in infectious disease (ID) in Kansas City, Missouri. To his great credit, he is one of a handful of ID specialists in the United States who diagnoses and treats chronic tick-borne infections. He also has a contingent of patients diagnosed with chronic fatigue syndrome. I asked Joe how he distinguishes patients with Lyme from those with CFS, since they present with the same symptoms. He answered that if they don't respond to treatment for Lyme, then they are diagnosed with CFS.

Joe was intrigued when one of his CFS patients presented him with a lab test that demonstrated elevated mold toxins in her urine, so he did a study. He tested 112 patients with CFS for urinary mold toxins, and 104 were positive. A control group of fifty-five people without CFS all tested negative.[9]

When Joe interviewed the patients who tested positive, 90 percent had a history of past or present exposure to water-damaged buildings. But some of these exposures occurred many years in the past. Joe wondered why patients with a history of mold exposure years ago would currently be eliminating mold toxins in their urine—why wasn't it all gone? He hypothesized that they had toxic mold colonized inside them. In other words, they had inhaled or perhaps ingested fungal spores (the terms *mold* and *fungi* are synonymous) that led to colonization of these fungi and the ongoing production of mold toxins internally. In a subsequent paper, Joe reviewed the medical literature that confirmed the presence of both fungal species and mold toxins in the sinus washings of patients with chronic sinusitis.[10] Dr. Brewer believes that mold colonization in the sinuses is a major source of ongoing mold toxin production.

I used to think that mold was an occasional issue in patients with Lyme disease complex, and would only consider mold as a possible complication when a patient wasn't responding to treatment. I now see mold problems as so prevalent that I search for signs of mold toxicity on every patient's initial visit, even though the majority of my patients are from Colorado, where the humidity is relatively low.[†] Symptoms of mold sensitivity and toxicity parallel those of persistent *Bb* infection, as detailed in Chapter 6. This is not surprising since both conditions result in systemic inflammation. But having mold toxins in addition to tick-borne infections can make recovery dramatically more difficult.

There are several ways that mold exposure can cause problems. People can be allergic to mold, with exposure resulting in nasal congestion, sinus problems, and asthma. But it turns out that some people have systemic reactions not usually categorized as allergic. These patients describe fatigue, migraine headaches, depression, and joint pain when exposed to moldy environments.

Mold can also lead to chronic illness, as Joe Brewer documented in his CFS patients. Mold toxins, a.k.a. mycotoxins, are released from a handful of fungi. The most common molds associated with indoor water damage, *Aspergillus, Penicillium,* and *Stachybotrys* (black mold), discharge some bad actors: aflatoxin, ochratoxin, gliotoxin, and tricothecenes. These poisons can be harmful through a number of mechanisms. They can damage DNA and thereby be carcinogenic; they do this by inhibiting protein synthesis, DNA synthesis, and DNA methylation, causing oxidative damage to cell membranes, and impairing mitochondrial energy production. Mycotoxins can also damage the liver, kidneys, and nerve cells and result in cardiovascular problems, nausea, vomiting, and diarrhea.[11]

Like Lyme disease complex, mycotoxins can cause immune suppression as well as systemic inflammation, making it more difficult to treat any coexisting infections. The impact of mycotoxins on the nervous system mimics that of tick-borne

---

†   The US Southwest is relatively dry but yet has a lot of mold problems. Mold spores abound regardless of geography and low humidity, and winds allow them to circulate widely. Furthermore, according to Wendy Bodin, BS, CPH, Ckt, "mold issues in the Southwest are primarily due to the construction methods and materials being used. Many newer buildings are overly insulated and trap moisture in the walls where it cannot escape, leading to mold growth. Most of this moisture is coming from ordinary bathroom showers and leaks in pipes, faucets, toilets etc. Other sources are doors, windows, and roofs that have not been sealed properly. In other words, the states that have the lowest construction standards have the highest rates of mold problems." (https://www.luminaryhealth.com/NM_Mold.html)

infections: pain syndromes, depression, movement disorders, balance issues, coordination difficulties, cognitive dysfunction, and outright dementia.[12] Mycotoxins are poisons; they have even been investigated as chemical warfare agents.[13]

Mycotoxins often cause endocrine disruption.[14,15,16] The vast majority of patients in my practice with pituitary and hypothalamic dysfunction have elevated urinary mycotoxins. The most common mold-associated pituitary abnormality is low ADH, or diabetes insipidus, resulting in excessive urination and thirst. (See Chapter 15.) This condition often remits after successful elimination of the toxins.

Many of my mold-toxic patients have depressed TSH levels even in the presence of low T4 and T3, again indicating low pituitary function. Similarly, low ACTH levels coincident with low morning cortisol also represent low pituitary output. Low testosterone in males is not uncommon in this setting; it is related to low FSH and LH production from the pituitary or diminished release of gonadotropin releasing hormone (GnRH) from the hypothalamus. (See Chapter 15 for a complete discussion of these hormone issues.)

Yet another potential problem is infection caused by the fungi themselves. Superficial infections, such as those found on the nails (onychomycosis) or skin (tinea versicolor) are not uncommon, even in otherwise healthy people. Fungi can also cause chronic sinusitis. Since yeast is a subset of fungi, chronic candidiasis sensitivity syndrome (discussed in Chapter 16) is often associated with these infections, which sometimes manifest as thrush or, in women, as vaginitis. However, most fungal infections of the internal organs occur in immunocompromised patients with conditions such as leukemia or AIDS.

There is a fourth way that mold can cause problems in patients with tick-borne infections: because these species can trigger a cytokine cascade and systemic inflammation,[17] exposure to mold will often exacerbate the symptoms of Lyme disease complex, causing a flare or even a relapse of previously-treated tick-borne infections. Molds can trigger mast cell degranulation.

TESTING FOR MOLD

The first step in dealing with mold begins with a thorough inspection of the home and workplace. This is more difficult than it sounds—there is no consensus as to the best method to test for mold. The sensitivity of air testing using mold plates available at hardware stores is low, and can be influenced by multiple variables such as room size or occupancy at time of testing. I have seen many instances of serious black mold infestations in homes in which these plates were negative.

Several labs perform fungal analysis via PCR (DNA) testing on dust samples, which is a more sensitive test; it is called an environmental relative mold index (ERMI) test. An abbreviated ERMI test is the HERTSMI assay, which tests for the five most common toxin-producing molds. These tests can also yield false negative results, although not false positives. Real Time Laboratory in Carrollton, Texas, offers EMMA testing, which identifies ten environmental molds and sixteen mycotoxins.

The best mold detection is obtained with a careful visual inspection accompanied by checking for humidity on all wall surfaces, infrared scanning for moisture behind walls, then testing any suspicious areas for mold as well as volatile organic compounds (VOCs). VOCs are noxious, harmful gasses that are emitted from molds as well as a long list of indoor products including paints, cleaning agents, air fresheners, dryer sheets, scented candles, dry-cleaned clothes, new carpeting and upholstery, copy machines, permanent markers, and so forth. The primary causes of sick building syndrome are molds and VOCs.

Most people with mold in their homes are totally unaware of a mold problem; their houses are clean and usually don't smell. But all it takes is trapped moisture behind a wall or bathroom tile to develop mold, which can happen even in the driest climates. Once the source of the moisture has been identified and fixed, mitigation can proceed.

Unfortunately, there is no consensus as to what constitutes adequate mitigation. In general, any mold-contaminated structures would be removed; then the premises can be fogged with a citrus extract that kills mold spores. Many mitigation specialists also suggest wiping down all surfaces—including ceilings— to remove mold spores and mold toxins.

Some experts claim that while hard surfaces can be cleaned, soft surfaces such as carpeting, upholstered furniture, mattresses, and clothes will continue to harbor mold toxins that cannot be eliminated. These experts suggest getting rid of all these "soft" items. Though there is no clear data guiding this recommendation, mold spores and toxins can be absorbed through the skin,[18] so I suggest that the premises be tested for both mold spores and mold toxins after mitigation is completed. As noted above, Real Time Laboratory performs residential mold toxin testing.

Three labs in the United States perform urine mycotoxin testing: Real Time Laboratory, Great Plains Laboratory, and Vibrant America. Each lab uses a different methodology to quantitate mycotoxins. Real Time uses ELISA and tests fifteen mycotoxins; Great Plains uses spectrophotometry and tests eleven; and Vibrant America tests thirty-one and uses liquifluorescence. Vibrant America is the newest of these labs and therefore has the shortest track record of accuracy.

Dr. Lisa Nagy performed a pilot study in which patients were tested before and after a sauna, and Nagy found a tenfold increase in urine mycotoxin levels after sauna.[19] Saunas mobilize mycotoxins from tissues and increase their excretion in the urine. Nagy's research findings can be used to increase the accuracy of testing; I routinely recommend that patients empty their bladders, then sit in a sauna for about twenty minutes, then collect the next urine. It is important not to drink a lot of water prior to the sauna, as this will dilute the urine. (Sauna therapy is discussed in more detail later in this chapter.)

THE MOLD CONTROVERSY

There is considerable controversy in the biotoxin community regarding the how and why of mycotoxins continuing to be a toxic burden long after exposure. Dr. Ritchie Shoemaker claims that patients with mold toxin problems suffer from genetic issues that hamper their capacity to excrete these toxins, and he disputes the existence of endogenous mycotoxin production by internal molds.[20] This assertion is not borne out by patients who are actively excreting high levels of mycotoxins in the urine even when they test positive for the so-called "dreaded gene," the unfortunate designation that Shoemaker labeled as the one responsible for an individual's body failing to target and eliminate these toxins.‡

Shoemaker claims that mycotoxins in the urine are from dietary contamination, but the high levels often documented in urine tests are not consistent with dietary mold intake. This is not to say that genetics and epigenetic issues do not play a role in susceptibility to illness caused by exposure to molds and mycotoxins; we know that certain genotypes increase the risk of autoimmunity. But it is more likely that many of these patients have endogenous mold colonization that continue to generate mycotoxins, as Dr. Brewer has documented.

Shoemaker makes other claims regarding biotoxins that are not consistent with my clinical experience. For example, he maintains that certain laboratory values, such as low melanocyte-stimulating hormone (MSH), high matrix metalloproteinase-9 (MMP-9), high transforming growth factor beta 1 (TGF-β1), and elevated C4a complement protein indicate biotoxin induced illness. However, these abnormalities also occur with other inflammatory conditions and are neither sensitive nor specific for biotoxin illness. On the other hand, I have found that low C3a complement protein and low vascular endothelial growth factor (VEGF) are usually associated with mycotoxin illness.

Shoemaker employs a low-tech screening test called a visual contrast study (VCS) to screen for biotoxin illness. This easy-to-do test examines the ability to distinguish gray lines on a white background, and is available online as well as in some doctors' offices. However, an abnormal VCS test can be related to issues other

---

‡   My own test for mycotoxins was quite high. I took binders, nasal spray, and saunas without any change in urinary mycotoxins, but when I added a systemic antifungal, itraconazole, the levels came down quickly. Shoemaker also claims that Lyme disease complex is caused by an inability to excrete Lyme toxins; there is no evidence for this claim.

than mycotoxins; some eye pathologies will also skew the results. In addition, I have seen patients with severe mycotoxin illness who have normal VCS test results.

TREATMENT OF MYCOTOXIN ILLNESS

Once the source of the exposure has been identified and remediated, the treatment of mycotoxin illness consists of using three primary interventions: toxin binders, systemic antifungals, and antifungal nasal sprays.

Toxin binders

Mycotoxins can be sequestered in a variety of tissues, but once they enter the circulation they will be excreted through the liver into the bowels. From there they may be reabsorbed back into the body in a process called enterohepatic circulation. Binders will adhere to the toxins in the bowels and prevent reabsorption.

The medical literature does not clarify which binder is most adherent to which mycotoxin. Therefore I recommend taking two different binders simultaneously, as tolerated.[21] Other medications and supplements need to be taken away from binders, or they will be bound, preventing their absorption. Ideally binders are taken one hour before and two hours after medications, supplements, and food. People with chronic constipation will need to maintain an even greater interval. The most common side effect of the binders is constipation; adding or increasing supplemental magnesium can help maintain normal bowel movements.

Most patients space dosing to mid-morning and mid-afternoon, and also in the evening if they stay up late enough. Taking binders three to four times daily is optimal, but twice daily is more realistic for most people.

Binders occasionally cause a Herxheimer type reaction, perhaps because additional toxins are released from the tissues as some exit the circulation. It is best to start slowly and increase the dose as tolerated.

The following are recommended mycotoxin binders:

- **Cholestyramine** (CSM) has been prescribed to decrease cholesterol since it works by decreasing fat absorption. It binds effectively to most mycotoxins, but there are a few downsides. The normal pharmaceutical CSM comes with either sugar or aspartame, an artificial sweetener. While it is also available as a pure resin through compounding pharmacies, it is expensive, and some patients find the smell and taste objectionable. In addition, CSM often causes gastrointestinal distress, particularly constipation. Most patients start at low doses such as ¼ teaspoon once daily, and increase gradually up to one tablespoon (4 grams) two to three times daily.

- **Activated charcoal** also binds to most toxins. The standard capsule is 280 mg, and patients typically start at two capsules daily, then progress to six capsules two to three times daily. Activated charcoal derived from coconut is composed of smaller granules and therefore has more surface area and increased binding capacity. These capsules are 500–600 mg, with typical doses of up to four capsules two to three times daily. As with CSM, charcoal can cause gastrointestinal upset, particularly constipation.
- **Bentonite clay** comes in powder and in suspension, but I highly recommend the latter since the powder tends to float rather than mix in liquids. Clay is usually better tolerated than CSM or charcoal by patients with constipation issues. Most people start with two tablespoons daily, working up to four tablespoons two to three times daily.
- **Welchol** has been recommended as a mycotoxin binder. It has a mechanism similar to CSM, but is not as powerful. There are no research studies that have documented its efficacy in binding mycotoxins, but anecdotal reports suggest that it is effective and better tolerated than CSM. Welchol comes as tablets or as a powder, and typical doses are 1875 mg (three tablets) two to three times daily.
- **Chlorella** is a blue-green algae and as such is a rich source of chlorophyll. It is recommended for detoxification of heavy metals and other pollutants and has been suggested as a mycotoxin binder. It is a good source of protein and several vitamins, boosts immune function,[22] is anti-inflammatory[23] and is anti-carcinogenic.[24]

  There is strong evidence that chlorophyll prevents the absorption of aflatoxins in foods.[25] It is important to obtain a pure source of chlorella, as its affinity for toxins often leads to contamination. Chlorella has the advantage of not needing to be spaced away from foods, medications, or supplements.

Antifungals

If a patient is colonized with toxic molds, it is crucial to eradicate this source of mycotoxin production.

- **Intranasal antifungals** are recommended to decrease colonization in the sinuses.[26] Compounding pharmacies can formulate nasal sprays with itraconazole, voriconazole, nystatin, or amphotericin B, usually in a solution with a biofilm buster such as EDTA, by prescription. Mupirocin is often added for antibacterial activity as well as for its action as a biofilm buster.[27]
- **Over-the-counter nasal sprays** have also been effective. These include oregano oil, olive leaf extract, and grapefruit seed extract. Nasal silver

has also been effective and can be compounded with EDTA, a biofilm buster. The prescription agents appear to be stronger, since they are more likely to precipitate a strong Herxheimer response. As with everything else, it is best to start slowly.

Intranasal ozone has been effective for some patients who could not tolerate any of the other nasal sprays.

- **Prescription systemic antifungals** will decrease the colonization of fungi elsewhere in the body. Itraconazole and voriconazole are the agents of choice. Other prescription medications include posiconazole and terbinafine. Be aware of drug interactions when using these medications. Nystatin will act against yeast and other fungi in the intestines, but is not absorbed systemically. Fluconazole, which is an excellent drug for *Candida* issues, does not treat the broader spectrum of fungi responsible for mycotoxin production.

- **Natural systemic antifungals** include A-FNG (Byron-White), Mycoregen and Pro-Myco (Beyond Balance), and Biocidin (Bio-Botanical Research). Some people have benefited from oregano oil and olive leaf extracts as well as from garlic concentrates, e.g. Allimax, and from Coptis rhizome extracts. All the antifungals can result in Herxheimer reactions, so it is best to proceed slowly.

- **Biofilm busters**. It is important to add a biofilm buster to any antifungal regimen since fungi have a strong predilection to colonize in biofilm communities.[28] (A discussion of biofilm busters can be found in Chapter 8.)

Antioxidants

- **Glutathione** is important when dealing with mold toxicity. Glutathione is a powerful antioxidant and will quench free radical damage. It also is crucial in the detoxification of fat-soluble compounds. Deficiency of glutathione is associated with oxidative damage to mitochondria.[29]

Glutathione can be administered via a number of routes. These include oral, sublingual, inhaled via a nebulizer, nasal, transdermal, and intravenous. If taken orally the liposomal form is preferred, as this will improve assimilation. Transdermal glutathione is practical for children who reject oral medication. Inhaled glutathione via a nebulizer has been beneficial in patients with asthma, cystic fibrosis, and chronic lung disease. Nasal glutathione rapidly crosses the blood-brain barrier and enters the cerebrospinal fluid, which may be particularly helpful in improving cognitive function. Intravenous glutathione yields the highest blood levels and presumably the best cellular penetration.

Glutathione may be problematic in patients who react to sulfur. Adding molybdenum (500 mcg twice daily) will decrease sulfur sensitivity, and glutathione can subsequently be started in low doses.

- **Additional antioxidants** like vitamin C, vitamin E, and selenium protect membranes from oxidative damage, and also help restore levels of reduced glutathione.

Probiotics

- **Probiotics** are also beneficial when treating mold toxicity. Research studies have demonstrated that gut microflora both degrade and bind aflatoxin and ochratoxin. This has been documented with *Lactobacillus rhamnosus, Lactobacillus plantarum*, and *Saccharomyces boulardii*.[30,31]

It is important to recognize that toxin binders, glutathione, and other antioxidants are beneficial in the treatment of other biotoxin and inflammatory issues. These binders adhere to inflammatory cytokines as well as to numerous other toxins, especially those found in sick buildings. In other words, these interventions are recommended for chronically ill people, even those without evidence of mold toxicity.

Dr. William Rea and colleagues at the Environmental Health Center in Dallas, Texas, have reported success doing provocative-neutralization immunotherapy to molds and mycotoxins in patients with mycotoxin illness.[32] This technique essentially messages the immune system to not react when exposed to these antigens. Dr. Rea reported on a series of twenty-eight patients with mycotoxin toxicity who underwent sauna treatments in addition to immunotherapy, physical therapy with massage, immune stimulation, toxin binders, antifungal agents, and intravenous antioxidants. They all improved, and twenty-seven returned to work.

Chris was forty-one years old and living in Boulder, Colorado, when I first saw him. He had suffered from frequent sore throats, nasal congestion, and cough throughout his thirties. Immunotherapy seemed to help, and he maintained an active lifestyle, working as a high-powered executive and competing in hundred-mile bike races until he was thirty-nine years old. Then one day, while he was visiting friends in Arizona, he physically crashed

Chris had medical evaluations with multiple providers to determine the cause of his symptoms, but nothing was found. At his initial visit with me he complained of severe fatigue, shortness of breath, impaired cognition, chronic sinus congestion, frequent sore throats, sore soles, leg cramps, moodiness, balance issues, unrefreshing sleep, neck pain and stiffness, recent onset motion sickness, polyuria (excessive urination), polydipsia (excessive thirst), and heartburn.

Chris's labs were significant for the following abnormalities:

Test	Result	Interpretation
Vitamin B$_{12}$	263 pg/ml	Low—consistent with pernicious anemia and failure to absorb vitamin B12 in a non-vegan
Free Testosterone	8.7 pg/ml	Low—probably secondary to low pituitary function
Fasting ADH	<0.8 pg/ml	Low— diabetes insipidus secondary to low pituitary function
Homocysteine	10.4	High—consistent with methylation mutations
MTHFR A1298C	+/+ homozygous	Methylation mutation with decreased conversion of folate to 5-MTHF
AM Cortisol	10.4 mcg/ml	Low—consistent with adrenal insufficiency
DHEA-S	106.6 mcg/dl	Low—consistent with adrenal insufficiency
1,25 diOH-vitamin D	127.0 pg/ml	High—secondary to inflammation resulting from increased extra-renal hydroxylation
25-OH-vitamin D	28.0 ng/dl	Low —suppressed by the elevated 1,25 diOH vitamin D
Urine Tricothecenes	.99 ppb	High—toxins from black mold
Total T3: Reverse T3	7	Borderline—thyroid action decreased by excessive conversion of T4 to reverse T3
Co-infection testing	Negative	Low sensitivity test—does not rule out co-infections

Chris's Lyme Western Blot:

Band	IgM	IgG
18 kDa	+	-
23–25 kDa	IND	IND
28 kDa	-	-
30 kDa	-	++
31 kDa	++	-
34 kDa	IND	-
39 kDa	++	IND
41 kDa	+++	++
45 kDa	-	-
58 kDa	+	-
66 kDa	-	-
83–93 kDa	+	-

A mold inspection of Chris's house revealed Stachybotrys in the basement, Penicillium and Aspergillus in the kitchen, and Alternaria and Cladisporium in the master bathroom. The latter two molds are common in the outdoor environment and do not produce mycotoxins, but their high levels in the master bathroom reflect increased humidity in that space.

Subsequent testing revealed that Chris had low testosterone and diabetes insipidus, both consistent with suppressed pituitary output. (See Chapter 15.) It has been my experience that the vast majority of patients with low pituitary function have mold toxins.

Although co-infection testing was negative, Chris was also suffering from babesiosis and bartonellosis. These infections were initially missed because blood testing was negative and Chris did not have a Herxheimer reaction when challenged with A-Bab and A-Bart; he was one of those few who do not experience die-off reactions. But ongoing symptoms led to trials with anti-microbials that target these infections, and his response was consistent with these diagnoses.

The arc of Chris's illness started with genetic mutations resulting in methylation issues and compromised cellular detoxification. It is unclear when Chris developed pernicious anemia; this may have been hereditary, but it could also have been an autoimmune reaction triggered by his infections or the mycotoxins. He had been living with mold in his house, which was causing respiratory symptoms, but he continued to feel well in general and lead a high-functioning lifestyle. It appears that he did not become ill even when he had an unobserved tick attachment leading to infection with Bb, Bartonella, and Babesia; his immune system competently kept these bugs in check. But his body was under stress, and he was accumulating mold toxins.

It turns out that the house in Arizona in which Chris was staying when he "crashed" had a large mold infestation, and the exposure triggered Chris's "illness." Mycotoxins suppressed his pituitary gland, he was no longer making ADH (diabetes insipidus), and he experienced low pituitary secretion of FSH and LH, resulting in low testosterone. Then his adrenal glands lost their reserve, and he developed adrenal insufficiency. His elevated reverse T3 and low T3 to reverse T3 ratio were consistent with inflammation, and further contributed to his fatigue.

Chris was treated with multiple interventions: antibiotic medications and herbs for his tick-borne infections, B_{12} injections for pernicious anemia, betaine hydrochloride supplements with meals for low gastric acid output associated with pernicious anemia, methylation support supplements to bypass his MTHFR mutation, DHEA and low-dose hydrocortisone to support adrenal function, liothyronine (T3) to offset the high reverse T3, hCG injections to *raise testosterone, and a pituitary glandular to treat diabetes insipidus. The mold in his home was mitigated and he took toxin binders, systemic antifungals, and nasal antifungals to treat his mold issues.*

Chris responded wonderfully. He was back to full energy, sleeping well, and doing his hundred-mile bike rides. But then he crashed again—and most of his initial symptoms returned. The first relapse was after visiting the same house in Arizona where he had stayed when he initially became ill. It took him a couple of months to regain his health. The second time was when he spent a night in a cabin in the mountains. Needless to say, both these structures had serious mold contamination.

Most people don't experience the black-and-white scenarios that Chris did; he felt great and then suddenly relapsed after a mold exposure. A more common scenario is for people to notice they feel better after being away from home for a week or more, but their symptoms gradually worsen on returning. There are a number of possible reasons that patients relapse. These include emotional stress, trauma, surgery, high-dose cortisone intake, another tick attachment with infection, a Herxheimer reaction, or falling off their diet or medical regimen. But I always put mold exposure high on the list of possibilities.

Remember Brad from Chapter 10, the eleven-year-old who became asymptomatic after treatment for tick-borne infections? Suddenly Brad relapsed, with severe intrusive thoughts, irritability, and episodic rage. Brad's father thought he was distressed by the death of a neighbor, and I thought that he had had a flare from the A-Bab he was taking, but he continued to worsen after discontinuing the herbal formula. It took a while to solve the mystery. It turns out that shortly before Brad relapsed, the family had gone swimming and had left the wet towels and bathing suits in their minivan for a week, by which point the vehicle was quite moldy. This was confirmed with an air sample mold test. The mold exposure had destabilized his immune system and led to a relapse.

HEAVY METALS

There are several heavy metals that negatively impact cellular physiology, but of these mercury and lead pose the most common threats. Perhaps that is because they have become ubiquitous in our environment. Mercury is an industrial pollutant, a byproduct of the manufacture of insecticides, fungicides, and chlorine. Another contributor is the burning of coal, which contains mercury; its combustion puts millions of pounds of mercury vapor into the atmosphere each year. Mercury is also a component of the fluid used in fracking, so the switch from coal to natural gas extraction can result in mercury being released into groundwater rather than the air. Medical waste incinerators also release tons of mercury into the air. Even volcanoes contribute mercury into the atmosphere. Much of this mercury ends up in our oceans, where it accumulates in fish. The larger the fish, the higher up on the food chain, and the more likely they are to carry high mercury levels.

These same sources have led to environmental lead contamination of many communities like Flint, Michigan.

Even more ominous is the risk of mercury exposure to unborn children, since mercury can cross the placental barrier. The National Research Council of the National Academy of Sciences and the EPA both describe problems in fetal development associated with mercury exposure. These reports led the FDA to issue an advisory recommending that pregnant women and *women who may become pregnant* avoid fish with the highest average amounts of mercury: tuna, bluefish, tilefish, grouper, king mackerel, orange roughy, marlin, shark, and swordfish.[33]

Mercury exposure doesn't end there. Thimerosol, a preservative that is 50 percent ethyl-mercury by weight, was used in childhood vaccines from the 1930s until 1999. A child who received four to five vaccines at one time could have received over forty times the level considered safe by the EPA.[34] It wasn't until July 1999 that the American Academy of Pediatrics and the Public Health Service, citing the possibility of neurodevelopmental damage in children, recommended that manufacturers remove thimerosol as quickly as possible, and the EPA and FDA directed the vaccine manufacturers to remove mercury from childhood vaccines. But those who received childhood vaccines one or two generations ago may still have that mercury in their tissues.

Perhaps the biggest and most controversial source of mercury is dental amalgams. Silver amalgam fillings are 50 percent mercury, while the rest is primarily silver and tin. This elemental form of mercury is quite volatile, and can be transformed into vapor by agitation and compression, which is a good description of chewing and grinding your teeth. The vapor is then inhaled and assimilated through the lungs as well as swallowed and absorbed through the gastrointestinal tract. From there it circulates in the blood and diffuses into tissues and across cell membranes.

While the American Dental Association continues to advocate the use of silver amalgams, and denies their potential for toxicity,[35] studies have demonstrated that these fillings contribute measurably to the accumulation of mercury in our bodies.§[36] Table 19–1 contains a list of problems associated with mercury overload.

---

§   Two books on this dental hazard are *The Toxic Time Bomb* by Sam Ziff (Aurora Press, NY, 1984), and *Amalgam Illness: Diagnosis and Treatment* by Andrew Hall Cutler (Sammamish, WA, 1999).

SIGNS AND SYMPTOMS OF MERCURY TOXICITY
Systemic
Fatigue
Drowsiness
Insomnia
Psychological disturbances
Personality changes, mood swings, irritability, excitability, fits of anger
Nervousness, anxiety
Depression
Neurological disturbances
Headaches
Dizziness
Tinnitus (ringing in the ears)
Tremors
Cognitive disturbances
Memory loss
Attention and concentration difficulties
Altered sensation (heightened or reduced taste, touch, vision, and hearing)
Numbness and tingling
Visual disturbances
Incoordination
Speech disorders
Oral cavity disorders
Bleeding gums
Alveolar bone loss
Loosening of teeth
Increased salivation
Metallic taste
Stomatitis (inflammation of the tongue)
Ulceration of gingivae, palate, tongue
Burning in mouth or throat
Leukoplakia (white deposits in the mouth)
Gastrointestinal
Loss of appetite
Abdominal pain/cramping
Diarrhea

(Table continued on next page)

Immunological
Allergies
Autoimmune illnesses
Recurrent infections
Other
Joint pains
Hormone disorders
Rashes
Cardiovascular disease
Hypertension
Renal damage
Anemia
Cough, irregular respirations

Table 19–1. Signs and Symptoms of Mercury Toxicity

Mercury is not the only heavy metal that constitutes a threat to health; lead has also become a ubiquitous heavy metal in the air and water. You don't need to live in Flint, Michigan, to have issues with lead toxicity, although levels vary geographically. Other well-documented villains include cadmium, arsenic, and aluminum. Table 19–2 lists sources of these metals and some of the medical problems associated with them.

Research has demonstrated that there is no safe threshold level below which heavy metals are not toxic. These metals inhibit many enzymatic reactions, disrupt normal energy production, suppress methylation, and interfere with hormone binding. The clinical effects of heavy metal toxicity are systemic and far-reaching. The principal target of these metals is the nervous system, but low doses also disrupt endocrine and immune function.[37,38,39]

Toxic metals have been linked to autoimmune disease, chronic fatigue syndrome, fibromyalgia, and heart disease.[40,41,42,43] All patients with Lyme disease complex should consider appropriate testing for these toxins. Like mold and mycotoxins, the presence of heavy metals can sabotage the treatment of infections. Elevated levels of mercury and lead are the most common to find, although all heavy metals are implicated in health problems, and most patients with elevated levels have no history of industrial exposure.

Unfortunately, simple blood tests do not provide a true assessment of heavy metal status because most metals accumulate in tissues and inside cells, not in the circulating blood. The most accurate results are therefore obtained using a provocation test, where a drug that binds with the metal in tissues and then delivers it to the kidneys or bowels for excretion is used prior to testing. The stool or urine

HEAVY METALS: SOURCES AND TOXICITY		
Metal	**Sources**	**Toxicity**
Arsenic	Food, air, soil, and water contaminated from pesticides, herbicides, fungicides, industrial (smelting), paints, leaded gasolines, volcanoes	Fatigue, headaches, rashes, loss of hair and nails, weakness, hyperpigmentation of skin, anemia, increased salivation, neuropathy, vascular disease
Lead	Air pollution from leaded gasoline and industrial sources; water from contaminated sources, plumbing fixtures; paints, cans, improperly glazed ceramics, lead crystal, vegetables grown in lead-contaminated soil	Children: delayed mental development, delayed learning, behavioral problems, hyperactivity. Children and adults: Fatigue, anemia, loss of appetite, weight loss, abdominal pain, vomiting, headaches, insomnia, nervousness, cognitive difficulties, impaired fertility
Cadmium	Food, air, water, soil contaminated from cigarette smoke, mining, coal burning, industrial pollution (batteries), plastics, fertilizers, fungicides, and pesticides	Loss of sense of smell, anemia, dry scaly skin, hypertension, emphysema, kidney disease, bone fractures, hair loss, cancer
Aluminum	Antiperspirants, toothpaste, baby powder, cosmetics, cigarette filters, antacids, contaminated water and foods, foods cooked in aluminum pots and pans, and aluminum foil	Toxicity primarily documented in people with renal failure. There are studies linking aluminum with learning and behavioral abnormalities in children, and Alzheimer's disease.

Table 19-2. Heavy Metals: Sources and Toxicity

is collected over the next six to twenty-four hours and analyzed for metals. These drugs, known as chelating agents, are listed in Table 19-3. Treatment utilizes these same drugs, administered either orally or intravenously. There are also many nutritional supplements that can mobilize and promote elimination of heavy metals—these are listed in Table 19-4.

Removal of silver amalgam fillings is imperative, particularly for anyone with chronic illness. However, it is important to use a dentist who specializes in mercury removal, because if not done properly, mercury vapor will be inhaled and ingested during the process, leading to exacerbation rather than alleviation of the problem.

Another method for relieving the body burden of heavy metals is to sweat them out. Infrared saunas are an excellent tool to facilitate release of these toxins.

PHARMACEUTICAL CHELATING AGENTS TO REMOVE HEAVY METALS		
Agent	**Also Known As**	**Comments**
DMPS	Dimercaptopropane sulfate	Administered intravenously, orally, and transdermally; long history of safety in Germany; removes mercury, lead, arsenic and other heavy metals; not FDA approved but available from compounding pharmacies. Occasional severe reactions in chemically sensitive individuals.
	Unathiol	
	Dimaval	
DMSA	Dimercaptosuccinic acid	Administered orally; FDA approved for use in children and adults; removes mercury, lead, arsenic, and other heavy metals. Available from overseas pharmacies.
EDTA	Ethylene-diamine-tetra-acetate	Administered intravenously; the calcium salt can be given rapidly and binds many heavy metals; it can also be given orally and rectally but is less effective. Sodium EDTA needs to be given slowly intravenously; it is used to treat cardiovascular disease as well as heavy metal poisoning.
	Calcium disodium EDTA	
	Sodium EDTA	
Penicillamine	Cuprimine	Administered orally; has been primarily used for the treatment of copper overload (Wilson's disease) and lead toxicity, but now being used to remove other heavy metals as well
	Depen	

Table 19–3. Pharmaceutical Chelating Agents to Remove Heavy Metals

NATURAL AGENTS THAT BIND HEAVY METALS AND PROMOTE DETOXIFICATION		
Category	**Agent**	**Comments**
Herbs	Cilantro	Mobilizes heavy metals from tissues
	Chlorella	Binds heavy metals for excretion
	Garlic	Freeze-dried or high allicin content most effective
Antioxidants	Vitamin C	Either oral or intravenous
	Glutathione	Intravenous preferred
	Selenium	Binds mercury
	Alpha lipoic acid	Protects cells from heavy metal toxicity
Accessory nutrients	MSM	Source of sulfur, which is incorporated into amino acids that bind mercury
	N-Acetylcysteine	Precursor to glutathione and sulfur-containing amino acids, which bind mercury
Amino acids	Methionine	Binds mercury
	Cysteine	Binds mercury

Table 19–4. Natural Agents That Bind Heavy Metals and Promote Detoxification

SAUNAS

Many cultures incorporate saunas into their lifestyle or religious rituals, but saunas have also been adapted for detoxification and general health. Recall that Dr. Lisa Nagy documented a tenfold increase in urinary mycotoxin excretion after a single sauna.[44] Saunas help mobilize a wide variety of foreign substances for elimination, and are recommended for general detoxification as well as for the treatment of sick building syndrome.[45,46]

Saunas have also been successful in alleviating muscle pain and fatigue[47,48] and in decreasing inflammation in patients with rheumatoid arthritis.[49] In addition, saunas have documented utility in patients with congestive heart failure and high blood pressure, although cardiac patients should get medical clearance before embarking on sauna therapy.[50]

Whereas a traditional sauna uses heat to produce profuse sweating, the same result can be achieved at a lower temperature using infrared energy. I was introduced to infrared saunas by Dr. Erica Elliot, a physician in Santa Fe, New Mexico, who specializes in environmental illness. Dr. Elliot had many patients with multiple chemical sensitivity syndrome (MCS) who improved with long-term sauna therapy. Since then I have met several MCS patients who have experienced decreased reactivity to chemicals and improved well being with sauna detoxification."

Infrared is part of the electromagnetic spectrum that is being investigated for multiple medical applications.[51] Infrared in saunas appears to facilitate mobilization of toxins. This can sometimes happen too rapidly: serious toxicity can result if toxins are mobilized faster than the body's capacity to excrete them. I have seen patients take daily saunas and become quite ill. One patient in my practice developed the sudden onset of diabetes insipidus, presumably due the impact of mobilized toxins on his pituitary gland.

For this reason, I suggest patients start at low exposures and progress slowly, particularly those with fragile health status. Benefit will be seen starting at 100 degrees Fahrenheit for five minutes twice weekly, increasing by five degrees and five minutes every week up to 130 degrees for thirty minutes twice weekly. Maximum sauna exposure is 140 degrees for thirty minutes every other day. It is important to shower immediately after the sauna even if there is no sweat, since toxins on the skin can be reabsorbed.

It is also important to support the liver, kidneys, and lymphatics. I recommend glutathione, as described above, as well as other liver support supplements such as silymarin, NAC (N-acetyl cysteine), and ALA (alpha lipoic acid). There

---

** Two companies, Heavenly Heat and High Tech Health, make infrared saunas without glue, which is important for patients with chemical sensitivities.

are many supplement companies that distribute combined liver support nutrients such as Detox Formula by Vital Nutrients. It is also important to drink lots of water with added electrolytes when doing saunas regularly. In addition, it makes sense to take the Pekana basic detox homeopathic drainage remedies Apo-Hepat, Renelix, and Itires, as described in the treatment of Herxheimer reactions in Chapter 8.

INTRAVENOUS PHOSPHATIDYLCHOLINE

Dr. Patricia Kane pioneered the application of IV phosphatidycholine (PC) in the treatment of a long list of neurological and autoimmune disorders, and standardized its use in what she designated as "the PK protocol." As described earlier in this chapter, PC is important for methylation, specifically in the synthesis of methionine and SAMe. PC is a major component of cell membranes, facilitating transport of essential lipids; it is also a constituent of surfactant, a substance that protects the lungs and gastrointestinal tract; it is a major ingredient of bile, which is necessary for fat absorption; it protects the liver and promotes detoxification; and it is a precursor for acetylcholine, a neurotransmitter essential for cognition. PC has been demonstrated to improve memory,[52] reduce inflammation,[53] and protect the liver.[54] Dr. Kane uses the PK protocol for neurodetoxification and the treatment of neurodegenerative diseases such as Parkinson's, multiple sclerosis, and ALS, although no controlled clinical studies have yet documented the benefit of intravenous PC for these conditions.

The PK protocol is mainly used in integrative medicine practices to facilitate detoxification. It is often administered back-to-back with intravenous glutathione. The physiological basis for this is sound, and hopefully future clinical studies will corroborate the benefits of this treatment.

OTHER DETOXIFICATION CONSIDERATIONS

It is important to be eating a "clean" diet, which means consuming mainly whole foods, preferably ones which are organic, along with quality proteins and healthy fats. Some foods such as parsley, cilantro, garlic, lemon, dandelion greens, and cruciferous vegetables facilitate detoxification. Alcohol creates its own toxins and should be avoided.

The chemical burden on our bodies comes not only from heavy metals, mold spores, and toxins that contaminate the air and the water. Chemical herbicides and pesticides don't just impact their intended victims; they affect the user as well. VOCs from indoor products were mentioned above, and a longer list can be found at health.ny.gov/publications/6513. Every effort should be made to limit exposure.

Technological "progress" has resulted in a toxic environment even within our homes. Throwing away air fresheners, scented candles, and dryer sheets, and using cleaning agents, shampoos, and detergents that are labeled "Free and Clear" of fragrances is often essential for reclaiming health.

There is a long list of detox interventions that many people claim to be beneficial but have not undergone scientific scrutiny. These include, but are not limited to, skin brushing, foot detox baths, lymphatic massage, and coffee enemas. I am not an advocate of fasting if a patient is in a weakened state, but good sleep, exercise, and sunlight are always a good idea.

TAKE-HOME POINTS

1. Detoxification is complicated, involving cells, lymphatics, the gut, liver, kidneys, and skin. Adequate detoxification is essential in the treatment of Lyme disease complex.

2. Chronic physiologic stress can overwhelm the body's innate capacity for detoxification.

3. Genetic mutations can impact methylation pathways involved in intracellular detoxification. These can be identified, and targeted nutritional supplementation can bring these pathways into balance.

4. Mold can cause problems a number of ways: allergic reactions that can result in local and systemic symptoms; infections that are usually limited to the skin, scalp, and mucous membranes; mold toxins that can cause dysfunction in the immune, nervous, and endrocrine systems; and mold toxins that can compromise a person's capacity to clear infection.

5. The best way to assess mold toxins is with a urine assay provoked by a sauna. The presence of mycotoxins may represent ongoing exposure or a previous exposure in which spores were inhaled or ingested, setting up endogenous colonization of fungi that continue to manufacture toxins.

6. Treatment of mold toxins involves mitigating any exposure, then using toxin binders, and systemic and nasal antifungals.

7. Heavy metals, particularly mercury and lead, can also compromise immune, nervous, and endocrine function and can impede a person's capacity to clear infection.

8. Glutathione, other antioxidants, and phosphatidylcholine are particularly important in promoting proper detoxification.

9. Saunas facilitate mobilization of toxins as well as excretion through the skin.

10. Accumulation of toxins can cause many symptoms, particularly fatigue and impaired cognition.

Chapter 20

Diet and Nutrition

There is no one diet or set of supplements for everyone. In general, the longer a person has been ill, the more likely there has been immune and endocrine disruption leading to increasingly prevalent insulin resistance and food sensitivities. These issues have been discussed in Chapters 15 and 16 respectively.

DIET

There are two dietary "absolutes" for people with Lyme disease complex: avoid sugar and avoid alcohol. Sugar means all sugar, whether it's table sugar, brown sugar, honey, agave, maple syrup, high fructose corn syrup, molasses, coconut sugar, fruit juice, or even a lot of fruit. Sugar suppresses the immune system; drinking a one-liter bottle of soda will depress white blood cell reactivity by 40 percent.[1] Sugar also stimulates yeast growth and increases the risk of developing SIBO (see Chapter 16). Sugar intake can lead to wide swings in blood sugar, with an initial high glucose level followed by reactive hypoglycemia. High sugar intake not only leads to obesity, but also to insulin resistance with fatigue, inflammation, and increased risk of both heart disease and AODM—adult onset diabetes mellitus (see Chapter 15).

The most addictive substances are those that get into the bloodstream the fastest. Heroin and other opiates top the list, but the top contenders among foods are sugar, alcohol, and caffeine. People who have sugar cravings and cannot resist finishing that pint of ice cream usually have candidiasis sensitivity syndrome (CSS), discussed in Chapter 16. The treatment is to eliminate sugar cold turkey, since ongoing ingestion will only make the cravings worse.

A cautionary tale arises from a scenario I have seen repeated hundreds of times: the patient with a sugar habit stops sugar and goes through withdrawal—they feel awful and their cravings go wild; sometimes they dream of shooting people for a doughnut. After about two weeks these cravings go away and they begin feeling better. After a month they are at a party and eye some cookies, and think, "Just one bite won't hurt." They take the bite, and the cookie now tastes sickeningly sweet. Their first instinct is to put it down, but instead they take a second bite—and they're gone. In fact, the whole tray of cookies is gone, and they have fallen off the wagon.

People habituated to sugar need to stay off it 100 percent. Sugar needs to be out of the house; family members need to get their treats elsewhere and not bring them home. Chromium picolinate supplements can be helpful during the weaning process, both in stabilizing blood sugar levels and decreasing sugar cravings. Doses are 200–500 mcg twice daily.[2] I do not recommend using sugar substitutes. For one thing, many of them contain polyols that alter bowel flora and may increase the risk of AODM. In addition, consuming sweets can maintain the habit of craving sweets.

Most alcoholic beverages have sugar and yeast, especially wine and beer. But alcohol by itself also poses an issue. Many patients with Lyme disease complex have minimal tolerance for alcohol with immediate adverse reactions or terrible hangovers. Alcohol adds to the detoxification load of the liver and will worsen problems such as CSS, insulin resistance, and SIBO. Alcohol also stimulates the release of heat shock proteins, which contribute to inflammation.[3]

Beyond the sugar and alcohol prohibitions, the next dietary steps should be tailored to the individual. Identifying and eliminating food allergens is discussed in Chapter 16. The most common problematic foods are gluten, dairy, and eggs. Patients with CSS need to avoid both sugar- and yeast-containing foods, and generally do better when they also limit carbohydrates.

A low-glycemic diet is also essential for anyone with evidence of insulin resistance. This means eliminating refined grains, rice, corn, white potatoes, and sugar. Ideally, it is best to stay off foods that have a glycemic index greater than fifty. The Harvard Health website "Glycemic Index for 60+ Foods" (health.harvard.edu/diseases-and-conditions/glycemic-index-and-glycemic-load-for-100-foods) provides a starting place to find the glycemic value of many common foods. There are also a number of cookbooks and recipes for those first venturing into low-glycemic eating.

What's left is a Paleolithic-like diet that focuses on meat, vegetables, fruits, and tubers—basically what we ate as hunter-gatherers before entering the agricultural age. Research has demonstrated that Paleo regimens are anti-inflammatory and can decrease autoimmune activity.[4]

Patients with SIBO need to eat a low-carb Paleo-type regimen, designed to starve the bacteria that contribute to their GI discomfort. The low-FODMAPS diet restricts short-chain carbohydrates that are easily fermented by gut bacteria, and is particularly helpful on a temporary basis. (FODMAPS is an acronym for fermentable oligosaccharides disaccharides monosaccharides and polyols. Polyols include many sugar substitutes.)

In addition to sugar, alcohol, and many grains, other foods that generate inflammation should also be avoided. These include trans fats, sugar substitutes, food additives (like MSG), processed meat, and many common cooking oils—the best choice is to use extra virgin olive oil when cooking. Many people find foods in the nightshade family (tomatoes, bell peppers, white potatoes, eggplant) to be pro-inflammatory. Patients with excessive mast cell activation may need to limit histamine-containing foods (see Chapter 18).

Finally, organic food is recommended whenever possible. In the first research study of its kind, investigators found that people who adhered to an organic diet had a lower incidence of some types of cancer.[5] While more research is necessary, it only goes to reason that consuming pesticides and herbicides is not healthy. Many chemicals have been shown to cause epigenetic changes that will impact future generations.[6]

NUTRITIONAL SUPPLEMENTS

As with diet, there is no "one size fits all," although there are some general recommendations that can help bring the body into balance, support immune function, decrease inflammation, afford protection from toxins, and improve energy production. Here are the basics:

- **Omega-3 essential fatty acids (Ω-3 EFAs):** These are derived mainly from fish oil, but other sources include flaxseeds and krill oil. Omega-3s have significant anti-inflammatory action and are concentrated in the brain, where they are important for cognitive function. The role of omega-3 fatty acids in decreasing risk of cardiovascular disease is well established. (EFAs are discussed in more detail in Chapter 18.)
- **Magnesium:** If someone told me he or she was only willing to take one supplement, I would suggest magnesium. Soil depletion and poor dietary habits have led to wholesale deficiencies in this important mineral, which is a cofactor in hundreds of enzymatic reactions in our bodies.

  Magnesium has particular utility in patients with Lyme disease complex, because it is relaxing: it relaxes blood vessels, thereby improving circulation and normalizing high blood pressure; it calms nerves, decreasing anxiety and helping sleep; it can alleviate depression; it eases muscle tension, decreasing twitching, muscle cramping, muscle jerking, and restless legs; it improves peristalsis, relieving constipation; and it sometimes alleviates cardiac rhythm abnormalities, asthma, and migraines.

  Routine blood testing is not a sensitive indicator of magnesium adequacy. Serum magnesium levels are almost useless since most magnesium is concentrated inside cells. Red blood cell magnesium is a better test, but it still lacks sensitivity.

Magnesium glycinate, malate, and citrate are well absorbed. Magnesium oxide is not well absorbed, although it can effectively help with constipation. ReMag is a solution of pico-sized magnesium chloride that is exceptionally well absorbed. A lot of patients take magnesium at bedtime to help sleep. Magnesium is also available as a topical gel, which is particularly useful for muscle spasms, as described in Chapter 17.

- **Multivitamin**: A good multivitamin and multimineral will supply B complex, trace minerals, and antioxidants including vitamins C and E.
- **Coenzyme Q10**: Also known as ubiquinol, this nutrient is essential for mitochondrial energy production and is particularly important for cardiac function. CoQ10 should be avoided if taking atovaquone, as it may interfere with this drug's action against *Babesia*.
- **Vitamin D**: By definition a vitamin is a compound essential for normal growth and nutrition that is required in the diet because it cannot be synthesized by the body. Although small amounts of vitamin D are found in our diets (mainly from fish oil), technically it is not a vitamin, since humans have the capacity to manufacture it in skin exposed to sunlight. In addition, vitamin D acts like a hormone, since it not only regulates calcium absorption and bone metabolism, it also modulates immune function.

Vitamin D is initially metabolized in the liver into 25-hydroxyvitamin D, which is the storage form of vitamin D; this is the form measured in most assays for vitamin D adequacy. However, this is not the active form of the vitamin; 25-hydroxyvitamin D needs to be activated by the kidneys, where an additional hydroxy group is added to form 1,25-di-hydroxyvitamin D, commonly called calcitriol. (*Hydroxy* refers to a molecule that combines oxygen and hydrogen. The scientific nomenclature for hydroxy is OH.) Calcitrol is the form of vitamin D that does the work, and is what is found in supplements labeled vitamin D3.

A decrease in kidney function, which often occurs with aging, may result in a lack of activation of vitamin D, resulting in low vitamin D function even when 25-hydroxyvitamin D levels are normal. But there is another twist that often occurs in people in patients with Lyme disease complex: some immune cells called macrophages can do the same thing as the kidneys, i.e. add the second hydroxy group that activates vitamin D.[7] This extrarenal activation of vitamin D is not regulated by normal feedback control mechanisms, and therefore can generate high levels of active vitamin D even when the storage form of vitamin D is low. It is not uncommon for people with chronic inflammation to have high levels of the active 1,25-dihydroxy D, even when the storage form, 25-hydroxy D, is low. Abnormally high vitamin D may result in high serum calcium levels, nausea, vomiting, and weakness.

This means that it is important to measure 1,25-dihydroxyvitamin D in people with Lyme disease complex prior to deciding whether or not to recommend vitamin D supplements. Vitamin D is important for bone strength, muscle strength, and normal immune function,[8,9] and vitamin D levels, as measured by 1,25-dihydroxyvitamin D, are best maintained at the upper limits of normal. But those with high levels of 1,25-dihydroxyvitamin D should avoid supplementation.

Since inflammation is such a major issue in Lyme disease complex, anti-inflammatory agents are essential. These are detailed in Chapter 18 and include:

- Curcumin, the active form of the herb turmeric.
- Boswellia, also known as Indian frankincense.
- CBD from hemp oil, as described in Chapters 17 and 18.
- Proteolytic enzymes such as Wobenzym, bromelain, and papain. These need to be taken on an empty stomach to be effective.

Antibiotics knock microbes down, but it is up to the immune system to clear the infection. This became abundantly clear when physicians first began treating people with AIDS, who suffered from severe immune dysfunction. These patients became infected with opportunistic infections, and often succumbed regardless of aggressive antibiotic treatment.

Therefore it may seem evident to enhance immune function in people with Lyme disease complex, but this needs to be approached carefully. People suffering from autoimmune reactivity and systemic inflammation could experience an exacerbation of these symptoms, depending on which part of the immune system is dominant or hyperactive. For example, patients with an acute infection may benefit from adding nutraceuticals that enhance the Th1 arm of the immune system, like andrographis, echinacea, berberine, transfer factor, vitamin C, and beta-glucan. Once entering a chronic phase, the picture gets complicated. Some patients end up being stuck in an imbalance of Th1 dominance, and the supplements listed could potentially exacerbate inflammation. However, those patients who experience widespread autoimmune inflammation may have developed Th17 activation with suppression of Th1, and therefore suffer from Th2 dominance. These patients could benefit from Th1 boosters like transfer factor. (See Chapter 18 for a detailed explanation of the immune response, Th1, Th2, and Th17.)

Antioxidants help protect cells from damage by free radical oxidation, which occurs with systemic inflammation. These include:

- Vitamin C, particularly in its liposomal form
- Vitamin E as natural tocopherols, 200–400 iu daily
- Selenium, 200–400 mcg daily
- Glutathione, the most potent antioxidant in our bodies, is also essential for detoxification. The liposomal form is best assimilated through the GI tract and is best absorbed on an empty stomach. There are other methods of administration, including topical, nasal, and via nebulizer, but the best is intravenous. (See Chapter 19 for an extended discussion on glutathione.)

TAKE-HOME POINTS

1. People who suffer from chronic inflammatory conditions need to be attentive to their diet and additional needs for nutritional supplementation.
2. Anyone with Lyme disease complex should completely avoid sugar and alcohol.
3. Dietary recommendations need to be individualized. More specific recommendations are detailed in chapters that address the specific conditions that develop in patients with Lyme disease complex.
4. Those patients who have been ill for a long time often experience systemic inflammation, and are more likely to develop problems with food sensitivities, insulin resistance, MCAS, and gastrointestinal problems such as leaky gut and SIBO.

Chapter 21

Fatigue

Fatigue is the most common complaint for which patients see their physicians. Many don't have a chronic illness but simply lack the energy and vitality that is portrayed on TV commercials featuring sixty-five-year-old seniors riding their bicycles and taking Centrum Silver. On the other hand, there is fatigue, and then there is fatigue. People with Lyme disease complex sometimes lack the energy to take a shower, walk to the mailbox, or talk on the telephone. Generally, when physicians evaluate fatigue, they do routine testing to rule out anemia, low thyroid function, and liver and kidney disease. That's about it.

I separate fatigue into above the neck and below the neck. Above the neck manifests in sleepiness; the overwhelming need to close your eyes and take a nap. Below the neck is weakness and lethargy; when one flight of stairs is too daunting to take the first step.

In general, above-the-neck fatigue is caused by blood sugar issues, such as hypoglycemia and insulin resistance, food sensitivities, or sleep disorders. Below-the-neck fatigue is often caused by adrenal insufficiency, low thyroid function, sex hormone deficiencies, or mitochondrial disorders. Mitochondria are the energy manufacturing organelles inside your cells. Lyme encephalopathy, toxin overload, and allergies, including *Candida* sensitivity, usually cause a mixed bag.

Most people with Lyme disease complex have more than one of these conditions occuring simultaneously. Chronic infection with systemic inflammation can by itself result in severe fatigue. In addition, pain and depression can cause fatigue, although infection can drive all three—pain, depression, and fatigue.[1]

EVALUATING THE CAUSE OF FATIGUE

A workup for fatigue begins with an in-depth history and physical exam and may also include the following:

- Detailed dietary history
- Comprehensive history for mold, pesticide, and industrial and other chemical exposures
- Sleep history with or without a sleep study
- Glucose tolerance test with simultaneous insulin levels
- Thyroid evaluation (see Chapter 15)
- Elimination-Challenge diet testing and/or blood tests for food sensitivities (see Chapter 16)
- Adrenal evaluation (see Chapter 15)
- Allergy testing for molds, dust, dander, and pollens
- Testing for heavy metals (see Chapter 19)
- Testing for urine mold toxins (see Chapter 19)
- Testing for sex hormones, pituitary hormones and growth hormone (see Chapter 15)
- Testing for viral antibodies—Epstein-Barr virus, *Cytomegalovirus*, herpes simplex I and II, human Herpesvirus 6
- Testing for dysautonomia with postural vital signs or tilt table test
- Environmental mold testing at home, school, and at work (see Chapter 19)

We assess a symptom by the company it keeps. If fatigue is accompanied by postural light-headedness, low blood pressure, salt cravings, or post-exertional malaise, think adrenal insufficiency. If a patient is intolerant of the cold, has difficulty losing weight, and is constipated, suspect hypothyroidism. If sleepiness occurs after meals, suspect food sensitivities or insulin resistance. You get the idea.

Treatment obviously depends on the results of the evaluation. Sometimes cleaning up the diet by getting off caffeine, sugar, and alcohol can make a remarkable difference. *Candida* sensitivity can cause severe exhaustion and is particularly common in Lyme patients who have been on months of antibiotics without taking an anti-yeast agent (see Chapter 16).

MITOCHONDRIAL DYSFUNCTION

Through a process known as oxidative phosphorylation, mitochondria—the organelles in our cells that are responsible for energy production—produce ATP, an energy molecule. This process, also known as aerobic respiration, requires oxygen. If oxygen is not adequate, our bodies resort to anaerobic respiration. This occurs outside of mitochondria and produces lactic acid. The following neutraceuticals can improve mitochondrial function.[2]

- **Co-enzyme Q10**: a.k.a. ubiquinol, is important for oxidative phosphorylation. Doses from 50–500 mg twice daily can improve energy production, but should not be taken if a person is also on atovaquone for babesiosis, as it can intefere with this medication's action.
- **Carnitine**: this dipeptide made from lysine and methionine facilitates transport of fatty acids across mitochondrial membranes and is critical for mitochondrial function. Acetyl-L-Carnitine is more agile than carnitine at crossing the blood brain barrier and it can improve cognition as well as energy.[3] Doses are 500–1000 mg twice daily.
- **Alpha-lipoic acid:** a critical cofactor in mitochondrial function as well as a potent antioxidant and anti-inflammatory agent.[4] Doses are usually 600 mg once or twice daily.
- **Antioxidants:** Vitamin C, vitamin E, zinc, magnesium, and chromium also assist mitochondrial energy production. Nicotine adenine dinucleotide (NADH) is an antioxidant cofactor in more than two hundred reactions in the body; several studies have demonstrated its capacity to improve energy in patients with chronic fatigue syndrome.[5,6]

There are companies that incorporate these mitochondrial support nutrients into one formulation. For example, Researched Nutritionals offers ATP360.

Long term antibiotics can cause mitochondrial dysfunction leading to fatigue.[7] Patients who develop fatigue after initial improvement with antibiotics should consider a trial off their antibiotic regimen.

DIET AND FATIGUE

Peg moved to Colorado after living on the East Coast all her life. For the previous ten years she had been treated by two different prominent Lyme-literate physicians who appropriately diagnosed her with Lyme, Babesia, Bartonella, *and* Mycoplasma *infections. She was treated with a series of different antimicrobials and improved, but never achieved 100 percent remission. Whenever the medications were discontinued she would relapse. Neither of her physicians had discussed diet or mold.*

When I first saw Peg, she was fifty-seven years old, and had a long list of symptoms including severe lethargy and post-exertional malaise. I recommended she go on a no-sugar, low-glycemic, low-yeast diet. On her next visit her energy had improved at least 50 percent, and many other symptoms had improved. Lab results documented a number of other as yet untreated issues, all of which were suspicious from taking a detailed history: adrenal

insufficiency, high reverse T3, high fasting insulin (insulin resistance), detox-
ification issues (MTHFR mutations—see Chapter 19), active infection with
Epstein-Barr virus and markedly elevated mold toxins.

Peg's improvement with simple diet restrictions is significant, but clearly there are
a lot of other issues needing attention.

VIRAL INFECTIONS AND FATIGUE

Madeleine, born and raised in Colorado, had problems from a young age. She
suffered from eczema, asthma, and night terrors in addition to recurrent tonsil-
litis and strep throats. Even as a child she experienced anxiety and depression.

As Madeleine got older everything worsened. She developed fatigue, back
pain, headaches, migratory joint pains, recurrent shoulder dislocations, sleep
disorder, tremors, night sweats, and cognitive dysfunction. At eighteen years
old, she was put on doxycyline for acne and felt somewhat better. When doxy
was discontinued a year later, she crashed—more fatigue, headaches, joint
pains, and depression.

At twenty-one years old, Madeleine consulted with a physician who tested
her for Lyme:

Band	IgM	IgG
18 kDa	++	-
23–25 kDa	-	-
28 kDa	-	-
30 kDa	-	-
31 kDa	IND	-
34 kDa	IND	-
39 kDa	IND	+
41 kDa	IND	++
45 kDa	-	-
58 kDa	-	-
66 kDa	-	-
83–93 kDa	IND	-

Co-infection testing was negative as were antibodies to EBV and cytomegalo-
virus (CMV) at that time., Madeleine's physician started her on azithromycin
for Lyme and clindamycin for babesiosis. Each caused a mild Herxheimer

reaction followed by some improvement. A-Bart caused a die-off reaction, but A-Bab did not. She stayed on both A-Bart and A-Bab.

Five months after starting treatment, Madeleine was getting worse. Her fatigue was severe and she was sleeping eighteen hours a day. At that time, additional labs revealed the following:

Test	Result	Reference Interval
EBV Ab VCA IgM	>160.0	Positive >43.9
EBV Ab VCA IgG	149.0	Positive >21.9
HHV-6 IgG	35.97	Positive >0.99
CMV Ab IgM	47.5	Positive >34.9
HSV IgM I/II combination	2.06	Positive >1.09
HSV 2 IgG	<0.91	Positive >1.09

The presence of IgM antibodies to EBV, CMV, and HSV suggest active infection. The elevation in IgG antibodies to HHV-6 are consistent with either an old exposure or an active infection. Madeleine began intravenous Meyer's cocktails which helped her energy. Meyer's cocktails contain high doses of vitamin C as well as B vitamins and some minerals, and often benefit patients with viral infections. Samento and Banderol were added, which were of mild benefit.

A salivary cortisol test showed low cortisols on all four specimens, consistent with adrenal insufficiency. For unclear reasons, Madeleine was given a Medrol Dosepak (methylprednisolone, a potent corticosteroid) and her symptoms flared, which is typical in patients with chronic infections, since steroids suppress the immune system. Her ferritin (iron stores) were on the low side, as were her red blood cell counts, hemoglobin, and hematocrit, and she began iron supplementation. Rifampin caused a mild Herxheimer reaction, then mild benefit, consistent with Bartonella infection.

Two years into treatment, Madeleine began intramuscular injections of LA Bicillin, 1.2 million units twice weekly, and stopped the oral medications. She noticed almost immediate improvement in energy, cognition, and pain. When the dose was doubled, she suffered a severe Herxheimer reaction, and she returned to the previous dose.

When I initially evaluated Madeleine, it was clear from her history that she had multiple issues: Bb infection, Bartonella infection (Herx reaction to both A-Bart and rifampin), Babesia infection (her night sweats had remitted on clindamycin even though the A-Bab challenge was negative), viral activation, adrenal insufficiency, and low iron. She was on the LA Bicillin, Effexor (an antidepressant), and a lot of supplements.

Madeleine's biggest complaints were hand tremor, twitching and jerking muscles, leg shaking, fatigue, and weakness (she walked with a cane), memory and attention difficulties, migratory joint pains, neck pain, back and spine pain, daily headaches, anxiety with panic attacks, depression, sleep difficulty with nightmares, menstrual irregularity with ovulatory and menstrual pain and PMS, sharp chest pains, chronic cough with occasional air hunger, an internal sense of vibration, night sweats, light and sound sensitivity, tinnitus, intermittent blurry vision, palpitations, light-headedness when standing up, heat intolerance, nausea, belching, bloating, and the sensation of food sitting in her stomach after eating. She had lost fifteen pounds over seven months.

Physical examination was remarkable for the following: blood pressure was 114/74 with a pulse of 96—these did not change when she stood up. Weight was 120 pounds. Her neck had some small lymph nodes and the thyroid was diffusely enlarged. Musculoskeletal exam revealed that Madeleine was hyperflexible (double-jointed); there were pale white striae on her thighs and mottling of her legs consistent with Bartonella *infection. In addition, Madeleine had dermatographia—a light scratch on the skin led to a dark red line indicating excessive histamine. The remainder of the exam was noncontributory.*

An ultrasound of Madeleine's thyroid demonstrated a multinodular goiter. An ultrasound of her pelvis revealed ovarian cysts. Food allergy blood tests were positive for dairy, eggs, yeast, and peanuts. She had a heterozygous MTHFR mutation on the A1298C allele with a normal homocysteine. Serum cortisol level in the a.m. was low at 8.4 mcg/dl. A repeat salivary cortisol level documented a low level in the morning but elevated at midnight. A urine mycotoxin assay revealed an elevation in tricothecenes, a toxin from black mold.

People with Lyme disease complex typically suffer from both excessive inflammation and immune incompetence. Viruses that were dormant may become active, thereby contributing to chronic illness and severe fatigue. Some patients have a past history of infectious mononucleosis caused by the Epstein-Barr virus, but most of us have been exposed to this virus. In the presence of chronic tick-borne infections, EBV and other viruses can be reactivated and contribute to fatigue and other symptoms.

Conversely, I have also witnessed patients who appear to have had dormant tick-borne infections that became active after coming down with an acute EBV infection. We return to the beaker analogy described by the environmental medicine physicians: different issues pile up and at some point spill over. It's easy to blame the last insult as the cause of illness, when in reality it was only the trigger that put people over the top.

It is apparent that Madeleine was born with an MTHFR mutation, but it was not severe enough to increase her homocysteine. She also appears to have Ehler-Danlos syndrome (EDS), a congenital issue that results in ligamentous laxity—explaining her double jointedness and recurrent shoulder dislocations. It is noteworthy that *Bartonella* infection can also play a role in joint hypermobility.[8] The childhood history of eczema, asthma, and recurrent respiratory infections suggest food and inhalent allergies. It is likely that she acquired infections with *Bb*, *Babesia*, and *Bartonella* at a young age given the severity of her multiple symptoms, and it is likely that she was infected in utero since it turns out that her mother is also suffering from Lyme disease complex. At some point Madeleine was exposed to black mold, and over time the chronic inflammation resulted in adrenal dysregulation and dysautonomia with rapid pulse. Madeleine did not have mast cell activation syndrome, but she did have excessive histamine as demonstrated by her dermatographia.

Madeleine also had hypochlorhydria (low stomach acid), leading to some of her gastrointestinal complaints. There is an increased incidence of hypochlorhydria with Ehler-Danlos syndrome.[9] Madeleine's chronically low ferritin, an indicator of iron storage, was caused by her decreased capacity to absorb iron related to the low HCl.

Madeleine had a multinodular thyroid but normal thyroid function testing. She also had multiple ovarian cysts but no evidence of polycystic ovary syndrome (PCOS). These conditions are not uncommon in the non-Lyme population, but may be related to systemic inflammation.

It is noteworthy that Madeleine developed significantly elevated antibody levels to multiple viruses after starting treatment. Antibodies to both EBV and CMV were initially negative and subsequently turned strongly positive, suggesting activation of a dormant infection.

Madeleine went on a strict diet omitting dairy, eggs, sugar, yeast, and gluten. She took betaine hydrochloride supplements with meals as well as quercitin (which stabilizes mast cells) before meals, and her gastrointestinal complaints remitted. She added hydrocortisone, 5 mg in the morning and 2.5 mg at noon, which increased her energy. She also took phosphatidylserine and ashwaganda at bedtime to suppress her elevated nighttime cortisols, and her sleep markedly improved.

Madeleine stayed on the LA Bicillin and slowly added SMZ-TMP to go after Bartonella; she had to progress slowly due to die-off reactions. Mimosa pudica was added to address Babesia. Hemp oil CBD extract improved cognition. Evening primrose oil (a source of gamma-linolenic acid, an anti-inflammatory omega-6 fatty acid) and pyridoxal-5-phosphate *(activated vitamin B$_6$) significantly decreased her PMS and menstrual cramps. Valcyclovir, to treat the viral infections, caused an immediate Herxheimer reaction and she had to progress slowly, but she noted a significant improvement in energy with the antiviral.*

At the time of this writing, all Madeleine's symptoms have diminished considerably. Madeleine is still under treatment, but her mood is great. Most notably, she has graduated from college and went to Paris to visit the art museums. Her mother still recalls checking in on Madeleine when she was sleeping eighteen hours a day to make certain she was still breathing.

It has been well documented that viruses such as Epstein-Barr and human herpesvirus 6 are associated with chronic fatigue, although the causal relationship is not always clear. Most of us have been exposed to these viruses and carry antibodies to them. But the presence of IgM antibodies as well as high elevations in IgG levels suggest that these viruses may be active, and treatment often leads to symptom improvement. A trial of antiviral agents should be considered.

Valcyclovir and its cousins acyclovir and famcyclovir are used routinely to treat herpes simplex I and II (HSV, which cause oral and genital outbreaks) as well as herpes zoster, which causes shingles. Once infected with these viruses, they never leave—they just lie dormant but are prone to reactivation—not only with skin outbreaks but also with fatigue and malaise.

These same antiviral medications are often beneficial against EBV and CMV, which are also in the Herpes family. HHV-6 is harder to treat, but some patients do well on ganciclovir (Valcyte), which has also been used for chronic EBV infections.[10] Patients on ganciclovir need to be carefully monitored with routine blood counts and chemistries as it can cause bone marrow suppression and kidney failure.

There are natural remedies that are often beneficial in the treatment of viral infections. These include monolaurin; A-EB/H6, a Byron White extract that is particularly powerful against EBV, and HHV-6; and transfer factor, an immune stimulator derived from colostrum. Researched Nutritionals makes Transfer Factor Plas Myc, which messages the immune system to target several virus infections. High-dose intravenous vitamin C, as in a Meyer's cocktail with B vitamins and minerals, can be quite helpful in the treatment of viral infections, especially when administered on a weekly basis.

VITAMIN B12

High-dose vitamin B$_{12}$ injections often help energy, even in patients who do not suffer from a B$_{12}$ deficiency. It may also improve cognition, mood, and neuropathic pain. Doses range from 1,000 to 25,000 micrograms injected daily. Compounding pharmacies manufacture doses higher than 1,000 mcg/ml as both hydroxycobolamin and methylcobolamin. It is impossible to overdose on vitamin B_{12}, although it will turn urine pink. Fragile patients may find higher doses as too activating and become agitated.

THE BOTTOM LINE

Patients feel dramatically improved with a multifaceted approach. Remember what happens when you keep driving on that flat tire? Antimicrobials may reduce infection, but the entire body is under stress, and all systems need to be addressed to regain health. Peg's and Madeleine's stories clearly demonstrate the need for an integrative approach to treating Lyme disease complex. Anything less than that won't yield the results patients need.

TAKE-HOME POINTS

1. Fatigue takes on many shapes: profound sleepiness, body lethargy, weakness, and post-exertional malaise. The quality and pattern of fatigue hints at the underlying pathology.
2. Assess fatigue by the company it keeps. This goes for all symptoms —always look for patterns.
3. Patients with Lyme disease complex are usually suffering from multiple issues contributing to fatigue. It takes a multifaceted integrated approach and tenacious detective work to evaluate the underlying causes of fatigue.

Section Four

WHAT ELSE?

What else indeed? The human body is infinitely complex. As much as we now know, I believe we are just scratching the surface of the human condition. It is clear that year after year we will gain more answers to the how and why we become ill. In the meantime, Chapter 22 details a handful of conditions that may play a complicating role in Lyme disease complex but do not get much attention.

Chapter 23 details many of the alternative treatments that some patients have found beneficial. While there are no controlled studies to document their efficacy, the anecdotal reports on some of these interventions are impressive.

There are some questions that come up repeatedly in my practice. In Chapter 24, I have listed the most common ones my patients ask, with the best answers we have at this time.

Chapter 22

Other Considerations

The preceding chapters cover the most common problems associated with Lyme disease complex. This chapter will describe of a handful of other conditions experienced by some patients.

PORPHYRIA

Porphyria is the name given to a group of disorders related to problems in the production of heme, a component of hemoglobin, myoglobin, and some enzymes. Heme production occurs in the liver and bone marrow, where it is made from chemicals called porphyrins and from porphyrin precursors. There are eight different enzymes that are necessary for the production of heme. A deficiency in each particular enzyme will result in a different type of porphyria. Porphyrias fall into two categories: genetic and secondary, or acquired.

When there is a deficiency in an enzyme, the precursors accumulate and lead to toxicity, and the toxin buildup leads to symptoms. The major clinical manifestations of porphyria are neuro-visceral, meaning they affect the nerves and the abdominal organs, and cutaneous—i.e. affecting the skin. The former typically results in intermittent acute attacks, often triggered by drugs and other chemical exposures. The most common symptoms are abdominal pain, mental changes, mood disorders, palpitations, and high blood pressure, but may also include other neurological symptoms, nausea and vomiting, fatigue, shortness of breath, urinary burning, and chest pain. Attacks may be accompanied by red or brown urine.

The cutaneous porphyrias (porphyria cutanea tarda) can cause either continuous or intermittent symptoms. These manifest as severe photosensitivity, i.e. symptoms triggered by sun exposure with skin burning, blistering, itching, redness, and/or swelling. (The photosensitivity of this syndrome gave rise to the werewolf and vampire myths in Balkan folklore.)

Chronic viral infections, particularly HIV and hepatitis C, have been implicated in acquired cutaneous porphyria. There are claims that infection with *Bb* can precipitate acute porphyria in genetically disposed individuals, but I have not seen data to confirm this.

Diagnosis of neuro-visceral porphyria is based on urine testing for porphyrin precursors PBG and ALA. However, this testing is only accurate if urine is collected during an acute attack, the sample protected from light with aluminum foil, then refrigerated until brought to the lab. The cutaneous porphyrias can be diagnosed by detection of elevated plasma or urine porphyrins.

Patients with porphyria require a diet high in carbohydrates and sugar, and feel much worse on a Paleo-type regimen. This is particularly challenging when patients have yeast or mold problems, as they need to walk a culinary tightrope. Hydroxychloroquine is the drug of choice for porphyria, and supplementation with folic acid and vitamin B_{12} can be helpful.

KRYPTOPYRROLURIA

Kryptopyrroluria (KPU), also known as pyroluria, is another disorder of hemoglobin production and is related to porphyria. In this condition the body produces excess amounts of hydroxyhemopyrrolin-2-one (HPL), which is excreted by the kidneys. HPL binds with zinc and vitamin B_6 and pulls them out of the body, creating a deficiency of these nutrients. This may result in a variety of neurological, mood, and behavioral symptoms.

Orthomolecular psychiatrists, who address mental illness by correcting underlying biochemical imbalances, claim that KPU is an organic marker for schizophrenia. However, research studies have failed to document a consistent correlation, and KPU is still not considered to be a genuine disease in the mainstream medical literature. On the other hand, functional medicine physicians have found that testing and treating for this disorder can facilitate significant health benefits.

KPU can be triggered by a variety of stresses, both emotional and physical, including infection. Dr. Dietrich Klinghardt claims that over 70 percent of his patients with Lyme disease have KPU.[1] Treatment includes replacement of vitamin B_6 and zinc plus other nutrients.

Dr. Klinghardt and Scott Forsgren have published a detailed description of KPU, its history, pathophysiology, associated conditions, diagnosis and treatment, and interested readers can refer to their article for more information: townsendletter .com/July2017/krypto0717.html.

MORGELLONS DISEASE

Morgellons disease is a condition characterized by small fibers or other particles emerging from skin sores. Because it is so poorly understood and outside the usual presentation of illness, doctors have at times resorted to labeling patients with this illness as delusional.[2] Sadly, it is quite real.

The skin lesions may be fibrous, sand- or seed-like, black specks, or crystallized particles. Morgellons patients describe intense itching, with crawling and stinging sensations under the skin. They also complain of fatigue, joint pains, muscle pains, impaired cognition, sleep disturbances, gastrointestinal symptoms, blurred vision, neuropathic pain, and mood and behavioral disorders—anxiety, depression, and personality changes. The skin lesions appear spontaneously and are slow to heal. These fibers have been evaluated with microscopy and spectroscopy, but have yet to reveal their composition.[3]

The majority of patients with Morgellons have antibodies to *Bb* on Western blot testing. Many also have antibodies to co-infections including *Babesia*, *Ehrlichia*, *Anaplasma*, and *Bartonella*.[4,5,6] Consistent with an infectious etiology, patients usually respond to antimicrobials to these pathogens.[7] In addition, anti-helminthic agents often decrease the outbreak of skin lesions.[8] Palliative treatment with anti-itching topical medications and other supportive measures affords some relief.

Morgellons disease is often disfiguring and debilitating. Hopefully new insights will soon lead to improved treatment outcomes.

ELECTROMAGNETIC FIELD ISSUES

Have you heard of the body electric? It is literally true. Normal body functions are the result of chemical reactions which generate the movement of electrons, inducing a nearly infinite number of tiny electric currents. Exposure to low frequency electromagnetic fields (EMFs)* can induce circulating currents within the human body, which can interfere with the body's own electrical signals, stimulate muscles and nerves, and interfere with other bodily functions. [9,10,11,12]

The number of EMF sources has increased exponentially due to industrialization and the technological revolution. All electric devices generate EMFs, but high sources of radiofrequency radiation include cell phones, smart meters, cordless phones, Wi-Fi routers, and laptop computers. High-voltage power lines emit particularly strong magnetic fields, and children living nearby have been shown to have an increased risk of leukemia and brain cancer.[13,14,15]

---

* EMF is also referred to as electromagnetic radiation (EMR) and radiation frequency (RF).

While it is not disputed that EMFs above certain levels can trigger biological effects, there has been skepticism in the medical community about low-level exposure causing problems. However, there are an increasing number of studies documenting the ill effects of lower levels of exposure. These problems include but are not limited to headaches, mood disorders, impaired cognition, fatigue, sleep problems, neuropathic pain, testosterone suppression, reproductive toxicity in females, cardiovascular disease, dysautonomia, and immune dysfunction.[†16,17,18,19,20,21,22,23,24,25] I have seen patients who cannot hold a cell phone to their ear because it causes buzzing inside their heads.

There is an increasing number of people worldwide who are reporting symptoms due to low levels of exposure. A worst-case scenario for these individuals occurs when servers or entire cities go to a 5G network, which is more pervasive and at higher frequencies than 4G. While not yet documented in double-blinded provocation studies, EMF sensitivity parallels the status of food sensitivities forty years ago and multiple chemical sensitivity syndrome twenty years ago: the pathophysiology of these conditions are still not well understood, but they are increasingly accepted as real.[‡]

Treatment is exceedingly difficult. The primary step is to reduce exposure, which is not easy. The International Institute for Building-Biology and Ecology maintains a list of certified consultants who can assess EMF exposure in a home and make recommendations for remediation.[§]

It is quite plausible that people suffering from Lyme disease complex who develop widespread hypersensitivity conditions would be particularly susceptible to the ill effects of EMFs. Any patient who continues to be symptomatic after trying every other course of action should investigate whether EMF reduction provides relief. On the other hand, it is a good idea for everyone to become aware of the insidious nature of this increasing problem of the twenty-first century and take steps to reduce their exposure.

DENTAL CAVITATIONS

Infections following dental work, particularly root canals, can result in areas of dead jawbone called cavitations. These represent breeding grounds of bacteria that

---

†   The Biointiative Report 2012 is a lengthy review of EMFs, their biological effects, and a rationale for imposing standards on EMF exposure: http://www.bioinitiative.org/ (Accessed October 23, 2018).

‡   The incidence of anxiety and depression in teenagers has increased significantly, and suicide is now the number two cause of death in this population. One wonders how much the excessive use of smartphones are contributing to this problem, not only because of its implications regarding poor socialization but also because of excessive EMF exposure.

§   See https://hbelc.org/find-an-expert/environmental-consultants.

resist treatment. Ozone injections into the surrounding gums can be beneficial, but patients typically require surgery. There are numerous claims that the presence of cavitations impairs immune competence and compromises the ability to effectively treat Lyme disease. No controlled studies on this issue are available, but it makes sense that a pocket of untreated infection inaccessible to antibiotics would compound the difficulty of treating Lyme disease complex.

WHAT ELSE?

I can guarantee that more imbalances, more dysregulation, and more pathology will come to light with the increasing prevalence of patients with chronic inflammatory disorders. Stay tuned.

Chapter 23

Alternative Treatments

H ealth-care providers and researchers in the field of chronic Lyme are continually searching for answers. What additional factors beyond the infections may be contributing to symptoms in chronically ill people? Are there innovative ways to address these problems? Many LLMDs integrate alternative medical treatments into their practices, while others will only do so after studies provide conclusive proof of benefit.

My criteria for assessing a treatment modality is, first of all, does it work? Second, what are the risks? And only third, how well do we understand the underlying mechanism of action? The history of medicine is full of examples of therapies that were first applied and only later understood. Aspirin was used quite effectively for a long time before researchers uncovered how it exerts its anti-inflammatory actions. I will recommend an intervention if it benefits patients without harm, trusting that we will gain more understanding at some future date.

A number of the treatments in this section meet these criteria—although most are lacking controlled studies that document efficacy, they have shown promise, and I have recommended some of them. This chapter also reviews treatment modalities that I do not use, as they don't meet my criteria, and I deem them "not ready for prime time."

OXIDATIVE THERAPIES

Welcome to the world of free radicals and oxidative therapies. In the 1960s and 1970s the free radicals were the hotheads on college campuses who stirred up the student body, organized sit-ins at the dean's office, and managed to generate enough chaos that classes were sometimes canceled before final exams. Free radicals in the human body play a similar role. They are oxygen-containing molecules with an uneven number of electrons spinning in their outer orbit, making them highly charged and unstable. A free radical avidly seeks out vulnerable molecules in order to steal an electron. This process, called oxidation, creates a new free radical molecule with an unpaired electron, which then goes on to repeat the felony. Unless checked, one free radical can generate a string of hundreds of additional free-radical reactions.

Nature, of course, provides an antidote. Free radical oxidation is balanced with antioxidants. Antioxidants are free radical quenchers—molecules that can sacrifice an electron, thereby satisfying the free radicals' hunger. Vitamin C, vitamin E, selenium, copper, manganese, and carotenoids like beta-carotene are nutritional antioxidants. Green and yellow vegetables are replete with antioxidant nutrients that afford protection against unchecked free-radical activity.

However, free radicals are not just found in the body; they are in cigarette smoke, exhaust fumes, air pollution, herbicides, pesticides, industrial wastes, food additives, radiation, and heavy metals such as mercury, cadmium, lead, and even iron. When free radicals get the upper hand, undesirable consequences ensue. Left unchecked, free radical activity results in damage to cell membranes, mutation of genetic material, and inflammation. Free radical damage has been linked to cardiovascular disease, cancer, diabetes, allergies, cataracts, mental disorders, immune disorders, arthritis, and aging.

However, free radicals are not necessarily bad. Just as inflammation can provide protection from infection, free radicals play a part in normal cellular metabolism, delivering energy to cells. They can also kill germs and get rid of toxins. Free radicals help regulate numerous chemicals such as hormones. Healthy oxidation as well as antioxidation needs to be supported—it's about balance.

This provides the rationale for oxidative therapies. It appears that as long as the body's antioxidant requirements have been met, adding certain oxidative agents can be therapeutic. Oxidative therapies have been documented to exert the following actions:[1]

- Modulate immune function by balancing inflammatory and anti-inflammatory cytokines; in particular they have been effective in treating autoimmune disorders
- Increase the delivery of oxygen from the blood to the cells, and improve tissue oxygenation
- Inactivate bacteria, viruses, fungi, yeast, and protozoa
- Stimulate endogenous anti-oxidant activity
- Inhibit tumor growth
- Increase red blood cell membrane flexibility, which improves circulation[2]

There are four types of oxidative therapies currently available: hyperbaric oxygen, ozone, hydrogen peroxide, and ultraviolet blood irradiation. As with the different antibiotics, they share similarities and differences.

Hyperbaric Oxygen

Oxygen is a powerful antibiotic. It is particularly effective against anaerobic bacteria, which thrive in low-oxygen environments. The Lyme spirochete is a facultative anaerobe, meaning that it thrives when oxygen tension is low. *Bb* will not survive when the partial pressure of oxygen is high. Sitting in a hyperbaric oxygen chamber with the pressure near 2.5 atmospheres and breathing 100 percent pure oxygen increases tissue oxygen to 200–300 mm mercury.[3] This level is theoretically lethal to the spirochetes. Hyperbaric oxygen therapy (HBOT) may also enhance antibacterial action by generating free radicals that are directly capable of killing the microbes, as well as by enhancing the effect of other antibiotics. An added benefit is that HBOT has been shown to suppress inflammation and autoimmunity.[4]

There is only one report in the medical literature on HBOT in a series of patients with Lyme disease. Dr. William Fife treated ninety-one patients, all of whom met the CDC criteria for Lyme. Nine of these could not complete their treatments for a variety of reasons, leaving 82 in the study. Differing HBOT protocols were tried, ranging from ten to thirty treatments, although one patient received 145 treatments over the course of nine months.

Overall, 85 percent showed significant improvement, and only 13 percent claimed no benefit at all. Virtually all patients described Herxheimer reactions, which sometimes persisted throughout the series of "dives" (the name given to each session, due to HBOT's use in treating diving-related illness), and sometimes continued for up to a month after cessation of treatments. Most of the subjects did not experience any significant improvement until after completing the therapy.[5]

Unfortunately this study did not have a control group for comparison, and there was no long-term follow-up. Despite these limitations, HBOT has been recommended as an adjunct to antibiotics in the treatment of Lyme disease complex. There are some risks, as with any medical procedure, but they are minimal. The primary danger is to the ears; the pressure is likened to descending in an airplane. This generally causes only minor discomfort, but those who cannot pop their ears and equalize the pressure during-treatment can experience severe pain and even permanent damage.

I interviewed patients at the Chico Hyperbaric Clinic in Chico, California, in 2002.* Most patients felt better after a month of intensive HBOT administered twice daily for five days per week. As with other treatments, those who were sickest the longest were the least likely to respond, and those that were also on aggressive antibiotic regimens did the best; however, the relapse rate was high.

---

*   The Chico Hyperbaric Clinic formerly run by Mitch Hoggard is now part of Enloe Medical and no longer treats patients with Lyme disease.

HBOT is not a panacea for people stricken with Lyme. The time commitment, cost, and availability will prevent most people from getting HBOT, and my experience is that other oxidative interventions are more effective.

Ozone

Ever notice the fresh air smell during a lightning storm or after it rains? That's ozone, generally found high in the stratosphere acting as an ultraviolet shield; in fact, storms bring ozone down to earth. Whereas the normal oxygen molecule is very stable, with two atoms of oxygen (designated O_2), ozone is made up of three oxygen atoms (O_3), and is not stable. It is, in fact, a powerful oxidizer. It can kill viruses, bacteria, fungi, and parasites, and it can detoxify pesticides, detergents, chemical manufacturing wastes, and other harmful chemicals. Since a low concentration of ozone is not harmful to people or pets but is damaging to microbes, ozone generators have been used by municipalities, private companies, and individuals to purify air and treat odors.[6]

When given to an individual, ozone increases the amount of oxygen in the blood and enhances the delivery of oxygen to the tissues, making it a useful medical tool. It accelerates wound healing, modulates the immune system, and induces enzyme production. It also kills bacteria, viruses, fungi, and parasites, and helps eliminate toxic chemicals.[7,8]

There are a number of different methods for getting ozone into the place where it will do the most good. It can be injected directly into joints, which can bring rapid relief in acute arthritis. It can be injected into the gums to treat a dental infection. It can also be injected directly into a vein, although this procedure is potentially dangerous and must be done carefully. The most common methods of ozone administration for systemic problems are via rectal insufflation, in intravenous fluids, and using a specialized steam cabinet.

In rectal insufflation, a mixture of oxygen and ozone is given like an enema over a few minutes, then retained for ten to twenty minutes. There are several advantages to this method. The intestinal surface is filled with fingerlike projections called villi, which create a large surface area. This facilitates absorption of the ozone into the bloodstream. The intestines also contain a huge network of lymphatic and immune cells that respond to ozone stimulation. Additional benefits are that bacteria in the intestines are brought into balance by exposure to the ozone, and the portal blood flow from the intestines carries ozone rapidly to the liver, where it can assist in detoxification. Rectal ozone has been particularly helpful in colitis, and it has been widely used for systemic illnesses such as cancer, AIDS, and other infections including Lyme disease.[9]

Major autohemotherapy (MAH), a form of IV ozone therapy, has also been used for these conditions. During MAH, blood is first withdrawn using a technique similar to that used to collect blood donations. Once 100 to 250 mls of blood has been withdrawn, an equal amount of ozone gas is injected into the drainage bottle. The gas bubbles through the blood and dissolves. The bottle is then hung upside down, and the ozonated blood is reinfused. The entire process usually takes about half an hour.

Steam cabinets are a popular method of administering ozone since their use is less invasive than the other options. The patient sits in a specially designed steam cabinet that has an inflow of steam mixed with ozone and oxygen from separate tanks. There is a seal around the person's neck so the ozonated steam will not be inhaled. Instead the ozone is absorbed through the skin, and makes its way through the blood to tissues throughout the body. There are fringe benefits: the steam heat aids in detoxification and increases the antimicrobial effectiveness of any antibiotics being taken at the time.

Despite extensive experience utilizing ozone in Europe, Russia, and Cuba,[10] there are no studies, controlled or otherwise, that document ozone's efficacy against Lyme. As with many of the interventions discussed in this chapter, there are only anecdotal reports by doctors and testimonials by patients. To add my own anecdote, I have found ozone to be an effective adjunct when treating patients with Lyme disease complex. In my experience the most impactful administration of ozone is when MAH is combined with ultraviolet blood irradiation, described below.

Ultraviolet Blood Irradiation

The industrial world has been sterilizing with ultraviolet light for decades. Most bacteria are susceptible to the killing effect of this ionizing radiation. Niels Ryberg Finsen began treating various skin conditions with UV light in the late 1800s, with his success winning him the 1903 Nobel Prize for medicine. Thirty years later, Emmett Knott first applied this technology to blood irradiation, removing about 250 mls of blood, passing it through a radiation chamber, and then transfusing it back into the patient. His first patient was a woman who had become septic following an abortion. This was in 1933, before the widespread introduction of antibiotics, and the mortality rate for septic abortions at that time was virtually 100 percent. Knott's patient promptly recovered and went on to have more children.[11]

By the 1940s many American hospitals were successfully using UV blood irradiation (UVBI) for a variety of infectious conditions including sinusitis, abscesses, pneumonia, wound infections, and peritonitis.[12] As with the other oxidative modalities, the use of UVBI became overshadowed by the dominance of antibiotics in Western medicine. Currently the FDA has only approved the use of UVBI in the treatment of cutaneous T-cell lymphoma, a rare form of cancer.

Like the other oxidative therapies, UVBI appears to do a lot more than kill bugs. It also boosts oxygen delivery to the cells, improves circulation, modulates immune function, and augments energy production.[13] In my experience, the patients who have had the most success clearing their Lyme symptoms with oxidative therapies have had ozone and UVBI treatments simultaneously. Blood passes through the UV light chamber as it is being withdrawn into a bottle, where it is mixed with ozone, then reinfused back through the UV chamber and into the patient. There has been no documented downside to this treatment other than Herxheimer reactions; it is limited, however, by access to good veins and to doctors who are willing to implement a treatment that is frowned upon in conventional medical circles.

Hydrogen Peroxide

Most people are aware that peroxide can be used as a disinfectant and as a bleach. What they may not know is that these applications are directly attributable to its potent oxidizing abilities. Even less known is that the immune system produces its own hydrogen peroxide as a first line of defense against microbes, and that our bodies manufacture hydrogen peroxide to metabolize proteins, carbohydrates, and fat. Peroxides also regulate hormone production and blood sugar levels, increase oxygen delivery to the tissues, and enhance the enzymes necessary to burn oxygen in the production of energy.

On the other hand, too much of a good thing can be had. Excess peroxide results in excess production of hydroxyl free radicals, which damage cell membranes, mutate genetic materials, and provoke inflammation. Therefore, for hydrogen peroxide therapy to be beneficial, it needs to be administered under carefully supervised conditions.

There have been even fewer studies done on hydrogen peroxide than on ozone. Anecdotal reports from doctors indicate that intravenous infusions of dilute hydrogen peroxide have helped patients with a variety of chronic illnesses, including chronic fatigue syndrome, fibromyalgia, cancer, HIV, hepatitis, and chronic infection with Bb.[14] I have witnessed the benefits of intravenous hydrogen peroxide in acute and chronic viral infections.

Hydrogen peroxide suffers from the same political issues as ozone—mainstream medicine maintains there is no scientific evidence documenting its efficacy.[15] Since the NIH has not approved funding for studies and drug companies would rather keep these inexpensive, unpatentable agents off the market, the scientific evidence will most likely be a long time in coming.

RIFE TECHNOLOGY

In the early 1900s, Royal P. Rife set out to find a cure for cancer, which he thought to be caused by a virus. No one knows what inspired Rife to build an electromagnetic field (EMF) generator, but he spent thousands of hours watching organisms under the microscope while he exposed them to different EMF frequencies. He found specific frequencies that killed the smallpox virus, the tuberculosis mycobacterium, and the typhoid bacillus. Rife did eventually isolate a virus he believed triggered the growth of tumors, and it is reported that he had success in treating some patients with cancer with his EMF generator.

The story of Rife's discoveries and their eventual suppression by the National Cancer Institute and by Dr. Morris Fishbein, then president of the AMA, is detailed in Barry Lynes's book *The Cancer Cure That Worked.*[16] Rife died after his laboratory was burned to the ground and lengthy court battles had broken his spirit. However, he left behind copious notes, leaving others the ability to duplicate his work, given that the technology behind his EMF generator is actually quite simple.

Rife's EMF machine is based on the principle of harmonic resonance. This principle can be demonstrated by banging one tuning fork near a second of the same frequency. The sound vibrations emitted by the first will induce the second tuning fork to sing as well. If the EMF generator emits a frequency that is resonant with the cell wall of a bacterium, then the cell wall will vibrate. If it does this long and hard enough, the cell wall will shatter—much like the soprano hitting high C and breaking a crystal wineglass.

Doug MacLean was the first person to explore the use of Rife technology to treat Lyme disease. He built an EMF generator in the early 1980s, got a microscope, procured a culture of *Bb*, and observed the microbes while exposing them to different frequencies. He then used the EMF generator on himself to treat his own chronic Lyme.

Researchers at the University of Washington have rediscovered the utility of using electromagnetic fields to treat infectious diseases. In 2000, Henry Lai, a research professor of bioengineering, found that the malaria parasite appeared to lose vigor and die when exposed to oscillating magnetic fields.[17] This information is of particular interest to those treating tick-borne infections, since *Babesia* is a protozoa similar to malaria.

More recently, researchers at UT Southwestern Medical Center have shown that high-frequency alternating magnetic fields—the same principle used in induction cooktops—can be used to destroy bacteria that are encased in a slimy "biofilm" growing on metal surfaces such as prosthetic joints.[18]

There is a growing subculture of enthusiasts using Rife technology to treat a number of conditions. Several different machines are available on the Internet, and some people build their own. In one configuration, the user puts a coil on or near a part of his body, as with Doug MacLean's device. Others use a paddle placed on one part of the body, with a foot pad to ground the circuit. Most of the machines, however, generate an EMF field using a light source. The frequency of the EMF field can be changed by dials that regulate the amount of electrical current, similar to a dimmer on an electric light. The treatment is delivered by having the patient simply sit in front of the light.

Rife machines contain frequency designations for different bacterial infections, yeast, toxins, viruses, parasites, and so forth. Patients will often Herx from treatments, so they should be spread out accordingly. While I don't recommend it as a stand-alone treatment, I have witnessed Rife technology benefit patients with Lyme disease complex, and consider it an option for patients who don't tolerate any antimicrobial herbs or pharmaceuticals.

STEM CELL THERAPY

Stem cells are special; they have the capacity to divide indefinitely, and produce cells that can differentiate into any cell type in the body. There are two main types, embryonic and adult stem cells. These progenitor cells can restore the function of tissues lost due to injury or disease. They also have the capacity to modulate inflammatory and immune responses to tissue injury associated with infections. However, the therapeutic potential of their use in the treatment of Lyme disease is questionable and has not yet been demonstrated.

As of 2019, the FDA has only approved stem cell therapy for bone marrow replacement to treat cancers of the blood and of the bone marrow, and a number of clinics offering stem cell treatment for other indications have been shut down by FDA injunctions.[19] Although there are a number of international clinics touting use of stem cell therapy, I consider it premature in the treatment of Lyme disease complex.

SILVER

Silver has been used as an antimicrobial for a long time. King Cyrus of Persia put boiled water for his troops in flagons of silver when going to war in the fifth century BCE.[20] More recently, silver has found a variety of applications in human health care: for burn treatment, bone prostheses, and in cardiac devices. Dilute silver nitrate was used from the 1880s until the 1980s for prevention of neonatal conjunctivitis. The bioactive silver ion interacts with bacterial, fungal, viral, and protozoal cell walls and denatures key enzyme systems, but it has low toxicity in the human body. Silver is also an effective biofilm buster.[21]

There are numerous anecdotal reports on the benefits of colloidal silver in the treatment of Lyme disease. Since the antimicrobial properties of silver are dependent on size and surface area, silver nanoparticles are theoretically the most effective.[22] When taken orally, silver has wide distribution in the body and is excreted via the urine and bile. It can also be administered intravenously in small amounts and intranasally to treat sinusitis and fungal colonization. Several of my patients have improved with intravenous silver.

Silver has a high margin of safety, but there is a potential for toxicity in the skin, where trapped particles induce a blue-gray discoloration called argyria.[23] It should be noted that it takes truly heroic doses of silver over time to develop this unsightly and permanent condition. Nano-sized particles are less likely to cause side effects.

I have definitely seen patients benefit from silver. I do not consider it to be a stand-alone treatment, but it can be an effective adjunct to other antimicrobial therapy.

BEE VENOM THERAPY

Bee venom therapy (BVT) is even older than silver. There are images on rocks drawn by early hunter-gatherers depicting the honeybee as a source of medical treatment. BVT has documented antioxidant and anti-inflammatory effect.[24] It has been recommended for arthritic conditions with some benefit,[25] and for multiple sclerosis, where benefit has not been documented.[26]

Bee venom contains mellitin, which has been shown to have significant antimicrobial activity against *Bb* in cell cultures.[27] However, in vitro activity does not necessarily translate to in vivo effectiveness. My clinical experience is that bee venom does have anti-inflammatory action in some patients, evidenced by a reduction in joint pain. However, I have not seen it impact the infection itself. In addition, people with bee sting allergy could potentially have severe reactions to BVT.

LOW-DOSE IMMUNOTHERAPY

In general, chronic tick-borne infections don't attack hardware, they disrupt software. Instead of invading tissue, the microbes trigger immune hyperreactivity with systemic inflammation. It's the overreactive state that becomes the major driver of illness. What if the body of a patient with Lyme disease complex could be prompted to just ignore these bugs? Theoretically the disease process would be stopped in its tracks.

Low-dose immunotherapy (LDI) is the opposite of a vaccine. Rather than stimulate the immune system to attack pathogens, LDI messages the immune system to ignore them. The predecessor of LDI was LDA, low-dose antigen therapy.[†] I participated in a study conducted from 1993 to 2001, along with over 100 other physicians, that documented the clinical benefits of LDA in the treatment of allergies to inhalants, foods, and chemicals.[28] In many ways LDI is similar to allergy immunotherapy, a way of teaching the immune system not to overreact.

Conventional immunotherapy for allergies employs increasing doses of antigens—the substance to which a person is allergic—with the intent of stimulating blocking antibodies. This may be effective with conventional IgE mediated allergies, but can also cause severe reactions like anaphylaxis. In contrast, LDI utilizes antigen doses that are at least a million times lower, but paired with an enzyme, beta-glucuronidase, that stimulates the production of regulatory T cells (a type of immune cell that acts to suppress immune response). This induces tolerance to the accompanying antigens in the injection.

The question is, what happens if a person's immune system ignores these critters? Won't this lead to unopposed overwhelming infection? The answer is that this does not happen. For one thing, every person's body contains trillions of microbes with which we cohabitate. LDI only mutes the response to specific antigens. Secondly, while LDI can neutralize the response of the adaptive immune system, innate immune defenses remain intact. (See Chapter 18.) There are many people infected with *Bb*, *Babesia*, or *Bartonella* who are not ill; their immune systems keep the pathogens in check, because their software has not been reprogrammed.

Dr. Ty Vincent was the first physician to use immunotherapy to treat people with chronic tick-borne infections as well as other persistent infections. He maintains that people with Lyme disease complex no longer have active microbial infection, but rather have autoimmune hyperreactivity triggered by the microbes. Research demonstrating the benefit of repeated and/or prolonged antibiotic treatment demonstrates that he is mistaken about the former claim, but he is correct about the latter. He has been successfully administering LDI using infinitesimally small doses of dead microbes to message the immune system not to react.

Responses to LDI are dose specific, and it takes careful titration to find the correct dose for each person. Too strong a dose can result in severe Herxheimer reactions. LDI can be administered either by intradermal (under the skin) injection or sublingually, and doses need to be spaced carefully. Some patients don't tolerate even the most dilute doses.

I have found LDI to be a useful adjunct in my practice. However, I don't recommend it instead of antimicrobials and other supportive interventions. Rather, I have found it appropriate in patients who do not tolerate any antimicrobials or who continue to be symptomatic despite appropriate treatment. Note that LDI is

---

†   LDA was initially termed EPD, enzyme-potentiated desensitization.

not commonly offered as a component of treatment even within integrative Lyme practices, as most of the practitioners offering LDI are environmental physicians, not LLMDs.

LOW-DOSE NALTREXONE

Naloxone, the generic name for Narcan, has played a prominent role in the opioid crisis. Narcan attaches to opiate receptors in the brain and blocks opiate binding. It acts within minutes and lasts for about an hour, making it ideal for reversing narcotic overdoses. Naltrexone is a related drug with slower onset but longer-lasting action. Both drugs block the analgesic effects of exogenous opiate drugs as well as the pleasure response of endogenous endorphins.

Low doses of naltrexone (LDN) have effects that appear paradoxical; LDN can decrease both pain and inflammation. It was originally believed that a small and transient opioid blockade prompted the body to compensate by up-regulating both endogenous opioids (endorphins) and opioid receptors.[29] However, subsequent studies indicate that its activity may be unrelated to its effect on endorphins and opiate receptors. LDN's anti-inflammatory effects in the central nervous system appear to be mediated by its suppression of microglial cells, specialized white blood cells in the brain that activate immune defenses. There are reports of LDN decreasing symptoms in people with fibromyalgia, inflammatory bowel disease, and pain syndromes.[30]

Despite research studies and numerous websites expounding its efficacy, my experience of LDN has been underwhelming. An occasional patient may have noticable benefit, but often these are not sustained. Additionally, LDN can cause sleep problems, including nightmares, and for this reason I suggest starting it at doses of 1 mg at bedtime and slowly progressing the dose. The target dose hovers around 4.5 mg, but as with other interventions, ideal doses will vary from person to person. LDN is available at compounding pharmacies by prescription and is inexpensive, so it is worth trying. However, it should not be taken by anyone taking an opiate for pain, as it will block the narcotic's effect and could precipitate a withdrawal syndrome.

HYPERTHERMIA

Fever therapy goes back a long way. Ruy Díaz de Isla reported that fever had a beneficial effect on people with late-stage syphilis in the fifteenth century. Three hundred fifty years later, Juluis Wagner-Jauregg performed detailed experiments in which he induced fevers in syphilitic patients by injecting them with malaria. Some of his patients did well, and in 1927 he was awarded the Nobel Prize in medicine.[31]

Fever therapy is based on the concept that some microbes are killed at high temperatures. Allegedly, Lyme spirochetes will all perish at 106.9°F (41.6°C). Injecting malaria into patients has deservedly gone out of favor, so hyperthermia is now induced using infrared-A-irradiation in a specialized thermal chamber designed to safely increase body temperature, with the goal of reaching 107°F (42°C).[32]

Hyperthermia is currently employed at some medical centers as an adjunct to cancer treatment. It is also offered to patients with Lyme disease in Germany and Mexico, where it is administered along with aggressive antibiotics and detoxification therapies. Anecdotal reports suggest that some patients who have undergone hyperthermia have improved but have not been cured, and that some patients did not tolerate the treatment.[33,34] It is unclear what the impact of hyperthermia is on the various co-infections. Needless to say, it is a risky procedure, with potential complications such as febrile seizures.[35]

I do not recommend hyperthermia for the treatment of Lyme disease complex at this time. That said, there is evidence that raising core body temperature enhances the antimicrobial effects of antibiotics[36] and stimulates the action of T helper immune cells.[37] Sauna therapy, as detailed in Chapter 19, appears a safer means of raising core temperature without the risks posed by hyperthermia.

PEPTIDE THERAPY

Peptides are small proteins made up of a chain of amino acids. Peptides attach to specific receptors on the surface of cell walls and provide a signal that alters cellular function. Our bodies naturally produce over 7,000 peptides with a wide range of functions, including but not limited to hormone production, immune balance, reduction of inflammation, cognition, aging, and DNA repair.

There is a long list of peptides employed in peptide therapy, and some have been used in patients with Lyme disease complex with significant benefits. Thymosin alpha-1 is commonly prescribed for patients with chronic infection and inflammation because it helps restore normal Th1 and Th2 balance while also supporting immune capacity to fight infection. Another commonly prescribed peptide for patients with Lyme disease complex is BPC-157. In its oral form it has been effective at healing inflammation in the gastrointestinal tract. When given subcutaneously, it has been helpful at alleviating muscle and tendon pain.

Most of the peptides now being recommended for patients with Lyme disease complex have not been researched in long-term clinical studies, but their anecdotal success has led to their being employed by many LLMDs. While peptides continue to enter clinical development at a rapid pace, many are not yet FDA approved.[38] The International Peptide Society holds conferences and courses to learn more about using peptides in clinical practice.

FREQUENCY THERAPIES

There are a host of treatments that work on energetic levels. As with the other interventions in this chapter, no controlled studies on these treatments have been performed. On the other hand, there is growing use of these modalities, since patients who do not respond to conventional treatments often seek answers outside of mainstream medicine. Some of these therapies, like acupuncture and homeopathy, have been in use for centuries. Others are fairly new but gaining increasing application in the treatment of chronic infections.

Frequency specific microcurrent (FSM) is a physical therapy that applies low level electric currents to injured or inflamed tissues. It has been successful at relieving muscle and nerve pain as well as migraine headaches. There are no side effects associated with FSM although some patients notice short-term fatigue, drowsiness, or nausea after treatments.

The Ondamed is an electromagnetic device that delivers specific frequencies based on feedback from the patient's pulse. The manufacturer claims that it facilitates self-regulation in dysfunctional tissue with a host of physiologic benefits.[39] The benefits of this therapy are highly variable and appear to be practitioner-dependent, but I have personally seen patients who have done well using it as adjunctive treatment.

BRAIN RETRAINING

Brain neurofeedback utilizes EEGs to enable people to alter their brain waves. It is being used successfully to treat a number of neuropsychological conditions such as depression, anxiety, obsessive compulsive disorder, and attention deficit disorder.[40,41] Biofeedback has been used successfully to regulate the autonomic nervous system in patients with dysautonomic syndromes such as POTS.[42]

Both the Gupta Protocol and Annie Hopper's Dynamic Neural Retraining System are designed to quiet the limbic system of the brain. The limbic system is that part of the brain involved in behavioral and emotional responses and is designed for short-term survival. Any type of threat—not just physical and emotional trauma—but also chemicals, mold, infections, and systemic inflammation can trigger a limbic response that impacts the autonomic nervous system (including the fight-or-flight response), hormones, and immune regulation. Gupta's and Hopper's techniques have successfully helped bring patients into balance, including improving chronic fatigue and decreasing environmental sensitivities.

IN SUMMARY

The cumulative impact of epigenetic trauma appears to have compromised the antimicrobial resiliency of large swaths of the population. At the same time, reliance on antibiotics has increasingly been undermined by the resourcefulness of ever-evolving microbes. Given this, the best hope for recovery may lie in discoveries outside the realm of mainstream pharmaceuticals—those that seek to restore the body to balance.

MyLymeData, a project of Lymedisease.org, has collected data from more than 12,000 Lyme patients in the United States since its inception in 2015. Their 2019 report included the following outcomes for those patients who listed use of alternative treatment modalities:

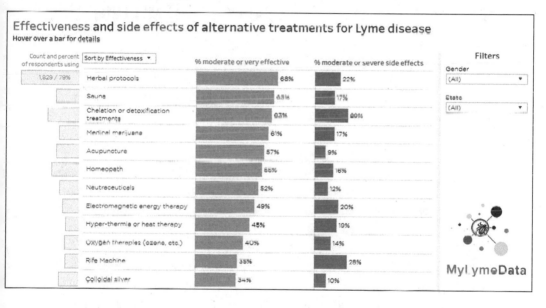

At present it appears that combining pharmaceutical treatment with appropriate alternative interventions has been most successful. This is consistent with my clinical experience. The entire report is free to the public, and can be downloaded at: lymedisease.org/mylymedata-alternative-lyme-disease-treatment.

Chapter 24

Frequently Asked Questions

CAN LYME DISEASE BE SEXUALLY TRANSMITTED?

The spirochete *Borrelia burgdorferi* is a cousin of *Treponema pallidum*, the bacteria that causes syphilis. This raises the question of whether Lyme disease can be sexually transmitted. Studies in animals have yielded conflicting results. Two separate reports demonstrated transmission of *Bb* from infected mice to uninfected mice, presumably through intercourse.[1,2] However, another study of rodents failed to show sexual transmission.[3]

In 2003, Harvey and Salvato speculated that Lyme disease could be sexually transmitted by virtue of epidemiological evidence of *Bb* infection occurence in the absence of infected ticks in Houston, Texas.[4] The most frequently discussed report on this subject was published in 2014 by Marianne Middelveen and colleagues, who demonstrated the presence of culture-proven *Bb* in the semen and vaginal secretions of human subjects diagnosed with Lyme disease.[5]

However, it is important to realize that the presence of *Bb* in semen and vaginal secretions does not prove that this microbe can be transmitted by sexual intercourse. And while Harvey and Salvato considered Houston an area where Lyme was not endemic, it turns out that this was a false assumption.[6] Some physicians believe that partners of people with Lyme disease should be treated simultaneously to avoid reinfections—a Ping-Pong back-and-forth scenario. But the bottom line is that we still do not have a definitive answer to this important question. In my medical practice, where I have seen thousands of patients with Lyme disease, I cannot say I have seen a clear-cut case of sexually transmitted infection, but it is difficult to make this assessment, since partners typically have similar environmental exposures.

CAN LYME DISEASE BE TRANSMITTED IN UTERO?

In 2001, Dr. Tessa Gardner authored a chapter in the fifth edition of *Infectious Diseases of the Fetus and Newborn Infant*, a textbook that is periodically updated.[7]

Gardner provided a magnificent, in-depth review of Lyme disease covering 124 pages. She described multiple reports documenting the evidence that maternal infection with *Bb* can be transferred to the unborn fetus, and that, among pregnant women with Lyme disease, there is a higher incidence of miscarriage, stillbirths, and neonatal deaths as well as children with congenital Lyme disease. Gardner described how some of these children showed evidence of infection early on, while others manifested symptoms much later. She also emphasized that infected newborns are often seronegative; i.e. antibody testing is not a reliable indicator of infection. Gardner's chapter was withdrawn from subsequent editions of the text, presumably because the topic of Lyme had become a controversial issue.

Babesia, *Bartonella*, and *Anaplasma* can also be transmitted in utero.[8,9,10] There is a case report of *Ehrlichia* transmitted via a blood transfusion,[11] which raises the possibility that this microbe can also be transferred from pregnant mother to fetus. Animal studies suggest that *Mycoplasma* species may also lead to neonatal infection.[12]

There is strong evidence that antibiotic treatment of pregnant women with Lyme disease decreases the incidence of maternal-fetal transmission and the associated negative outcomes. In a group of sixty-six mothers with Lyme disease who were treated with antibiotics prior to conception and during the entire pregnancy, all gave birth to normal, healthy infants. In contrast, there were eight pregnancies that resulted in *Bb*- or *Bartonella* positive placentas, umbilical cords, and/or foreskin remnants in the control group of untreated women.[13,14]

It has now become routine among LLMDs to treat pregnant women throughout gestation with antibiotics such as amoxicillin, cefdinir, and azithromycin. Atovaquone for babesiosis can also be prescribed during pregnancy. That said, caution is advised whenever prescribing medications for pregnant women. Most herbs have not been studied for their suitability in pregnancy, and are not recommended. It is important to also consider the fact that while congenital Lyme is real, we do not know its frequency; there are many actively infected women who give birth to healthy children with no subsequent evidence of infection. If a pregnant mother has tested positive for Lyme, it is recommended to test the cord blood at the time of delivery to determine if there is evidence of transmission to the newborn infant.

WHAT HAPPENED TO THE LYME VACCINE?

In 1998, SmithKline Beecham (SKB), now GlaxoSmithKline (GSK), released a vaccine for Lyme disease called LYMErix, but they withdrew it from the marketplace in 2002. LYMErix had an unusual method of action—it stimulated production of antibodies designed to attack *Bb* in the midgut of the tick, allegedly before the bacteria had a chance to enter the person's body. SKB claimed that the vaccine afforded 78 percent protection after three doses.

There were many problems with LYMErix. The vaccine was designed to stimulate antibodies to a single outer-surface protein of *Bb*, OspA. This particular protein had been identified as the one triggering arthritis. The vaccine was therefore developed to prevent Lyme arthritis, but not prevent the many other problems associated with Lyme disease such as fatigue and neurological issues.

It turns out that OspA stimulates antibodies in both joints and nerves in susceptible people and in animals.[15] The LYMErix vaccine therefore resulted in serious neurological syndromes in some people,[16] and some claims of chronic arthritis.[17] These were the basis for a successful class-action lawsuit against SKB in 2001, where the manufacturer was mandated to pay for a lifetime of IVIg (intravenous gamma globulin) treatment for victims.

The drug manufacturer subsequently claimed that LYMErix was withdrawn from the market because of poor sales. However, in reality the vaccine was not that effective to begin with, and SKB's costs went up considerably due to the lawsuit and judgment. In addition, by discontinuing LYMErix, SKB avoided having to release post-marketing data that likely would have shown higher rates of vaccine-related side effects than originally reported.[18,19]

Since LYMErix was designed to kill *Bb* in the midgut of ticks, it was premised on the (mistaken) assumption that prolonged tick attachment is needed for disease transmission. Thus it entirely missed preventing any infection transmitted by tick saliva in the very act of attachment.[20] An additional problem is that the vaccine afforded no protection for co-infections, which, in general, are harder to diagnose and treat than Lyme.

This hasn't stopped vaccine advocates from continuing to ply their lucrative trade. Stanley Plotkin, a pediatrician at the University of Pennsylvania, has been particularly public in his advocacy for return of the LYMErix vaccine. On September 18, 2013, he authored an op-ed in the *New York Times* entitled "Bring Back the Lyme Vaccine." And in August 2018, Plotkin referred to the withdrawal of LYMErix from the market as a "public health fiasco." It turns out that Plotkin is a paid consultant to vaccine manufacturers; it is patently misleading that this association was not disclosed when he was stating his opinion.

It is important to realize that while vaccines are considered "smart bombs" that work by stimulating antibodies to just one microbe such as influenza or pertussis, in reality vaccines contain adjuvants that can stimulate widespread immune activation. In other words, vaccines can precipitate a cytokine cascade and systemic inflammation. This may result in a relapse or exacerbation of symptoms in patients with Lyme disease complex.[21] I have witnessed several patients relapse after routine vaccinations.

Jane was seventy-seven years old and living in Denver when she became aware of an insect bite that developed into a two-inch round red rash with two rings; it itched a lot. Within a month she became aware of pain in her knees, hips, and thighs as well as the onset of muscle cramps.

Jane had a Western blot performed at LabCorp and it was negative for Lyme disease, with only the 41 band positive in the IgG assay. She was prescribed doxycycline 100 mg twice daily. She did not have a Herxheimer reaction, but her symptoms continued to progress, with diffuse joint pains, fatigue, and weakness. She had difficulty getting in and out of both bed and her car, and her balance was unsteady. Her itching became widespread.

On physical exam Jane appeared depressed. She had profound weakness with a slow gait, but the remainder of her examination was normal. I was suspicious of persistent infection with Bb despite the negative LabCorp Western blot, and her itching made me concerned about Bartonella. I explained to Jane that she could need aggressive antibiotics, and she demurred. She said, "I am old and have had a good life. Perhaps I should just let these infections kill me." My response was, "These infections probably won't kill you, but you'll feel like you want to die."

Before additional lab results were available, I asked Jane to start A-Bart, which provoked her joint pains and muscle cramps. But when the Herxheimer reaction subsided she was able to increase the dose to twenty drops twice daily, and she felt better. She had much the same response to A-L complex.

Jane's lab results demonstrated a positive Bartonella IgM at 1:160, a negative Bartonella IgG, and a positive Bartonella FISH, providing confirmation of a Bartonella infection. A Lyme Western blot performed at IGeneX showed the same negative result as the LabCorp sample. However, the EM rash and her response to A-L complex confirmed Lyme disease, despite the negative Lyme Western blot. (Recall that if antibiotics are started early, they can prevent an antibody response.)

When I saw Jane in follow-up she was in complete remission. Not only were her pains gone, but her energy and strength were restored. Jane did not want to add antibiotics, so I added Nutramedix's Samento and Banderol herbal extracts one at a time, and for the next year she remained asymptomatic.

Then Jane suddenly relapsed. All her symptoms returned; in fact they were much worse than the first time I saw her. After taking a detailed recent history, it turned out that her relapse began one day following her receiving two vaccinations: Shingles (herpes zoster) and influenza.

DOES TREATMENT OF LYME DISEASE WITH ANTIBIOTICS LEAD TO ANTIBIOTIC RESISTANCE?

There have been many studies on antibiotic susceptibility in different strains of *Bb*. The results are quite consistent: different strains of *Bb* have the same pattern of susceptibility and resistance to many antibiotics.[22,23] The same studies suggest that emergence of antibiotic resistance is unlikely. This is consistent with my clinical experience—once a patient has a good response to an antibiotic, it is rare that the antibiotic stops working. When a patient hits a downturn, it is likely due to another factor such as a mold encounter, diet indiscretions, a co-infection flare, or emotional distress.

WHAT SHOULD I DO IF I GET A TICK BITE?

The first step is proper removal of the tick. Any mishandling of the tick such as squeezing it, putting Vaseline over it, or holding a hot match to it will increase the chance of disease transmission. The tick should be removed with fine-point tweezers by grasping the tick where it meets the skin, then gently pulling until it releases. Ticks can also be removed using "tick keys" that scoop the tick off the skin. There are many websites that describe appropriate tick removal.

While it is true that the longer the tick is attached, the higher the risk of transmission, it is possible to get Lyme disease even if the tick is attached for less than twenty-four hours. A study at the Pasteur Institute documented that *Bb* can be transmitted within twelve hours in a mouse model.[24] The salivary juices of the tick, which contain anticoagulants, anesthetics, and immune suppressors, also contain microbes that can be injected at the time of attachment. It is well documented that other tick-borne infections including *Rickettsiae*, *A. phagocytophilum*, *B. miyamotoi*, *B. hermsii*, and Powassan virus can be transmitted in less than twenty-four hours, some even within minutes of attachment.[25]

It is essential to identify the tick—only the blacklegged tick reliably transmits *Bb*, although other ticks can transmit other infections. There are pictures online that can be used to identify ticks. It is a good idea to save the tick in case you want to get it tested for *Bb* or other pathogens; however, my experience is that tick testing is not reliable.

CAN LYME BE TREATED WITH A SINGLE DOSE OF DOXYCYCLINE?

In July 2001, Dr. Robert Nadelman and colleagues published an article in the *New England Journal of Medicine* suggesting that 200 mg of doxycycline given within seventy-two hours of a tick attachment provides effective prophylaxis for Lyme disease. Proof of efficacy was lack of an EM rash within four weeks of the bite. That was the endpoint of their study; there was no long-term follow up.[26]

Clearly, this study contains serious flaws. An EM rash does not occur universally in people who get Lyme disease. Some studies state it occurs in up to 70 percent of infected people, but others suggest that the incidence is much lower. Using the absence of a rash as proof that there is no infection is poor reasoning. Furthermore, the lack of long-term follow-up makes it impossible to determine whether participants went on to develop chronic symptoms of Lyme disease. Anecdotally, my medical practice is replete with patients who developed Lyme disease complex without ever having witnessed either a tick bite or an EM rash. Finally, a high proportion of ticks carry multiple microbes, some of which are not responsive to doxycycline. Even those microbes that are responsive to doxycycline will not be eradicated with a single dose of this antibiotic.

SHOULD ALL TICK BITES BE TREATED WITH PROPHYLACTIC ANTIBIOTICS?

There is no black-and-white answer as to whether or not to treat prophylactically if bitten by a blacklegged tick. Prophylactic treatment makes sense for those who live in an area highly endemic for Lyme disease, because a high percentage of ticks are infected. Treatment is the same as for a well-documented case of acute Lyme disease: antibiotics for at least four weeks. Be aware that early treatment will prevent the body from mounting an antibody response, and therefore subsequent testing for Lyme will be negative.

Antibiotic choice is also not black-and-white. Doxycycline has the advantage of treating tick-borne pathogens other than *Bb*, including *Ehrlichia*, *Anaplasma*, *Coxiella*, and *Rickettsiae*. The downside to doxycycline is that it causes significant sun sensitization, can be hard on the stomach, and the usual dosing of 100 mg twice daily may not reach therapeutic levels. Amoxicillin and cefuroxime are also commonly used for prophylaxis after a tick bite. While these antibiotics do not cover as wide a spectrum of infections as doxycycline, they are often better tolerated.

It is imperative to maintain vigilance for symptoms suggestive of active infection with *Bb* or a co-infection whether or not prophylactic treatment was initiated. For those who decide to delay treatment, Lyme testing should be performed two weeks after attachment. I also recommend that all patients be tested for co-infections at least two weeks after attachment even if prophylactic antibiotics are initiated.

DOES STEVIA TREAT LYME?

In 2015, investigators reported that the popular sugar substitute stevia exhibited antibiotic activity against *Bb*. Their study tested antimicrobial action in vitro; that is, stevia's capacity to kill *Borrelia* spirochetes in cell cultures in the laboratory.[27] In vitro studies do not necessarily translate to efficacy in treating Lyme disease—there is a wide discrepancy between in vitro susceptibility and in vivo effectiveness.[28] At this time there is no data or clinical experience to suggest that stevia should be used to treat Lyme disease.

SHOULD PATIENTS WITH LYME DISEASE EXERCISE?

Dr. Joseph Burrascano posted "Advanced Topics in Lyme Disease" guidelines online in 2008. In addition to many treatment and dietary recommendations, he described the need for adequate rest, and he also outlined an exercise protocol to facilitate healing. Exercise is not only important in enhancing muscle tone and cardiovascular fitness, it is also essential for competent immune function.[29] This excellent summary can be accessed at lymenet.org/BurrGuide200810.pdf.

SHOULD PATIENTS WITH LYME DISEASE BREASTFEED?

In the aforementioned publication, Dr. Burrascano also mentions that spirochetes have been cultured from breast milk. However, in personal communication on this topic, he clarified that the culture he referenced was performed on breast milk of untreated women infected with Lyme. Given that breastfeeding provides passive and likely long-lasting active immunity, and that human milk protects against infections in the breastfed infant via secretory IgA antibodies as well as several other factors like bactericidal lactoferrin, breastfeeding by women with Lyme is recommended.

Section Five

LAST THOUGHTS

As I write this section, I am sitting in a hospital room with my wife. She had the sudden onset of severe chest pain and neurological symptoms and was admitted through the emergency room.

The tests showed evidence of cardiac stress but, gratefully, no heart damage. However, she also has multiple neurological deficits, the worst being that her left leg is paralyzed. When I asked the cardiologist what could account for simultaneous cardiac stress and severe neurological deficits, he said he didn't deal with the nervous system. When I asked the neurologist about the connection, he had a similar response: he wasn't interested in heart problems.

I should not be surprised. But the lack of intellectual curiosity concerning what would cause the simultaneous occurrence of cardiac and neurological symptoms was, to put it mildly, stunning. They never asked, "What is the underlying pathophysiology that would explain what has happened here?"

It is a perfect metaphor for, and sad commentary on, the direction of Western medicine today: a reductionist approach that compartmentalizes the body into parts and fails to appreciate that everything is connected. The evaluation of patients is divvied up to specialists and sub-specialists, each with their own areas of competence, but none with the whole picture. In theory, primary care practitioners (PCPs) assemble the specialists' reports and put it all together. In practice, PCPs see twenty to forty patients a day; they have neither the time nor the expertise to connect the dots. It's like the blind men and the elephant—none of these physicians sees the whole patient.

Our work as physicians and healers is to see the whole patient. Instead of focusing on one organ system, I want to know everything. The diagnostic challenge is to discern patterns of insults, symptoms, and lab tests that correlate with specific microbes, specific organ dysfunction, specific diet issues, and environmental exposures. We keep asking questions until we detect patterns in the chronically ill patient that correlate with any number of overlapping issues such as infections, hormone deficiencies, immune dysregulation, toxic exposures, and diminished capacity to detoxify. And then we explore the interrelationship of all these problems. Differentiation then integration.

I think of these overlapping patterns on the physiological level as horizontal issues. But there are also vertical issues: emotional health, support networks, resource capacity, belief systems, and spiritual well-being. As I described in Chapter 1, the concept of mind-body connection is a misnomer; the mind and body are one universe, and our perception of self in the world is a template on which we manifest all levels of being.

We who are blessed with the opportunity to help others are obliged to be objective and discerning, but also to hold a space of safety, acceptance, compassion, and respect. As I watch the nurses' interactions with my wife in this hospital, I appreciate their competence, but I am awed at their depth of caretaking, their kindness, and their humanity. My prayer is that we physicians can dissolve our headstrong egos and be fully present with our patients.

Chapter 25

The Challenge

My colleagues and I agree: diseases are getting more complicated, people are getting sicker, and they are more difficult to treat. Thirty years ago, when I was practicing environmental medicine, I primarily saw kids who presented with food sensitivities, and 95 percent were sensitive to one or more of perhaps a half dozen foods. It was rare to see a senior citizen with food issues. Now people of all generations are reacting to anything and everything, including low doses of perfumes, exhaust fumes, and cleaning agents. Mold has preceded us on this planet, and our exposure to it has been with us as long as the human race has existed—but mold is now generating more and more illnesses. Growing numbers of people are having difficulties with autoimmune problems and detoxification. In the past, Lyme disease was much easier to treat. Now it causes increasing debilitation.

As is clear from the length of this book, the complexity of illness is expanding. The medicine bag of practitioners has grown substantially over the past decades, as has their ability to intercede in arenas that were previously poorly understood, such as methylation and mycotoxins. Yet about 10 percent of patients continue to elude treatment.

There are multiple factors that precipitated the Lyme disease epidemic, tipping it from a simple infection into a major health conundrum. The final issue is that *we* have changed. Our resilience, our ability to bounce back, our resistance to infection, and our capacity to tolerate exposures to toxins have all declined. Mutations in the DNA of genetic inheritance have always been present, but now it seems that many people's metabolic pathways are increasingly overwhelmed.

As I have stated repeatedly in this book, the problem is in our software, not our hardware. Human regulatory systems are designed to maintain homeostasis, but increasing numbers of people are experiencing chaos—with immune systems that are hypervigilant and flailing at real and unreal threats; nervous systems that are unstable and unreliable; endocrine systems that fail to maintain adequate hormone production; and gastrointestinal systems that fail to digest foods or to maintain healthy boundaries with food-borne toxins and pathogens.

The increasing number of people experiencing internal chaos are the result of the cumulative stresses bequeathed from previous generations. Sadly, a newborn no longer begins life with a clean slate. The epigenetic transmission of insults that are passed down and accumulate with each generation have resulted in an ever lower capacity to deal with life in the twenty-first century. The multiple affronts that have led to these epigenetic changes, particularly since the technological revolution, include changes in diet, soil depletion of nutrients, exposure to hundreds of thousands of xenobiotic agents, increasing levels of EMF exposure, as well as the disintegration of supportive communities.

The past century has witnessed the devolution of living in tight-knit communities with extended families to nuclear families and then to single families, and, more and more, single individual households, and even some without a home at all. The dissolution of community support impacts not only our mental well-being, but also our physical health. Chapter 1 described the ACE study, in which adults with a history of childhood trauma had a substantially higher risk of lung disease, heart disease, and immune disorders.[1] Cumulative childhood stress is associated with inflammation and autoimmunity.[2,3] And this psychological trauma, which impacts physiology, is also passed on epigenetically.[4]

A review paper by Rachel Yehuda and Amy Lehrner on intergenerational transmission of trauma and the role of epigenetic mechanisms states, "There is now converging evidence supporting the idea that offspring are affected by parental trauma exposures occurring before their birth, and possibly even prior to their conception. On the simplest level, the concept of intergenerational trauma acknowledges that exposure to extremely adverse events impacts individuals to such a great extent that their offspring find themselves grappling with their parents' post-traumatic state."[5]

PTSD is not only a psychological disorder, it is also biological. Alexander McFarlane, a professor at the University of Adelaide in Australia who studies PTSD, clarifies that, "The development of traumatic memories at the time of stress exposure represents a major vulnerability through repeated environmental triggering of the increasing dysregulation of an individual's neurobiology."[6] Our understanding is coming full circle: the mind-body is one organism, the psychological and biological are intertwined.

These accumulated physical and emotional multigenerational traumas are manifesting in a tsunami that is destabilizing individuals' core regulatory systems. Increasingly, people respond as if they have continuous PTSD—their nervous and immune systems going haywire at both real and imagined threats, with all the downstream consequences evident in an increasingly sick population.

The growing prevalence of anxiety and depression in the US population is particularly evident among teens and young adults, but all age groups are affected. There was a 64 percent increase in the number of Americans of all ages taking antidepressants between 1999 and 2014;[7] 9 percent of children and adolescents in the United States were taking psychotropic medications in 2014;[8] a study three years later found that 19 percent of adults over sixty were taking antidepressants.[9] The life span of Americans is now decreasing, in part due to the rising incidence of addiction and suicide in middle-aged white men.[10] This epidemic of mental illness is not distinct from the epidemic of Lyme disease—in fact, they overlap in many people. The same destabilizing, multigenerational factors are at the heart of both of these afflictions.*

Dr. Nancy Brown and I performed a pilot study in 2018, which has yet to be published. We tested ten adolescents in a Colorado residential treatment center who were suffering from anxiety and depression severe enough that they could no longer live at home or go to school.** The teens did not have any known organic disorders. Laboratory testing revealed evidence of tick-borne infections in six, and was highly suspicious in another three. There were elevated levels of anti-neuronal antibodies in nine of ten subjects, consistent with pediatric acute-onset neuropsychiatric syndrome (see Chapter 15 for a discussion of PANS.) The presence of anti-neuronal antibodies is consistent with autoimmune inflammation of the brain, causing severe mental health disorders. These numbers astounded us, and we are now planning a larger study with a control population. Nevertheless, these preliminary data suggest that a significant factor in the alarming increase in mental health disorders in adolescents may be due to organic issues, and autoimmune inflammation in particular.

Where do we go from here? That's a great question, and I don't pretend to have all the answers. But I do have a few ideas.

The first step is to acknowledge the genesis of what is happening. If we are suffering from a cumulative, collective PTSD, we need to find safety—and by this I mean safety on all levels. I'm talking about a New Deal for Health and Well-being that confronts the "progress" of the technological revolution with its unintended consequences. We clearly need to improve the macro-environment—the air we breathe, the water we drink, the food we eat, and the ubiquity of toxic chemicals. We obviously need to reverse the forces that are leading our planet to become increasingly uninhabitable. We need to become more knowledgeable about unseen forces like EMFs. We need to challenge our addiction to cell phones and social

---

*   These data all preceded the coronavirus pandemic, which is destined to leave its own PTSD/ epigenetic mark on this and subsequent generations.

**   IRB Tracking Number: 20180603.

media. We need to discard the myth of the rugged individual and embrace the notion of mutual interdependence. We need to slow down. We need to connect with one another and experience belonging. We actually feel safer and happier when we open up and become vulnerable, and when we are willing to suspend some of our individual needs to serve the wider community.

Addressing our micro-environments, we need to find better ways to signal or train our internal regulatory systems to feel safe, to decrease hypervigilance and hyperreactivity—to calm our immune and nervous systems. This could be in the form of yet-to-be discovered medications, but just as likely it will take the form of energetic or biofeedback techniques.

Let's hope we find more answers soon.

Appendix A

Lyme Disease Complex: Anatomy of an Illness*

Antecedents

Genetic / epigenetic / congenital factors
   Predisposition to allergy,
      autoimmunity, celiac
   Methylation/detoxification mutations
   Ehler Danlos Syndrome
   Hypogammaglobulinemia
Intrauterine trauma
Ancestral trauma

Developmental Factors

Diet / nutritional status
Toxin exposure
   Mold toxins
   Heavy metals
Other environmental toxins
Trauma/stress—adverse childhood
   experiences
   Physical injuries
   Emotional trauma
Licit / illicit drug use / alcohol
Infections
Physical conditioning

Triggering Event

Tick attachment → tick-borne
   infections
Note: a tick attachment with microbial
transmission may have occurred
much prior to the illness, but a healthy
immune system kept the infections in
check until another stressor became
the triggering event.

Consequences—Downstream issues

Immune disruption
   Immune hyperreactivity → systemic
      inflammation
   Immune suppression
   Acquired hypogammaglobulinemia
   Multiple allergies
   MCAS—Mast Cell Activation
      Syndrome
Endocrine disruption
   Adrenal
   Thyroid

---

* This breakdown of the genesis of disease is based on Leo Galland's description of the
patient-centered diagnosis in his book *The Four Pillars of Healing*. New York: Random
House, 1997.

Pituitary
Gonadal
Insulin resistance
Overload of detox pathways
Methylation mutations
Liver / kidney / lymphatic compromise
Gastrointestinal dysfunction
Digestion/absorption issues
Dysbiosis / fungal / parasitic infections
SIBO—Small Intestinal Bowel
Overgrowth
Leaky gut syndrome
Gastroparesis
Neurological dysregulation
Cognitive dysfunction
Neurological deficits
Neuropathy

Dysautonomia
Neuropsychiatric issues
Sleep disorders
Autoimmune encephalopathy/
Pediatric Acute-onset
Neuropsychiatric Syndrome

Complicating issues

Viral activation
Porphyria
Kryptopyrroluria
MCS—Multiple Chemical Sensitivity
Syndrome
Electromagnetic field exposure/
sensitivity

Appendix B

Symptom Check-off List

Symptom Or Sign	CURRENT SEVERITY				CURRENT FREQUENCY				
	None	Mild	Moderate	Severe	NA	Never	Occasional	Often	Constant
Persistent swollen glands									
Sore throat									
Fevers									
Sore soles, esp. in the a.m.									
Joint pain									
Fingers, toes									
Ankles, wrists									
Knees, elbows									
Hips, shoulders									
Joint swelling									
Fingers, toes									
Ankles, wrists									
Knees, elbows									
Hips, shoulders									
Unexplained back pain									
Stiffness of the joints or back									
Muscle pain or cramps									
Obvious muscle weakness									
Twitching of the face or other muscles									
Confusion, difficulty thinking									
Difficulty with concentration, reading, problem absorbing new information									
Word search, name block									

Symptom Or Sign	CURRENT SEVERITY				CURRENT FREQUENCY				
	None	Mild	Moderate	Severe	NA	Never	Occasional	Often	Constant
Forgetfulness, poor short-term memory, poor attention									
Disorientation: getting lost, going to wrong places									
Speech errors—wrong word, misspeaking									
Mood swings, irritability, depression									
Anxiety, panic attacks									
Psychosis (hallucinations, delusions, paranoia, bipolar)									
Tremor									
Seizures									
Headache									
Light sensitivity									
Sound sensitivity									
Vision: double, blurry, floaters									
Ear pain									
Hearing: buzzing, ringing, decreased hearing									
Increased motion sickness, vertigo, spinning									
Off-balance, "tippy" feeling									
Light-headedness, wooziness, unavoidable need to sit or lie									
Tingling, numbness, burning or stabbing sensations, shooting pains, skin hypersensitivity									
Facial paralysis—Bell's Palsy									
Dental pain									
Neck creaks and cracks, stiffness, neck pain									
Fatigue, tired, poor stamina									
Insomnia, fractionated sleep, early awakening									
Excessive nighttime sleep									
Napping during the day									
Unexplained weight gain									

Symptom Or Sign	CURRENT SEVERITY				CURRENT FREQUENCY				
	None	Mild	Moderate	Severe	NA	Never	Occasional	Often	Constant
Unexplained weight loss									
Unexplained hair loss									
Pain in genital area									
Unexplained menstrual irregularity									
Unexplained milk production; breast pain									
Irritable bladder or bladder dysfunction									
Erectile dysfunction									
Loss of libido									
Queasy stomach or nausea									
Heartburn, stomach pain									
Constipation									
Diarrhea									
Low abdominal pain, cramps									
Heart murmur or valve prolapse?									
Heart palpitations or skips									
"Heart block" on EKG									
Chest wall pain or ribs sore									
Head congestion									
Breathlessness, "air hunger," unexplained chronic cough									
Night sweats									
Exaggerated symptoms or worse hangover from alcohol									
Symptom flares every four weeks									
Degree of disability									

Appendix C

Initial Laboratory Testing on Most New Patients

P lease note that all new patients have previously been tested and screened for Lyme disease with a Western Blot or Immunoblot. The following tests should be drawn before 9:00 a.m. and fasting.

CBC	Babesia microti IgM & IgG*
CMP	Babeisa duncani IgG
MTHFR	Bartonella henslae IgM & IgG†
Homocysteine	Anaplasma phagocytophila IgM & IgG
Vitamin B12	Ehrlichia chaffensis IgM & IgG
Pregnenolone	RMSF IgM & IgG
Cortisol AM	Mycoplasma pneumonia IgM & IgG‡
DHEA-S	CMV IgM & IgG
TSH	EBV profile
Free T4	HHV-6 IgM & IgG
Free T3	VEGF
Reverse T3	

---

*   If the patient has Medicare I will order a comprehensive tick-borne disease panel at IGeneX which will be covered: TBD6. This includes testing for both *B.microti* and *B.duncani*.

†   IGeneX offers an IgXSpot test for *Bartonella* that is more sensitive and tests for four *Bartonella* species. Test panel BART3 includes the IgXSpot, W.Blot IgM & IgG and *Bartonella* FISH and PCR.

‡   It is important to get quantitative assays of antibodies rather than positive or negative. Labcorp does a quantitative assay.

On the basis of history and physical exam, I may include:
Antidiuretic hormone (fasting/no fluids for 12 hours)
Insulin (fasting)
HgBA1C
Testosterone, Free
Estradiol
Progesterone
RBC Magnesium
Quantitative immunoglobulins with IgG subsets
CD57[§]
ANA

Test kits: Salivary cortisol levels x 4
Urinary mycotoxins

[§]   If CD57 is very low (<20 at LabCorp), this level suggests active *Babesia* infection.

Guidelines for Patients Taking Disulfiram

D isulfiram is an incredibly powerful tool to treat tick-borne infections, but it also has the potential to cause problems. If we are careful with the way it is taken, then the risk is limited. Here are guidelines to ensure its safety.

It is imperative to avoid alcohol as well as topical products containing alcohol. Also, avoid fermented foods such as kombucha, pickles, sauerkraut, olives, soy sauce and vinegar as well as all sugar products and green tea.

The first and most common issue is Herxheimer reactions. If the Herxheimer reaction is severe, we decrease the dose. If the Herxheimer reaction is mild, then we wait until it has resolved before increasing the dose.

We treat Herxheimer reactions the same way we treat Herx reactions from other antimicrobials:

1. Binders, e.g. charcoal
2. Alkalinazation with lots of water and lemon as well as Alka Selzer Gold or Tri-Salts
3. Hot baths with Epsom salt and baking soda
4. Detox and drainage remedies
5. Glutathione

Disulfiram can cause "minor" side effects in some patients. These include constipation and bloating, acne, bad breath, body odor, nausea, weight gain, metallic taste, headaches and fatigue. Unless severe, these symptoms are not reason to stop the medication.

Disulfiram can cause neurotoxicity. At times this can be difficult to distinguish from a Herxheimer reaction. These drug reactions typically occur at higher doses, often right after a dose increase, but some patients experience neurotoxicity at lower doses. If symptoms of pins and needles, numbness, stabbing, shooting, or burning pain develop, this could represent disulfiram induced neuropathy. If symptoms of brain fog/impaired cognition, headache, mood changes or vision issues develop, this could represent toxic encephalopathy, which is brain toxicity. There are reports that it can cause hypertension and even psychosis, as well as irritation of the liver. It is important to get blood tests monthly to monitor liver function.

If the disulfiram dose is lowered or if the drug is stopped within days of the onset of neurotoxic symptoms, they typically remit quickly. It is essential that you contact me immediately if any of these symptoms develop.

Most of my patients do not suffer from these neurotoxic drug reactions. But because disulfiram has this potential, I am now recommending the following supplements which can protect the nervous system:

- Zinc
- Alpha Lipoic Acid
- Melatonin
- Vitamin C

Take disulfiram only at the recommended dose, and check in every two weeks. The check in should include the following:

- DSF dose, frequency, and duration
- Any changes noticed on that dosing schedule
- A complete updated med list

In addition, keep all emails in a chain with my responses so that I can easily refer to your past history as needed.

Appendix E

Resources*

Lyme education, advocacy, support, and fundraising organizations

Bay Area Lyme Foundation Raises money to fund research into better diagnosis and treatment for Lyme disease. bayarealyme.org

Children's Lyme Disease Network Dedicated to raising awareness of how Lyme and other tick-borne illnesses affect children specifically. Website includes information about PANS/PANDAS. childrenslymenetwork.org

Family Connections Center for Counseling Website of family therapist Sandra Berenbaum, LCSW, BCD. Information for families dealing with Lyme disease, as well as first-person accounts of children with Lyme disease. lymefamilies.com

Project Lyme's mission is to eradicate the epidemic of tick-borne diseases through awareness and education, support of cutting-edge science, and advocacy for solutions to end the suffering. Projectlyme.org

Global Lyme Alliance Recently formed by the merger of the Tick-Borne Diseases Association and Lyme Research Alliance, GLA raises money for Lyme disease research and has an informative website. globallymealliance.com

International Lyme and Associated Diseases Society (ILADS) Professional organization for physicians and other healthcare providers who treat Lyme disease. Sponsors medical and scientific conferences in the US and abroad. The ILADS website is a useful source of Lyme-related information, including downloadable brochures. ilads.org

---

* Many thanks to Dorothy Leland for sharing this document.

LymeDisease.org This national advocacy organization is a leading source for news, information, and analysis in the Lyme community. Website gives info about ticks, Lyme disease, co-infections, prevention, risk maps, and more. Digital quarterly journal, *The Lyme Times*, is available free to members. Free email newsletters, Facebook and Twitter updates, as well as the *Lyme Policy Wonk* and *Touched by Lyme* blogs. lymedisease.org

Lyme Disease Association Raises funds for research, works to promote Lyme-related legislation on both the federal and state level, has chapters and affiliates in many states, cosponsors patient education workshops, and puts on an annual scientific conference in conjunction with Columbia University. Website has a doctor referral tool. lymediseaseassosciation.org

National Capitol Lyme and Associated Diseases Education and support activities, primarily focused in the greater Washington DC area. natcaplyme.org

Financial grants for children with Lyme disease

LymeAid4Kids

For those under age 21 without insurance coverage for Lyme disease, this program provides up to $1,000 toward diagnosis and treatment. Created by author Amy Tan in conjunction with the Lyme Disease Association. See lymediseaseassociation.org for an application package.

Lymelight Foundation

Financial grants for Lyme treatment for patients from birth to age 25, up to a lifetime maximum of $10,000. Grants cover expenses relating to the treatment of Lyme disease, including medication, supplements, doctor visits, lab testing, alternative practitioners such as acupuncturists and chiropractors, and transportation to and from an out-of-area doctor or lab. lymelightfoundation.org

LymeTAP

Lyme Testing Access Program. Financial assistance for Lyme and tick-borne disease diagnostic testing. Will reimburse up to 75 percent of out-of-pocket costs of testing from a qualified CLIA/Medicare-approved laboratory of your choice. (US residents only.) lymetap.com Not limited to children.

Other financial assistance

NeedyMeds

This website offers free information on programs that help people who can't afford medications and healthcare. Financial assistance for prescription medicines, low-cost medical and dental clinics, drug discount cards, and information about Medicare and Medicaid. needymeds.org

Prescription Hope
You pay a monthly fee for this service, which helps you obtain low-cost medications. prescriptionhope.com

Information about PANS/PANDAS
PANDAS Resource Network, pandasresourcenetwork.org
PANDAS Network, pandasnetwork.org
Latitudes, latitudes.org
International OCD Foundation, www.iocdf.org

Online support groups
Lyme and pregnancy Facebook group, facebook.com/groups/492653780749584/
LymeDisease.org's network of state-based support groups, lymedisease.org/lyme -disease-support-groups/
Lymenet.org online discussion groups
MDJunction has a variety of online health support groups, including Lyme disease and Parents of Children with Lyme, MDJunction.com
Facebook has hundreds of Lyme-related pages and groups

Books about Lyme disease and related topics

The Beginner's Guide to Lyme Disease by Nicola McFadzean, ND. (Biomed Publishing, 2012.) An overview of the illness, the controversy, and treatment options.

Coping with Lyme Disease: A Practical Guide to Dealing with Diagnosis and Treatment by Denise Lane, with Kenneth Liegner, MD. (Hot Paperbacks, 3rd Edition, 2004)

Cure Unknown: Inside the Lyme Epidemic by Pamela Weintraub. (St. Martin's Griffin, 2nd Edition, 2013.)
A medical journalist whose whole family has had Lyme disease delves into the scientific, medical, and political turmoil surrounding the illness.

Digging Deep: A Journal for Young People Facing Health Challenges by Rose Offner and Sheri Sobrato Brisson. (Resonance House, 2014.)

Infusing for Lymies, free online book with lots of information about IV drugs and PICC lines. issuu.com/lymeunderground/docs/infusingforlymies

The Lyme Diet by Dr. Nicola McFadzean. (Biomed Publishing, 2010.)

Nutritional strategies for healing from Lyme disease. What to eat while healing from Lyme.

The Lyme Disease Solution by Dr. Kenneth Singleton. (Booksurge, 2008.)
An introduction to the medical aspects of Lyme diagnosis and treatment.

My Lyme Guide by Marjorie MacArthur Veiga and Sarah Fletcher, MD. (My Lyme Guide, 2013.) This book provides organizational tools for patients and caregivers, for tracking symptoms, medications, insurance records, and more. MyLymeGuide .com.

Out of the Woods: Healing from Lyme Disease for Body, Mind and Spirit by Katina Makris. (Helios Press, 2015) This memoir, written from an adult perspective, includes a lot of information about integrative and alternative methods of healing.

Suffering the Silence: Chronic Lyme Disease in an Age of Denial by Allie Cashel. (North Atlantic Books, 2015.) Written by a young woman who became infected with Lyme when she was seven years old.

Susanbarnett: When Your Child Has Lyme Disease: A Parent's Survival Guide by Sandra K. Berenbaum and Dorothy Kupcha Leland. (Lyme Literate Press, 2015.) Excellent support for parents negotiating the difficult terrain of sick children with advice on how to deal with those who are not Lyme literate.

Why Can't I Get Better? Solving the Mystery of Lyme and Chronic Disease by Dr. Richard Horowitz. (St. Martin's Press, 2013.) A review of Lyme disease and co-infections.

Videos

Under Our Skin & Under Our Skin 2: Emergence

These two documentaries demonstrate the profound effect of Lyme disease on patients and explain the complex politics of tick-borne illness in the United States. The original one can be viewed online for no charge on Hulu and YouTube. The sequel can be viewed online for a small charge. Details at underourskin.com

EDUCATING YOUR CHILD WITH LYME DISEASE

Council of Parent Attorneys and Advocates (COPAA) is a nonprofit network of attorneys, advocates, parents, and related professionals to protect the legal and civil rights of students with disabilities.

CHADD Children and Adults with Attention-Deficit/Hyperactivity Disorder provides education, advocacy, and support for individuals with ADHD. Informative website and a variety of printed materials.

Home School Legal Defense Association is a nonprofit advocacy organization providing homeschooling-related legal advice and resources. Includes a clickable map of the US, with information about homeschooling laws in each state. hslda.org

Homeschool.com Resources, information, message boards.

OnlyPassionateCuriosity.com Homeschooling blog with lots of advice and resource links.

Specialeducationguide.com This website includes a useful "Special education dictionary," explaining terms parents may need to know in dealing with schools.

Wright's Law Information about special education law, education law, and advocacy for children with disabilities.

Other resources
Direct Access Labs
Most states allow direct access testing (DAT), which allows you to obtain standard
   lab tests without a doctor's order and pay substantially less than you might otherwise pay. More information at the following websites:
accesalabs.com
directlabs.com
privatemdlabs.com
walkinlab.com
health-tests-direct.com

Disability-related resources
Beach wheelchairs in California: coastal.ca.gov/access/beach-wheelchairs.html
Beach wheelchairs on East Coast and other places: beachwheelchair.com/rentals.
   htm
United Disability Services offers lots of information about how to modify a home
   for various disabilities. estore.udservices.org
US government's website on resources and services for those with disabilities.
   Includes information about modifying homes for accessibility. Disability.gov

Food allergies
Food Allergy Research and Education (FARE) foodallergy.org
Celiac Disease Foundation offers extensive information about gluten-free diets,
   including menu plans. Celiac.org

Lyme-related vision problems

The Padula Institute of Vision's website provides information about visual processing disorders and other eye problems related to Lyme disease. padulainstitute.com.

Smartphone Apps

Medications: Pillboxie, Pill Reminder, Drugs.com

Symptom trackers: My Pain Diary, Symple, iMoodJournal, Period Tracker

Other record keeping: Paperless, Keep

Gluten-free Restaurants: Find Me Gluten Free, iEatOut Gluten and Allergen Free

Public Restrooms: The Bathroom Map, Where to Wee

Acknowledgments

I n the 1950s, my mother, Jane Kinderlehrer, believed sugar, white bread, and margarine were bad for you, organic food was good, and nutritional supplements could prevent illness. She was considered a "health nut," but she was completely undeterred. She walked her talk and became food editor of *Prevention* magazine for twenty-five years and wrote a dozen cookbooks that pioneered a healthy kitchen. My mother was an icon—she never wavered in speaking her truth and cooking her love. She lived long enough to witness her practices become mainstream, and she serves as a role model for me.

I sit on the shoulders of many people. When I began practicing what was called holistic medicine more than forty years ago, there were iconoclastic doctors and nutritional biochemists who were elucidating the role of nutrition in health and disease. Jonathan Wright, Alan Gaby, Jeffrey Bland, Neil Orenstein, Leo Galland, and Sidney Baker were particularly important in my education. Environmental medicine was another area that my internal medicine training did not prepare me for. Trailblazing physicians in that arena were Theron Randolph, William Rea, William Crook, and Doris Rapp.

A few brave physicians have documented the role of Lyme disease in chronic illness, and handed off tools to the rest of us—Paul LaVoie and John Masters did groundbreaking work and Joseph Burrascano, Jr. published his guidelines on the Internet, updating them regularly so that physicians just getting their feet wet could have a foundation of where to start. Joe introduced most of us to the variegated presentations of *Bartonella* infection, and Richard Horowitz did the same with *Babesia*. Robert Bransfield has spearheaded the education of physicians on the neuropsychiatric aspects of tick-borne infections. Ray Stricker and Lorraine Johnson have been fearless in their documentation of the persistence of active infection in chronically ill people with Lyme disease. Other practitioners who have been important colleagues and teachers include Amiram Katz, Steve Bock, Wayne Anderson, Joe Brewer, Neil Nathan, and Kathleen Gedroic.

I am grateful for the support and feedback of many people. My brother Bob is the first to review everything I write. He and I appear to have inherited the writing gene from my mother, and his word-smithing has been a major contribution to this book. I am also grateful to a handful of practitioners and laypeople who have unselfishly taken the time to review and give me helpful feedback on selected chapters. These include Ken Liegner, Kristine Gedroic, Robert Bransfield, Michael Zona, Joseph Burrascano, Jr., Ramzi Asfour, Joe Brewer, Julie Barter, Peter Van Etten, and Erica Roush. Hillary Schlinger stands out as a Lyme literate professional who did a superlative job in editing this book. And I am indebted to my professional editors, Kimberly Peticolas, Mark Amundsen, and Leah Zarra, who have chaperoned this book into the professional text I hoped it would be.

Special thanks Emilie Hagny-Downs, the graphic artist who was able to translate my scrawls into easily readable figures.

My agent, Jennifer Weis, has been a great source of support and guidance. I am indebted to her for her faith in me and my work.

And a special thanks to June Anderson, my secretary, office manager, bookkeeper, computer maven, and everything support person without whom I cannot imagine having a medical practice.

I want to thank my patients, whose trust in me has allowed me to live my passion. A while back I had dinner with some physician friends who practice mainstream medicine. I asked how their day at the office was, and they said "boring—same old patients." I do not have any boring patients. I love my patients and I love what I do. I am grateful beyond measure that I have landed in the role of witnessing long-suffering people become well.

Finally, I could not have persisted when I was in the throes of Lyme hell were it not for the unconditional love of my three daughters, Hannah, Eliana, and Tovah, as well as my wife, Carolyn. Their love and support have been the biggest blessings in my life.

Notes

PREFACE

1. Ronald Rosenberg et al., "Vital Signs: Trends in Reported Vectorborne Disease Cases—United States and Territories, 2004–2016," *MMWR Morbidity and Mortality Weekly Report* 67, no. 17 (April 2018): pp. 496–501, https://doi.org/10.15585/mmwr.mm6717e1.
2. "Recent Surveillance Data," Centers for Disease Control and Prevention (Centers for Disease Control and Prevention, November 7, 2019), https://www.cdc.gov/lyme/datasurveillance/recent-surveillance-data.html.
3. Christina A. Nelson et al., "Incidence of Clinician-Diagnosed Lyme Disease, United States, 2005–2010," *Emerging Infectious Diseases* 21, no. 9 (2015): pp. 1625–1631, https://doi.org/10.3201/eid2109.150417.
4. "Lyme Disease—United States, 2003–2005," *MMWR Morbidity and Mortality Weekly Report* 56, no. 23 (June 15, 2007): pp. 573–576.
5. J. M. Boltri, R. B. Hash, and R. L. Vogel, "Patterns of Lyme Disease Diagnosis and Treatment by Family Physicians in a Southeastern State," *Journal of Community Health* 27 (2002): pp. 395–402, https://doi.org/10.1023/a:1020697017543.
6. S. Hook, C. Nelson, and P. Mead, "Self-Reported Lyme Disease Diagnosis, Treatment, and Recovery: Results from 2009, 2011, & 2012 HealthStyles Nationwide Surveys," in *13th International Conference on Lyme Borreliosis and Other Tick-Borne Diseases* (Boston, MA, 2013).
7. Catharine I. Paules et al., "Tickborne Diseases—Confronting a Growing Threat," *New England Journal of Medicine* 379, no. 8 (2018): pp. 701–703, https://doi.org/10.1056/nejmp1807870.
8. Nancy A. Shadick et al., "The Long-Term Clinical Outcomes of Lyme Disease: A Population-Based Retrospective Cohort Study," *Annals of Internal Medicine* 121, no. 8 (October 15, 1994): pp. 560–567, https://doi.org/10.7326/0003-4819-121-8-199410150-00002.
9. E. S. Asch et al., "Lyme Disease: An Infectious and Postinfectious Syndrome," *Journal of Rheumatology* 21, no. 3 (March 1994): pp. 454–461.
10. Raphael B. Stricker and Lorraine Johnson, "Persistent Infection in Chronic Lyme Disease: Does Form Matter?," *Research Journal of Infectious Diseases* 1, no. 2 (2013), https://doi.org/10.7243/2052-5958-1-2.

CHAPTER 1

1. Leo Galland, *The Four Pillars of Healing: How the New Integrated Medicine—the Best of Conventional and Alternative Approaches—Can Cure You* (New York: Random House, 1997), pp. 3–24.

2. Vincent J. Felitti et al., "Relationship of Childhood Abuse and Household Dysfunction to Many of the Leading Causes of Death in Adults," *American Journal of Preventive Medicine* 14, no. 4 (1998): pp. 245–258, https://doi.org/10.1016/s0749-3797(98)00017-8.

CHAPTER 2

1. Stephen S. Hall, "Unfrozen," *National Geographic*, November 2011, https://www.national geographic.com/magazine/2011/11/iceman-autopsy/.
2. Nicholas Summerton, "Lyme Disease in the Eighteenth Century," *BMJ* 311, no. 7018 (December 2, 1995): p. 1478, https://doi.org/10.1136/bmj.311.7018.1478.
3. Arvid Afzelius, "Erythema Chronicum Migrans," *Acta Dermato-Venereologica* 2 (1921): pp. 120–125, https://doi.org/10.2340/0001555521120125.
4. A. G. Hoen et al., "Phylogeography of Borrelia Burgdorferi in the Eastern United States Reflects Multiple Independent Lyme Disease Emergence Events," *Proceedings of the National Academy of Sciences* 106, no. 35 (September 14, 2009): pp. 15013–15018, https://doi.org/10.1073/pnas.0903810106.
5. W. F. Marshall et al., "Detection of Borrelia Burgdorferi DNA in Museum Specimens of Peromyscus Leucopus," *Journal of Infectious Diseases* 170, no. 4 (January 1994): pp. 1027-1032, https://doi.org/10.1093/infdis/170.4.1027.
6. R. J. Scrimenti, "Erythema Chronicum Migrans," *Archives of Dermatology* 102, no. 1 (January 1970): pp. 104–105, https://doi.org/10.1001/archderm.102.1.104.
7. Polly Murray, *The Widening Circle: A Lyme Disease Pioneer Tells Her Story* (New York: St. Martin's Press, 1996).
8. Allen C. Steere et al., "Lyme Arthritis: An Epidemic of Oligoarticular Arthritis in Children and Adults in Three Connecticut Communities," *Arthritis & Rheumatism* 20, no. 1 (1977): pp. 7–17, https://doi.org/10.1002/art.1780200102.
9. "Fact Check: Are There Really More Trees Today Than 100 Years Ago?," tentree, accessed July 1, 2018, https://www.tentree.com/blogs/posts/fact-check-are-there-really-more-trees-today-than-100-years-ago.
10. Jed Kolko, "How Suburban Are Big American Cities?," FiveThirtyEight, May 21, 2015, https://fivethirtyeight.com/features/how-suburban-are-big-american-cities.
11. Koryos, "White-Tailed Deer Overpopulation in the United States," Koryos Writes, December 17, 2014, http://www.koryoswrites.com/nonfiction/white-tailed-deer-overpopulation-in-the-united-states.
12. Mary Beth Pfeiffer, *Lyme: The First Epidemic of Climate Change* (Washington, DC: Island Press, 2018).
13. Mary Beth Pfeiffer, "How Migratory Birds Are Moving Lyme Disease to New Places and Peoples," EHN, April 27, 2018, https://www.ehn.org/migratory-birds-are-moving-lyme-disease-to-new-places-and-peoples-2561494303.html.
14. Malcolm Gladwell, *The Tipping Point: How Little Things Can Make a Big Difference* (Boston: Little, Brown & Company, 2000).
15. R S Beach, M E Gershwin, and L S Hurley, "Persistent Immunological Consequences of Gestation Zinc Deprivation," *American Journal of Clinical Nutrition* 38, no. 4 (January 1983): pp. 579–590, https://doi.org/10.1093/ajcn/38.4.579.
16. Jianghong Liu, Sophie Zhao, and Teresa Reyes, "Neurological and Epigenetic Implications of Nutritional Deficiencies on Psychopathology: Conceptualization and Review of Evidence," *International Journal of Molecular Sciences* 16, no. 8 (May 2015): pp. 18129–18148, https://doi.org/10.3390/ijms160818129.
17. Simon C. Langley-Evans and Beverly S. Muhlhausler, "Early Nutrition, Epigenetics, and Human Health," *Epigenetics of Aging and Longevity*, November 17, 2017, https://www.sciencedirect.com/science/article/pii/B9780128110607000115.

18. Liu, "Neurological and Epigenetic Implications of Nutritional Deficiencies on Psychopathology," 18129–18148.

19. M. Collotta, P. A. Bertazzi, and V. Bollati, "Epigenetics and Pesticides," *Toxicology* 307 (May 10, 2013): pp. 35–41, https://doi.org/10.1016/j.tox.2013.01.017.

20. Anne Steinemann, "Ten Questions Concerning Air Fresheners and Indoor Built Environments," *Building and Environment*, November 5, 2016, https://www.sciencedirect.com/science/article/pii/S0360132316304334.

21. "'Greener' Laundry by the Load: Fabric Softener versus Dryer Sheets," *Scientific American*, December 10, 2008, https://www.scientificamerican.com/article/greener-laundry.

22. Natalie Matosin, Cristiana Cruceanu, and Elisabeth B. Binder, "Preclinical and Clinical Evidence of DNA Methylation Changes in Response to Trauma and Chronic Stress," *Chronic Stress* 1 (2017): p. 10, https://doi.org/10.1177/2470547017710764.

23. Adnan Bashir Bhatti and Anwar Ul Haq, "The Pathophysiology of Perceived Social Isolation: Effects on Health and Mortality," *Cureus* 9, no. 1 (January 24, 2017): p. 994, https://doi.org/10.7759/cureus.994.

24. Huan Song et al., "Association of Stress-Related Disorders with Subsequent Autoimmune Disease," *JAMA* 319, no. 23 (2018): pp. 2388–2400, https://doi.org/10.1001/jama.2018.7028.

25. Daniel A. Notterman and Colter Mitchell, "Epigenetics and Understanding the Impact of Social Determinants of Health," *Pediatric Clinics of North America* 62, no. 5 (2015): pp. 1227–1240, https://doi.org/10.1016/j.pcl.2015.05.012.

CHAPTER 3

1. Adriana Marques, "Chronic Lyme Disease: A Review," *Infectious Disease Clinics of North America* 22, no. 2 (2008): pp. 341–360, https://doi.org/10.1016/j.idc.2007.12.011.

2. Alison W. Rebman et al., "The Clinical, Symptom, and Quality-of-Life Characterization of a Well-Defined Group of Patients with Posttreatment Lyme Disease Syndrome," *Frontiers in Medicine* 4 (2017): p. 224, https://doi.org/10.3389/fmed.2017.00224.

3. Nancy A. Shadick, "The Long-Term Clinical Outcomes of Lyme Disease: A Population-Based Retrospective Cohort Study," *Annals of Internal Medicine* 121, no. 8 (1994): pp. 560–567, https://doi.org/10.7326/0003-4819-121-8-199410150-00002.

4. E. S. Asch et al., "Lyme Disease: An Infectious and Postinfectious Syndrome," *Journal of Rheumatology* 21, no. 3 (March 1994): pp. 454–461.

5. S. Hook, C. Nelson, and P. Mead, "Self-Reported Lyme Disease Diagnosis, Treatment, and Recovery: Results from 2009, 2011, & 2012 HealthStyles Nationwide Surveys," in *13th International Conference on Lyme Borreliosis and Other Tick-Borne Diseases* (Boston, MA, 2013).

6. Lorraine Johnson et al., "Severity of Chronic Lyme Disease Compared to Other Chronic Conditions: a Quality of Life Survey," *PeerJ* 2, no. e322 (March 27, 2014), https://doi.org/10.7717/peerj.322.

7. Peter Novak et al., "Association of Small Fiber Neuropathy and Post Treatment Lyme Disease Syndrome," *PLoS One* 14, no. 2 (February 12, 2019), https://doi.org/10.1371/journal.pone.0212222.

8. Jennifer M. Coughlin et al., "Imaging Glial Activation in Patients with Post-Treatment Lyme Disease Symptoms: a Pilot Study Using [11C]DPA-713 PET," *Journal of Neuroinflammation* 15, no. 1 (2018): p. 346, https://doi.org/10.1186/s12974-018-1381-4.

9. Alison W. Rebman et al., "The Clinical, Symptom, and Quality-of-Life Characterization of a Well-Defined Group of Patients with Post-Treatment Lyme Disease Syndrome," *Frontiers in Medicine* 4 (2017), https://doi.org/10.3389/fmed.2017.00224.

10. Gary P. Wormser et al., "The Clinical Assessment, Treatment, and Prevention of Lyme Disease, Human Granulocytic Anaplasmosis, and Babesiosis: Clinical Practice Guidelines

by the Infectious Diseases Society of America," *Clinical Infectious Diseases* 43, no. 9 (2006): pp. 1089–1134, https://doi.org/10.1086/508667.

11. Mark S. Klempner et al., "Two Controlled Trials of Antibiotic Treatment in Patients with Persistent Symptoms and a History of Lyme Disease," *New England Journal of Medicine* 345, no. 2 (2001): pp. 85–92, https://doi.org/10.1056/nejm200107123450202.

12. B. A. Fallon et al., "A Randomized, Placebo-Controlled Trial of Repeated IV Antibiotic Therapy for Lyme Encephalopathy," *Neurology* 70, no. 13 (2007): pp. 992–1003, https://doi.org/10.1212/01.wnl.0000284604.61160.2d.

13. L. B. Krupp et al., "Study and Treatment of Post Lyme Disease (STOP-LD): A Randomized Double Masked Clinical Trial," *Neurology* 60, no. 12 (2003): pp. 1923–1930, https://doi.org/10.1212/01.wnl.0000071227.23769.9e.

14. Allison K. DeLong et al., "Antibiotic Retreatment of Lyme Disease in Patients with Persistent Symptoms: A Biostatistical Review of Randomized, Placebo-Controlled, Clinical Trials," *Contemporary Clinical Trials* 33, no. 6 (November 1, 2012): pp. 1132–1142, https://doi.org/10.1016/j.cct.2012.08.009.

15. Daniel J. Cameron, "Generalizability in Two Clinical Trials of Lyme Disease," *Epidemiologic Perspectives & Innovations* 3, no. 12 (October 17, 2006), https://doi.org/10.1186/1742-5573-3-12.

16. DeLong, "Antibiotic Retreatment of Lyme Disease in Patients with Persistent Symptoms: A Biostatistical Review of Randomized, Placebo-Controlled, Clinical Trials."

17. Wormser, "The Clinical Assessment, Treatment, and Prevention of Lyme Disease, Human Granulocytic Anaplasmosis, and Babesiosis: Clinical Practice Guidelines by the Infectious Diseases Society of America."

18. John P. A. Ioannidis, "Why Most Published Research Findings Are False," *PLoS Medicine* 2, no. 8 (2005): p. e124, https://doi.org/10.1371/journal.pmed.0020124.

19. Abdur Rahman Khan et al., "Quality and Strength of Evidence of the Infectious Diseases Society of America Clinical Practice Guidelines," *Clinical Infectious Diseases* 51, no. 10 (2010): pp. 1147–1156, https://doi.org/10.1086/656735.

20. Dong Heun Lee and Ole Vielemeyer, "Analysis of Overall Level of Evidence Behind Infectious Diseases Society of America Practice Guidelines," *Archives of Internal Medicine* 171, no. 1 (2011): pp. 18–22, https://doi.org/10.1001/archinternmed.2010.482.

21. Jeanne Lenzer et al., "Ensuring the Integrity of Clinical Practice Guidelines: A Tool for Protecting Patients," *BMJ*, September 13, 2013, p. 347, https://doi.org/10.1136/bmj.f5535.

22. Lorraine Johnson and Raphael B Stricker, "The Infectious Diseases Society of America Lyme Guidelines: A Cautionary Tale about the Development of Clinical Practice Guidelines," *Philosophy, Ethics, and Humanities in Medicine* 5, no. 9 (2010): p. 9, https://doi.org/10.1186/1747-5341-5-9.

23. Allan D. Sniderman and Curt D. Furberg, "Why Guideline-Making Requires Reform," *JAMA* 301, no. 4 (January 28, 2009): pp. 429–431, https://doi.org/10.1001/jama.2009.15.

24. "'Attorney General's Investigation Reveals Flawed Lyme Disease Guideline Process, IDSA Agrees to Reassess Guidelines, Install Independent Arbiter" (Connecticut Attorney General's Office, May 1, 2008).

25. Sniderman, "Why Guideline-Making Requires Reform," pp. 429–431.

26. Raphael B. Stricker and Lorraine Johnson, "The Infectious Diseases Society of America Lyme Guidelines: Poster Child for Guidelines Reform," *Southern Medical Journal* 102, no. 6 (2009): pp. 565–566, https://doi.org/10.1097/smj.0b013e3181a594e9; Daniel M. Keller, "'Infectious Disease Treatment Guidelines Weakened By Paucity of Scientific Evidence," *Medscape Medical News*, November 13, 2009, http://www.medscape.com/viewarticle/712341.

27. Sniderman, "Why Guideline-Making Requires Reform," 429–431.

28. "Attorney General's Investigation Reveals Flawed Lyme Disease Guideline Process, IDSA Agrees to Reassess Guidelines, Install Independent Arbiter," 2008.

29. Sniderman, "Why Guideline-Making Requires Reform," 429–431.

30. Sniderman, "Why Guideline-Making Requires Reform," 429–431.

31. "Attorney General's Investigation Reveals Flawed Lyme Disease Guideline Process, IDSA Agrees to Reassess Guidelines, Install Independent Arbiter," 2008.

32. "Classifying Recommendations for Clinical Practice Guidelines," *Pediatrics* 114, no. 3 (September 1, 2004): pp. 874–877, https://doi.org/10.1542/peds.2004–1260.

33. Wormser, "The Clinical Assessment, Treatment, and Prevention of Lyme Disease, Human Granulocytic Anaplasmosis, and *Babesiosis*," 1089–1134.

34. Bayer ME et al. "*Borrelia burgdorferi* DNA in the urine of treated patients with chronic Lyme disease symptoms: A PCR study of 97 cases,". *Infection*. 1996 Sep-Oct; 24(5): pp. 347–353.

35. Jarrno Oksi et al., "*Borrelia Burgorferi* Detected by Culture and PCR in Clinical Relapse of Disseminated Lyme Borreliosis," *Annals of Medicine* 31, no. 3 (June 1999): pp. 225–232, https://doi.org/10.3109/07853899909115982.

36. Brian A. Fallon et al., "A Reappraisal of the U.S. Clinical Trials of Post-Treatment Lyme Disease Syndrome," *Open Neurology Journal* 6, no. 1 (May 2012): pp. 79–87, https://doi.org /10.2174/1874205x01206010079.

37. DeLong, "Antibiotic Retreatment of Lyme Disease in Patients with Persistent Symptoms," 1132–1142.

38. M. B. Chancellor et al., "Urinary Dysfunction in Lyme Disease," *Journal of Urology* 149, no. 1 (1993): pp. 26–30, https://doi.org/10.1016/s0022-5347(17)35989-x.

39. Marianne Middelveen et al., "Persistent Borrelia Infection in Patients with Ongoing Symptoms of Lyme Disease," *Healthcare (Basel)* 6, no. 2 (2018): p. 33, https://doi.org /10.3390/healthcare6020033.

40. Allen C. Steere, Paul H. Duray, and Eugene C. Butcher, "Spirochetal Antigens and Lymphoid Cell Surface Markers in Lyme Synovitis. Comparison With Rheumatoid Synovium and Tonsillar Lymphoid Tissue," *Arthritis & Rheumatism* 31, no. 4 (1988): pp. 487–495, https:// doi.org/10.1002/art.1780310405.

41. Daniel F. Battafarano et al., "Chronic Septic Arthritis Caused a Chronic Septic Arthritis Caused by *Borrelia Burgdorferi*," *Clinical Orthopaedics and Related Research*, no. 297 (December 1993): pp. 238–241, https://doi.org/10.1097/00003086-199312000-00038.

42. Emir Hodzic et al., "Resurgence of Persisting Non-Cultivable *Borrelia Burgdorferi* Following Antibiotic Treatment in Mice," *PLoS One* 9, no. 1 (2014): p. e86907, https: //doi.org/10.1371/journal.pone.0086907.

43. Monica E. Embers et al., "Persistence of *Borrelia Burgdorferi* in Rhesus Macaques Following Antibiotic Treatment of Disseminated Infection," *PLoS One* 7, no. 1 (November 2012): p. e29914, https://doi.org/10.1371/journal.pone.0029914.

44. Monica E. Embers et al., "Variable Manifestations, Diverse Seroreactivity and Post-Treatment Persistence in Non-Human Primates Exposed to *Borrelia Burgdorferi* by Tick Feeding," *PLoS One* 12, no. 12 (2017): p. e0189071, https://doi.org/10.1371/journal.pone.0189071.

45. Hodzic, "Resurgence of Persisting Non-Cultivable Borrelia Burgdorferi Following Antibiotic Treatment in Mice," e86907.

46. Keith Berndtson, "Review of Evidence for Immune Evasion and Persistent Infection in Lyme Disease," *International Journal of General Medicine* 6 (2013): pp. 291–306, https: //doi.org/10.2147/ijgm.s44114.

47. E. Sapi and A. MacDonald, "Biofilms of *Borrelia Burgdorferi* in Chronic Cutaneous Borreliosis," *American Journal of Clinical Pathology* 129 (2008): pp. 988–989.

48. Eva Sapi et al., "The Long-Term Persistence of *Borrelia Burgdorferi* Antigens and DNA in the Tissues of a Patient with Lyme Disease," *Antibiotics* 8, no. 4 (November 2019): p. 183, https://doi.org/10.3390/antibiotics8040183.

49. Ø. Brorson and S. H. Brorson, "In Vitro Conversion of *Borrelia Burgdorferi* to Cystic Forms in Spinal Fluid, and Transformation to Mobile Spirochetes by Incubation in BSK-H Medium," *Infection* 26, no. 3 (1998): pp. 144–150, https://doi.org/10.1007/bf02771839.

50. Jing-Ren Zhang et al., "Antigenic Variation in Lyme Disease Borreliae by Promiscuous Recombination of VMP-like Sequence Cassettes," *Cell* 89, no. 2 (1997): pp. 275–285, https:// doi.org/10.1016/s0092-8674(00)80206–8.

51. Sunit Kumar Singh and Herman Josef Girschick, "Molecular Survival Strategies of the Lyme Disease Spirochete *Borrelia Burgdorferi*," *Lancet Infectious Diseases* 4, no. 9 (2004): pp. 575–583, https://doi.org/10.1016/s1473-3099(04)01132-6.

52. M. S. Klempner, R. Noring, and R. A. Rogers, "Invasion of Human Skin Fibroblasts by the Lyme Disease Spirochete, *Borrelia Burgdorferi*," *Journal of Infectious Diseases* 167, no. 5 (1993): pp. 1074–1081, https://doi.org/10.1093/infdis/167.5.1074.

53. Thomas Häupl et al., "Persistence of Borrelia Burgdorferi in Ligamentous Tissue from a Patient with Chronic Lyme Borreliosis," *Arthritis & Rheumatism* 36, no. 11 (1993): pp. 1621–1626, https://doi.org/10.1002/art.1780361118.

54. Y. Ma, A. Sturrock, and J. J. Weis, "Intracellular Localization of *Borrelia Burgdorferi* within Human Endothelial Cells.," *Infection and Immunity* 59, no. 2 (1991): pp. 671–678, https://doi.org/10.1128/iai.59.2.671-678.1991.

55. H. J. Girschick et al., "Intracellular Persistence of *Borrelia Burgdorferi* in Human Synovial Cells," *Rheumatology International* 16, no. 3 (1996): pp. 125–132, https://doi.org/10.1007/bf01409985.

56. Judith Miklossy et al., "Persisting Atypical and Cystic Forms of *Borrelia Burgdorferi* and Local Inflammation in Lyme Neuroborreliosis," *Journal of Neuroinflammation* 5, no. 1 (September 25, 2008): p. 40, https://doi.org/10.1186/1742-2094-5-40.

57. Berndtson, "Review of Evidence for Immune Evasion and Persistent Infection in Lyme Disease," 291–306.

58. Bijaya Sharma et al., "Borrelia Burgdorferi, the Causative Agent of Lyme Disease, Forms Drug-Tolerant Persister Cells," *Antimicrobial Agents and Chemotherapy* 59, no. 8 (2015): pp. 4616–4624, https://doi.org/10.1128/aac.00864-15.

59. Rafal Tokarz et al., "Assessment of Polymicrobial Infections in Ticks in New York State," *Vector-Borne and Zoonotic Diseases* 10, no. 3 (2010): pp. 217–221, https://doi.org/10.1089/vbz.2009.0036.

60. Leo M. Schouls et al., "Detection and Identification of Ehrlichia, *Borrelia Burgdorferi* Sensu Lato, and Bartonella Species in Dutch Ixodes Ricinus Ticks," *Journal of Clinical Microbiology* 37, no. 7 (July 1999): pp. 2215–2222.

61. E. K. Hofmeister et al., "Cosegregation of a Novel Bartonella Species with *Borrelia Burgdorferi* and Babesia Microti in Peromyscus Leucopus," *Journal of Infectious Diseases* 177, no. 2 (n.d.): pp. 409–416, https://doi.org/10.1086/514201.

62. D. Cameron, "Severity of Lyme Disease with Persistent Symptoms. Insights from a Double-Blind Placebo-Controlled Trial," *Minerva Medica* 99, no. 5 (2008): pp. 489–496.

63. Sam T. Donta, "Tetracycline Therapy for Chronic Lyme Disease," *Clinical Infectious Diseases* 25, no. s1 (1997): pp. S52–S56, https://doi.org/10.1086/516171.

64. P. Wahlberg et al., "Treatment of Late Lyme Borreliosis," *Journal of Infection* 29, no. 3 (November 1994): pp. 255–261, https://doi.org/10.1016/s0163-4453(94)91105-3.

65. J. Oksi, J. Nikoskelainen, and M. K. Viljanen, "Comparison of Oral Cefixime and Intravenous Ceftriaxone Followed by Oral Amoxicillin in Disseminated Lyme Borreliosis," *European Journal of Clinical Microbiology & Infectious Diseases* 17, no. 10 (1998): pp. 715–719, https://doi.org/10.1007/s100960050166.

66. Jie Feng, "Stationary Phase Persister/Biofilm Microcolony of *Borrelia burgdorferi* Causes More Severe Disease in a Mouse Model of Lyme Arthritis: Implications for Understanding Persistence, Post-Treatment Lyme Disease Syndrome (PTLDS), and Treatment Failure," *Discovery Medicine*, accessed August 27, 2019, http://www.discoverymedicine.com/Jie-Feng/.

67. David L. Sackett et al., "Evidence-Based Medicine: What It Is and What It Isn't," *BMJ* 312 (January 13, 1996): pp. 71–72, https://doi.org/10.1136/bmj.312.7023.71.

SECTION TWO

1. Allen C. Steere, Edward Dwyer, and Robert Winchester, "Association of Chronic Lyme Arthritis with HLA-DR4 and HLA-DR2 Alleles," *New England Journal of Medicine* 323, no. 4 (1990): pp. 219–223, https://doi.org/10.1056/nejm199007263230402.
2. R. A. Kalish, J. M. Leong, and A. C. Steere, "Association of Treatment-Resistant Chronic Lyme Arthritis with HLA-DR4 and Antibody Reactivity to OspA and OspB of Borrelia Burgdorferi.," *Infection and Immunity* 61, no. 7 (1993): pp. 2774–2779, https://doi.org/10.1128/iai.61.7.2774-2779.1993.
3. Alexis Lacout et al., "The Persistent Lyme Disease: 'True Chronic Lyme Disease' Rather Than 'Post-Treatment Lyme Disease Syndrome,'" *Journal of Global Infectious Diseases* 10, no. 3 (2018): pp. 170–171, https://doi.org/10.4103/jgid.jgid_152_17.

CHAPTER 4

1. Raphael B. Stricker and Lorraine B. Johnson, "Persistent Infection in Chronic Lyme Disease: Does Form Matter?," *Research Journal of Infectious Diseases* 1, no. 2 (2013), https://doi.org/10.7243/2052-5958-1-2.
2. Karen E. Tracy and Nicole Baumgarth, "Borrelia Burgdorferi Manipulates Innate and Adaptive Immunity to Establish Persistence in Rodent Reservoir Hosts," *Frontiers in Immunology* 8 (2017): p. 116, https://doi.org/10.3389/fimmu.2017.00116.
3. Rebecca A. Elsner et al., "Suppression of Long-Lived Humoral Immunity Following Borrelia Burgdorferi Infection," *PLoS Pathogens* 11, no. 7 (July 2, 2015), https://doi.org/10.1371/journal.ppat.1004976.
4. Gary P. Wormser et al., "Yield of Large-Volume Blood Cultures in Patients with Early Lyme Disease," *Journal of Infectious Diseases* 184, no. 8 (2001): pp. 1070–1072, https://doi.org/10.1086/323424.
5. Rafal Tokarz et al., "Assessment of Polymicrobial Infections in Ticks in New York State," *Vector-Borne and Zoonotic Diseases* 10, no. 3 (2010): pp. 217–221, https://doi.org/10.1089/vbz.2009.0036.
6. Sara Moutailler et al., "Co-Infection of Ticks: The Rule Rather Than the Exception," *PLoS Neglected Tropical Diseases* 10, no. 3 (2016), https://doi.org/10.1371/journal.pntd.0004539.
7. Maria A. Diuk-Wasser, Edouard Vannier, and Peter J. Krause, "Coinfection by Ixodes Tick-Borne Pathogens: Ecological, Epidemiological, and Clinical Consequences," *Trends in Parasitology* 32, no. 1 (2015): pp. 30–42, https://doi.org/10.1016/j.pt.2015.09.008.
8. P. J. Krause et al., "Concurrent Lyme Disease and Babesiosis. Evidence for Increased Severity and Duration of Illness," *JAMA* 275, no. 21 (June 5, 1996): pp. 1657–1660, https://doi.org/10.1001/jama.275.21.1657.
9. Kunal Garg et al., "Evaluating Polymicrobial Immune Responses in Patients Suffering from Tick-Borne Diseases," *Scientific Reports* 8, no. 1 (2018): p. 15932, https://doi.org/10.1038/s41598-018-34393-9.
10. Allen C Steere et al., "Autoimmune Mechanisms in Antibiotic Treatment-Resistant Lyme Arthritis," *Journal of Autoimmunity* 16, no. 3 (2001): pp. 263–268, https://doi.org/10.1006/jaut.2000.0495.
11. Trever M. Koester et al., "Infectious Mononucleosis and Lyme Disease as Confounding Diagnoses: A Report of 2 Cases," *Clinical Medicine & Research* 16, no. 3–4 (2018): pp. 66–68, https://doi.org/10.3121/cmr.2018.1419.
12. E. B. Breitschwerdt, S. Sontakke, and S. Hopkins, "Neurological Manifestations of Bartonellosis in Immunocompetent Patients: A Composite of Reports from 2005–2012," *Journal of Neuroparasitology* 3 (2012): pp. 1–15, https://doi.org/10.4303/jnp/235640.

13. Vincent J Felitti et al., "Relationship of Childhood Abuse and Household Dysfunction to Many of the Leading Causes of Death in Adults," *American Journal of Preventive Medicine* 14, no. 4 (1998): pp. 245–258, https://doi.org/10.1016/s0749-3797(98)00017–8.

CHAPTER 5

1. Michael Cook, "Lyme Borreliosis: A Review of Data on Transmission Time after Tick Attachment," *International Journal of General Medicine* 8 (2015): pp. 1–8, https://doi.org/10.2147/ijgm.s73791.
2. Natacha Sertour et al., "Infection Kinetics and Tropism of *Borrelia Burgdorferi Sensu Lato* in Mouse After Natural (via Ticks) or Artificial (Needle) Infection Depends on the Bacterial Strain," *Frontiers in Microbiology* 9 (2018): p. 1722, https://doi.org/10.3389/fmicb.2018.01722.
3. Robert P. Smith et al., "Clinical Characteristics and Treatment Outcome of Early Lyme Disease in Patients with Microbiologically Confirmed Erythema Migrans," *Annals of Internal Medicine* 136, no. 6 (2002): pp. 421–428, https://doi.org/10.7326/0003-4819-136-6-200203190-00005.
4. Gary P. Wormser et al., "Yield of Large-Volume Blood Cultures in Patients with Early Lyme Disease," *Journal of Infectious Diseases* 184, no. 8 (2001): pp. 1070–1072, https://doi.org/10.1086/323424.
5. M. E. Aguero-Rosenfeld et al., "Evolution of the Serologic Response to *Borrelia Burgdorferi* in Treated Patients with Culture-Confirmed Erythema Migrans," *Journal of Clinical Microbiology* 34, no. 1 (1996): pp. 1–9, https://doi.org/10.1128/jcm.34.1.1–9.1996.
6. Maria E. Aguero-Rosenfeld, "Lyme Disease: Laboratory Issues," *Infectious Disease Clinics of North America* 22, no. 2 (2008): pp. 301–313, https://doi.org/10.1016/j.idc.2007.12.005.
7. Vera Preac-Mursic et al., "Survival of *Borrelia Burgdorferi* in Antibiotically Treated Patients with Lyme Borreliosis," *Infection* 17, no. 6 (1989): pp. 355–359, https://doi.org/10.1007/bf01645543.
8. Aguero-Rosenfeld, "Lyme Disease: Laboratory Issues," 301–313.
9. "Signs and Symptoms of Untreated Lyme Disease," Centers for Disease Control and Prevention, August 15, 2019, https://www.cdc.gov/lyme/signs_symptoms/index.html.
10. "Tick Encounter Resource Center," Winter Tick Activity, accessed May 10, 2019, https://tickencounter.org/tick_notes/winter_tick_activity.
11. "Signs and Symptoms of Untreated Lyme Disease," Centers for Disease Control and Prevention, August 15, 2019, https://www.cdc.gov/lyme/signs_symptoms/index.html.
12. R. B. Stricker, "Counterpoint: Long-Term Antibiotic Therapy Improves Persistent Symptoms Associated with Lyme Disease," *Clinical Infectious Diseases* 45, no. 2 (2007): pp. 149–157, https://doi.org/10.1086/518853.
13. Martina H. Ziska, S. T. Donta, and F. C. Demarest, "Physician Preferences in the Diagnosis and Treatment of Lyme Disease in the United States," *Infection* 24, no. 2 (1996): pp. 182–186, https://doi.org/10.1007/bf01713336.
14. Akshita Datar et al., "In Vitro Effectiveness of Samento and Banderol Herbal Extracts on the Different Morphological Forms of *Borrelia Burgdorferi*," *Townsend Letter, the Examiner of Alternative Medicine*, July 2010.
15. Kati Karvonen and Leona Gilbert, "Effective Killing of *Borrelia Burgdorferi* in Vitro with Novel Herbal Compounds," *General Medicine Open* 2, no. 6 (2018): pp. 1–4, https://doi.org/10.15761/gmo.1000153.
16. Anna Goc and Matthias Rath, "The Anti-Borreliae Efficacy of Phytochemicals and Micronutrients: An Update," *Therapeutic Advances in Infectious Disease* 3, no. 3–4 (2016): pp. 75–82, https://doi.org/10.1177/2049936116655502.

17. Jie Feng et al., "Identification of Essential Oils with Strong Activity against Stationary Phase *Borrelia Burgdorferi*," *Antibiotics* 7, no. 4 (2018): p. 89, https://doi.org/10.3390 /antibiotics7040089.
18. Datar, "In Vitro Effectiveness of Samento and Banderol Herbal Extracts on the Different Morphological Forms of *Borrelia Burgdorferi*," 2010.

CHAPTER 6

1. Stephen F. Porcella and Tom G. Schwan, "*Borrelia Burgdorferi* and *Treponema Pallidum*: a Comparison Of Functional Genomics, Environmental Adaptations, and Pathogenic Mechanisms," *Journal of Clinical Investigation* 107, no. 6 (2001): pp. 651–656, https://doi .org/10.1172/jci12484.
2. David C. Owen, "Is Lyme Disease Always Polymicrobial? The Jigsaw Hypothesis," *Medical Hypotheses* 67, no. 4 (2006): pp. 860–864, https://doi.org/10.1016/j.mehy.2006.03.046.
3. P. J. Krause et al., "Concurrent Lyme Disease and Babesiosis. Evidence for Increased Severity and Duration of Illness," *JAMA* 275, no. 21 (June 5, 1996): pp. 1657–1660, https: //doi.org/10.1001/jama.275.21.1657.
4. Thomas Butler, "The Jarisch–Herxheimer Reaction After Antibiotic Treatment of Spirochetal Infections: A Review of Recent Cases and Our Understanding of Pathogenesis," *American Journal of Tropical Medicine and Hygiene* 96, no. 1 (2016): pp. 46–52, https://doi .org/10.4269/ajtmh.16–0434.
5. S. Humphreys et al., "The Effect Of High Altitude Commercial Air Travel on Oxygen Saturation," *Anaesthesia* 60, no. 5 (September 2005): pp. 458–460, https://doi.org/10.1111 /j.1365–2044.2005.04124.x.

CHAPTER 7

1. S. W. Luger and E. Krauss, "Serologic Tests for Lyme Disease. Interlaboratory Variability," *Archives of Internal Medicine* 150, no. 4 (1990): pp. 761–763, https://doi.org/10.1001 /archinte.1990.00390160039009)
2. Marc G. Golightly, Josephine A. Thomas, and Ana L. Viciana, "The Laboratory Diagnosis of Lyme Borreliosis," *Laboratory Medicine* 21, no. 5 (1990): pp. 299–304, https://doi .org/10.1093/labmed/21.5.299.
3. L. L. Bakken et al., "Interlaboratory Comparison of Test Results for Detection of Lyme Disease by 516 Participants in the Wisconsin State Laboratory of Hygiene/College of American Pathologists Proficiency Testing Program," *Journal of Clinical Microbiology* 35, no. 3 (1997): pp. 537–543, https://doi.org/10.1128/jcm.35.3.537–543.1997.
4. Allen C. Steere et al., "Prospective Study of Serologic Tests for Lyme Disease," *Clinical Infectious Diseases* 47, no. 2 (2008): pp. 188–195, https://doi.org/10.1086/589242.
5. A. C. Steere et al., "Lyme Arthritis: Correlation of Serum and Cryoglobulin IgM With Activity, and Serum IgG With Remission," *Arthritis and Rheumatism* 22, no. 5 (May 1979): pp. 471–483, https://doi.org/10.1002/art.1780220506.
6. J. E. Craft et al., "The Antibody Response in Lyme Disease," *Yale Journal of Biology and Medicine* 57, no. 4 (1984): pp. 561–565.
7. "Association of State and Territorial Public Health Laboratory Directors (ASTPHLD)," in *Second National Conference on the Serologic Diagnosis of Lyme Disease* (Dearborn, MI, 1994).
8. M. E. Aguero-Rosenfeld et al., "Evolution of the Serologic Response to *Borrelia Burgdorferi* in Treated Patients with Culture-Confirmed Erythema Migrans," *Journal of Clinical Microbiology* 34, no. 1 (1996): pp. 1–9, https://doi.org/10.1128/jcm.34.1.1–9.1996.

9.   Steven E. Schutzer et al., "Direct Diagnostic Tests for Lyme Disease," *Clinical Infectious Diseases* 68, no. 6 (March 5, 2019): pp. 1052–1057, https://doi.org/10.1093/cid/ciy614.

10. "Case Definitions for Infectious Conditions Under Public Health Surveillance," *MMWR Morbidity and Mortality Weekly Report* 46, no. RR-10 (1997).

11. S. W. Luger and E. Krauss, "Serologic Tests For Lyme Disease. Interlaboratory Variability," *Archives of Internal Medicine* 150, no. 4 (April 1, 1990): pp. 761–763, https://doi.org/10.1001/archinte.150.4.761.

12. J. S. Shah et al., "Improved Sensitivity of Lyme Disease Western Blots Prepared with a Mixture of Borrelia Burgdorferi Strains 297 and B31," *Chronic Diseases International* 1, no. 2 (December 10, 2014): p. 7.

13. Dr. Jyotsna Shah and Dr. Joseph Burrascano, personal communications with author.

14. Maria E. Aguero-Rosenfeld et al., "Diagnosis of Lyme Borreliosis," *Clinical Microbiology Reviews* 18, no. 3 (July 2005): pp. 484–509, https://doi.org/10.1128/CMR.18.3.484–509.2005.

15. Advanced Lab, accessed January 1, 2018, http://www.advanced-lab.com/news/comment-lyme-tierno.pdf.

16. Raphael B. Stricker and Edward E. Winger, "Decreased Cd57 Lymphocyte Subset in Patients with Chronic Lyme Disease," *Immunology Letters* 76, no. 1 (February 1, 2001): pp. 43–48, https://doi.org/10.1016/s0165-2478(00)00316-3.

17. Sam T. Donta, Richard B. Noto, and John A. Vento, "SPECT Brain Imaging in Chronic Lyme Disease," *Clinical Nuclear Medicine* 37, no. 9 (September 2012): pp. 219–222, https://doi.org/10.1097/rlu.0b013e318262ad9b.

18. Brian A. Fallon et al., "Functional Brain Imaging and Neuropsychological Testing in Lyme Disease," *Clinical Infectious Diseases* 25, no. s1 (1997): pp. s57–s63, https://doi.org/10.1086/516175.

19. A. Newberg, A. Hassan, and A. Alavi, "Cerebral Metabolic Changes Associated with Lyme Disease," *Nuclear Medicine Communications* 23, no. 8 (August 2002): pp. 773–777, https://doi.org/10.1097/00006231-200208000-00011.

CHAPTER 8

1.   Joseph Burrascano, "Advanced Topics In Lyme Disease: Diagnostic Hints and Treatment Guidelines for Lyme and Other Tick Borne Illnesses," Lymenet, accessed July 26, 2019, http://www.lymenet.org/BurrGuide200810.pdf.

2.   D. Terekhova et al., "Erythromycin Resistance in Borrelia Burgdorferi," *Antimicrobial Agents and Chemotherapy* 46, no. 11 (2002): pp. 3637–3640, https://doi.org/10.1128/aac.46.11.3637–3640.2002.

3.   Akshita Datar et al., "In Vitro Effectiveness of Samento and Banderol Herbal Extracts on the Different Morphological Forms of Borrelia Burgdorferi," *Townsend Letter, the Examiner of Alternative Medicine*, July 2010.

4.   Kati Karvonen and Leona Gilbert, "Effective Killing Of Borrelia Burgdorferi in Vitro with Novel Herbal Compounds," *General Medicine Open* 2, no. 6 (2018): pp. 1–4, https://doi.org/10.15761/gmo.1000153.

5.   Anna Goc and Matthias Rath, "The Anti-Borreliae Efficacy of Phytochemicals and Micronutrients: An Update," *Therapeutic Advances in Infectious Disease* 3, no. 3–4 (2016): pp. 75–82, https://doi.org/10.1177/2049936116655502.

6.   Venkata Pothineni et al., "Identification Of New Drug Candidates Against Borrelia Burgdorferi Using High-Throughput Screening," *Drug Design, Development and Therapy* 10 (2016): pp. 1307–1322, https://doi.org/10.2147/dddt.s101486.

7.   K. K. S. Lewis, "Lyme Disease in the Era of Precision Medicine," LymeMind, October 4, 2016, https://www.youtube.com/watch?v=aUlKTnrGPgc.

8.   Kenneth B. Liegner, "Disulfiram (Tetraethylthiuram Disulfide) in the Treatment of Lyme Disease and Babesiosis: Report of Experience in Three Cases," *Antibiotics (Basel)* 8, no. 2 (May 30, 2019): p. 72, https://doi.org/10.3390/antibiotics8020072.

9.   L. W. Scheibel, A. Adler, and W. Trager, "Tetraethylthiuram Disulfide (Antabuse) Inhibits the Human Malaria Parasite Plasmodium Falciparum," *Proceedings of the National Academy of Sciences* 76, no. 10 (January 1979): pp. 5303–5307, https://doi.org/10.1073/pnas.76.10.5303.

10. Olga M. Viquez et al., "Copper Accumulation and Lipid Oxidation Precede Inflammation and Myelin Lesions in N,n-Diethyldithiocarbamate Peripheral Myelinopathy," *Toxicology and Applied Pharmacology* 229, no. 1 (2008): pp. 77–85, https://doi.org/10.1016/j.taap.2008.01.005.

11. D. Ziegler et al., "Oral Treatment With Alpha-Lipoic Acid Improves Symptomatic Diabetic Polyneuropathy: The SYDNEY 2 Trial," *Diabetes Care* 29, no. 11 (2006): pp. 2365–2370, https://doi.org/10.2337/dc06-1216.

12. B. S. Alghamdi, "The Neuroprotective Role of Melatonin in Neurological Disorders," *Journal of Neuroscience Research* 96, no. 7 (January 2018): pp. 1136–1149, https://doi.org/10.1002/jnr.24220.

13. Richard Horowitz and Phyllis Freeman. (2016). The Use of Dapsone as a Novel "Persister" Drug in the Treatment of Chronic Lyme Disease/Post Treatment Lyme Disease Syndrome. *Journal of Clinical and Experimental Dermatology Research*. 07. 10.4172/2155–9554.1000345.

14. Richard Horowitz and Phyllis Freeman. Efficacy of Double-Dose Dapsone Combination Therapy in the Treatment of Chronic Lyme Disease/Post-Treatment Lyme Disease Syndrome (PTLDS) and Associated Co-infections: A Report of Three Cases and Retrospective Chart Review. *Antibiotics*. 2020, 9, 725.

15. Bijaya Sharma et al., "*Borrelia Burgdorferi*, the Causative Agent of Lyme Disease, Forms Drug-Tolerant Persister Cells," *Antimicrobial Agents and Chemotherapy* 59, no. 8 (2015): pp. 4616–4624, https://doi.org/10.1128/aac.00864–15.

16. Øystein Brorson and Sverre-Henning Brorson, "An in Vitro Study of the Susceptibility of Mobile and Cystic Forms of Borrelia Burgdorferi to Metronidazole," *APMIS* 107, no. 6 (June 1999): pp. 566–576, https://doi.org/10.1111/j.1699–0463.1999.tb01594.x.

17. Øystein Brorson and Sverre-Henning Brorson, "An in Vitro Study of the Susceptibility of Mobile and Cystic Forms of Borrelia Urgdorferi to Tinidazole," *International Microbiology* 7, no. 2 (July 2004): pp. 139–142.

18. Øystein Brorson and Sverre-Henning Brorson, "Grapefruit Seed Extract Is a Powerful in Vitro Agent Against Motile and Cystic Forms of *Borrelia Burgdorferi Sensu Lato*," *Infection* 35, no. 3 (June 2007): pp. 206–208, https://doi.org/10.1007/s15010-007-6105-0.

19. Raphael Stricker and E. Sapi, "Evaluation of In-Vitro Antibiotic Susceptibility of Different Morphological Forms of Borrelia Burgdorferi," *Infection and Drug Resistance* 4 (2011): pp. 97–113, https://doi.org/10.2147/idr.s19201.

20. Øystein Brorson and Sverre-Henning Brorson, "An in Vitro Study of the Susceptibility of Mobile and Cystic Forms of *Borrelia Burgdorferi* to Hydroxychloroquine," *International Microbiology* 5, no. 1 (2002): pp. 25–31, https://doi.org/10.1007/s10123-002-0055-2.

21. P. H. Klesius and J. J. Giambrone, "Adoptive Transfer of Delayed Hypersensitivity and Protective Immunity to Eimeria Tenella with Chicken-Derived Transfer Factor," *Poultry Science* 63, no. 7 (1984): pp. 1333–1337, https://doi.org/10.3382/ps.0631333.

22. P. L. Fidel, J. Cutright, and C. Steele, "Effects of Reproductive Hormones on Experimental Vaginal Candidiasis," *Infection and Immunity* 68, no. 2 (January 2000): pp. 651–657, https://doi.org/10.1128/iai.68.2.651–657.2000.

23. Jennifer M. Tung, Lisa R. Dolovich, and Christine H. Lee, "Prevention of Clostridium Difficile Infection with Saccharomyces Boullardii: A Systematic Review," *Canadian Journal of Gastroenterology* 23, no. 12 (December 2009): pp. 817–821, https://doi.org/10.1155/2009/915847.

24. E. Krajewska-Kułak, C. Krajewska-Kułak E Lukaszuk, and W. Niczyporuk, "Effects of 33% Grapefruit Extract on the Growth of the Yeast-Like Fungi, Dermatopytes and Moulds," *Wiadomosci Parazytologiczne* 47, no. 4 (2001): pp. 845–849.

25. Anna Goc and Matthias Rath, "The Anti-Borreliae Efficacy of Phytochemicals and Micronutrients: An Update," *Therapeutic Advances in Infectious Disease* 3, no. 3–4 (2016): pp. 75–82, https://doi.org/10.1177/2049936116655502.

26. Sam T. Donta, "Macrolide Therapy for Chronic Lyme Disease," *Medical Science Monitor* 9, no. 11 (November 2003): pp. PI136–PI142.

27. Thomas Butler, "The Jarisch–Herxheimer Reaction After Antibiotic Treatment of Spirochetal Infections: A Review of Recent Cases and Our Understanding of Pathogenesis," *American Journal of Tropical Medicine and Hygiene* 96, no. 1 (2016): pp. 46–52, https://doi.org/10.4269/ajtmh.16–0434.

28. Raphael B. Stricker and Lorraine B. Johnson, "Persistent Infection in Chronic Lyme Disease. Does Form Matter?," *Research Journal of Infectious Diseases* 1, no. 2 (2013), https://doi.org/10.7243/2052-5958-1-2.

29. Jennifer M. Tung, Lisa R. Dolovich, and Christine H. Lee, "Prevention of *Clostridium Difficile* Infection with *Saccharomyces Boullardii*: A Systematic Review," *Canadian Journal of Gastroenterology* 23, no. 12 (December 2009): pp. 817–821, https://doi.org/10.1155/2009/915847.

30. S. Kalghatgi et al., "Bactericidal Antibiotics Induce Mitochondrial Dysfunction and Oxidative Damage in Mammalian Cells," *Science Translational Medicine* 5, no. 192 (March 2013), https://doi.org/10.1126/scitranslmed.3006055.

31. Pamela Weintraub, *Cure Unknown: Inside the Lyme Epidemic* (New York: St. Martin's Griffin, 2013).

CHAPTER 9

1. Diane M. Gubernot et al., "Conference Report: Transfusion-Transmitted Babesiosis in the United States: Summary of a Workshop," *Transfusion* 49, no. 12 (October 2009): pp. 2759–2771, https://doi.org/10.1111/j.1537-2995.2009.02429.x.

2. P. J. Krause et al., "Concurrent Lyme Disease and Babesiosis, Evidence for Increased Severity and Duration of Illness," *JAMA* 275, no. 21 (June 5, 1996): pp. 1657–1660, https://doi.org/10.1001/jama.275.21.1657.

3. Peter J. Krause et al., "Disease-Specific Diagnosis of Coinfecting Tickborne Zoonoses: Babesiosis, Human Granulocytic Ehrlichiosis, and Lyme Disease," *Clinical Infectious Diseases* 34, no. 9 (2002): pp. 1184–1191, https://doi.org/10.1086/339813.

4. "Twelfth International Scientific Conference on Lyme Disease and Other Spirochetal & Tick Borne Disorders" (New York City/New Jersey, 1999).

5. Elizabeth Stein et al., "Babesiosis Surveillance—Wisconsin, 2001–2015," *MMWR Morbidity and Mortality Weekly Report* 66, no. 26 (July 2017): pp. 687–691, https://doi.org/10.15585/mmwr.mm6626a2.

6. Peter J. Krause et al., "Persistent Parasitemia after Acute Babesiosis," *New England Journal of Medicine* 339, no. 3 (1998): pp. 160–165, https://doi.org/10.1056/nejm199807163390304.

7. Evan M. Bloch et al., "A Prospective Evaluation of Chronicbabesia Microtiinfection in Seroreactive Blood Donors," *Transfusion* 56, no. 7 (2016): pp. 1875–1882, https://doi.org/10.1111/trf.13617.

8. Peter J. Krause et al., "Atovaquone and Azithromycin for the Treatment of Babesiosis," *New England Journal of Medicine* 343, no. 20 (2000): pp. 1454–1458, https://doi.org/10.1056/nejm200011163432004.

9. "Fact Sheet: World Malaria Report 2015," World Health Organization, April 19, 2016, https://www.who.int/malaria/media/world-malaria-report-2015/en.

10. Didier Ménard and David A Fidock, "Accelerated Evolution and Spread of Multidrug-Resistant Plasmodium Falciparum Takes Down the Latest First-Line Antimalarial Drug in Southeast Asia," *Lancet Infectious Diseases* 19, no. 9 (2019): pp. 916–917, https://doi.org/10.1016/s1473-3099(19)30394-9.

11. L. W. Scheibel, A. Adler, and W. Trager, "Tetraethylthiuram Disulfide (Antabuse) Inhibits the Human Malaria Parasite Plasmodium Falciparum," *Proceedings of the National Academy of Sciences* 76, no. 10 (January 1979): pp. 5303–5307, https://doi.org/10.1073/pnas.76.10.5303.

12. Kenneth B. Liegner, "Disulfiram (Tetraethylthiuram Disulfide) in the Treatment of Lyme Disease and Babesiosis: Report of Experience in Three Cases," *Antibiotics (Basel)* 8, no. 2 (May 30, 2019): p. 72, https://doi.org/10.3390/antibiotics8020072.

13. Venkata Pothineni et al., "Identification of New Drug Candidates Against Borrelia Burgdorferi Using High-Throughput Screening," *Drug Design, Development and Therapy* 10 (2016): pp. 1307–1322, https://doi.org/10.2147/dddt.s101486.

CHAPTER 10

1. E. B. Breitschwerdt, S. Sontakke, and S. Hopkins, "Neurological Manifestations of Bartonellosis in Immunocompetent Patients: A Composite of Reports from 2005–2012," *Journal of Neuroparasitology* 3 (2012): pp. 1–15, https://doi.org/10.4303/jnp/235640.

2. S. A. Billeter et al., "Vector Transmission of Bartonella Species with Emphasis on the Potential for Tick Transmission," *Medical and Veterinary Entomology* 22, no. 1 (2008): pp. 1–15, https://doi.org/10.1111/j.1365-2915.2008.00713.x.

3. Eugene Eskow, Raja-Vemkitesh S. Rao, and Eli Mordechai, "Concurrent Infection of the Central Nervous System by *Borrelia Burgdorferi* and *Bartonella Henselae*: Evidence for a Novel Tick-Borne Disease Complex," *Archives of Neurology* 58, no. 9 (January 2001): pp. 1357–1363, https://doi.org/10.1001/archneur.58.9.1357.

4. Leo M. Schouls et al., "Detection and Identification of Ehrlichia, Borrelia Burgdorferi Sensu Lato, and Bartonella Species in Dutch Ixodes Ricinus Ticks," *Journal of Clinical Microbiology* 37, no. 7 (July 1999): pp. 2215–2222.

5. M. E. Adelson et al., "Prevalence of *Borrelia Burgdorferi, Bartonella Spp., Babesia Microti,* and *Anaplasma Phagocytophila* in Ixodes Scapularis Ticks Collected in Northern New Jersey," *Journal of Clinical Microbiology* 42, no. 6 (January 2004): pp. 2799–2801, https://doi.org/10.1128/jcm.42.6.2799-2801.2004.

6. Nandhakumar Balakrishnan et al., "Vasculitis, Cerebral Infarction and Persistent *Bartonella Henselae* Infection in a Child," *Parasites & Vectors* 9, no. 1 (October 2016): p. 254, https://doi.org/10.1186/s13071-016-1547-9.

7. Despoina N. Maritsi et al., "Bartonella Henselae Infection: An Uncommon Mimicker of Autoimmune Disease," *Case Reports in Pediatrics* 2013 (2013): pp. 1–4, https://doi.org/10.1155/2013/726826.

8. E. B. Breitschwerdt et al., "Bartonella Species Bacteremia in Patients with Neurological and Neurocognitive Dysfunction," *Journal of Clinical Microbiology* 46, no. 9 (2008): pp. 2856–2861, https://doi.org/10.1128/jcm.00832-08.

9. M. D. Fried et al., "*Bartonella Henselae* Is Associated with Heartburn, Abdominal Pain, Skin Rash, Mesenteric Adenitis, Gastritis and Duodenitis," *Journal of Pediatric Gastroenterology and Nutrition* 35, no. 3 (2002): Abstract 158.

10. Volkhard A. J. Kempf et al., "Evidence of a Leading Role for VEGF in Bartonella Henselae-Induced Endothelial Cell Proliferations," *Cellular Microbiology* 3, no. 9 (2001): pp. 623–632, https://doi.org/10.1046/j.1462-5822.2001.00144.x.

11. Maritsi, "*Bartonella Henselae* Infection: An Uncommon Mimicker of Autoimmune Disease," 1–3.

12. Rosa Maria Chiuri et al., "*Bartonella Henselae* Infection Associated with Autoimmune Thyroiditis in a Child," *Hormone Research in Paediatrics* 79, no. 3 (2013): pp. 185–188, https://doi.org/10.1159/000346903.

13. A. Van Audenhove et al., "Autoimmune Haemolytic Anaemia Triggered by *Bartonella Henselae* Infection: A Case Report," *British Journal of Haematology* 115, no. 4 (2001): pp. 924–925, https://doi.org/10.1046/j.1365-2141.2001.03165.x.

14. M. Tsukahara et al., "Bartonella Infection Associated with Systemic Juvenile Rheumatoid Arthritis," *Clinical Infectious Diseases* 32, no. 1 (January 2001): pp. 22–23, https://doi.org/10.1086/317532.

15. E. Cozzani et al., "Onset of Cutaneous Vasculitis and Exacerbation of IgA Nephropathy After Bartonella Henselae Infection," *Clinical and Experimental Dermatology* 37, no. 3 (October 2011): pp. 238–240, https://doi.org/10.1111/j.1365-2230.2011.04177.x.

16. Laszlo Hopp and Stephen C. Eppes, "Development of IgA Nephritis Following Cat Scratch Disease in a 13-Year-Old Boy," *Pediatric Nephrology* 19, no. 6 (January 2004): pp. 682–684, https://doi.org/10.1007/s00467-004-1432-1.

17. Michael Giladi et al., "Cat-Scratch Disease—Associated Arthropathy," *Arthritis and Rheumatology* 52, no. 11 (October 27, 2005): pp. 3611–3617, https://doi.org/10.1002/art.21411.

18. Ricardo G. Maggi et al., "*Bartonella Spp.* Bacteremia and Rheumatic Symptoms in Patients from Lyme Disease–Endemic Region," *Emerging Infectious Diseases* 18, no. 5 (2012): pp. 783–791, https://doi.org/10.3201/eid1805.111366.

19. Areum Durey et al., "*Bartonella Henselae* Infection Presenting with a Picture of Adult-Onset Still's Disease," *International Journal of Infectious Diseases* 46 (2016): pp. 61–63, https://doi.org/10.1016/j.ijid.2016.03.014.

20. Maggi, "*Bartonella Spp.* Bacteremia and Rheumatic Symptoms in Patients from Lyme Disease–Endemic Region," 783–791.

21. B. Stockmeyer et al., "Chronic Vasculitis and Polyneuropathy Due to Infection with *Bartonella Henselae*," *Infection* 35, no. 2 (2007): pp. 107–109, https://doi.org/10.1007/s15010-007-6021-3.

22. Maggi, "*Bartonella Spp.* Bacteremia and Rheumatic Symptoms in Patients from Lyme Disease–Endemic Region," 783–791.

23. Francesco Massei et al., "*Bartonella Henselae* Infection Associated with Guillain-Barré Syndrome," *Pediatric Infectious Disease Journal* 25, no. 1 (2006): pp. 90–91, https://doi.org/10.1097/01.inf.0000195642.28901.98.

24. E. Cozzani et al., "Onset of Cutaneous Vasculitis and Exacerbation of IgA Nephropathy After *Bartonella Henselae* Infection," *Clinical and Experimental Dermatology* 37, no. 3 (October 2011): pp. 238–240, https://doi.org/10.1111/j.1365-2230.2011.04177.x.

25. Stockmeyer, "Chronic Vasculitis and Polyneuropathy Due to Infection with *Bartonella Henselae*," 107–109.

26. Emilio Palumbo et al., "Immune Thrombocytopenic Purpura as a Complication of *Bartonella Henselae* Infection," *Le Infezioni in Medicina* 16, no. 2 (July 2008): pp. 99–102.

27. P. Baylor et al., "Transverse Myelitis in Two Patients with *Bartonella Henselae* Infection (Cat Scratch Disease)," *Clinical Infectious Diseases* 45, no. 4 (2007): pp. e42–e45, https://doi.org/10.1086/519998.

28. Elia M. Ayoub et al., "Role of *Bartonella Henselae* in the Etiology of Henoch-Schönlein Purpura," *Pediatric Infectious Disease Journal* 21, no. 1 (2002): pp. 28–31, https://doi.org/10.1097/00006454-200201000-00006.

29. Joan L Robinson et al., "Bartonella Seropositivity in Children with Henoch-Schonlein Purpura," *BMC Infectious Diseases* 5, no. 1 (2005): p. 21, https://doi.org/10.1186/1471-2334-5-21.

30. Edward B Breitschwerdt et al., "*Bartonella Henselae* Bloodstream Infection in a Boy With Pediatric Acute-Onset Neuropsychiatric Syndrome," *Journal of Central Nervous System Disease* 11 (2019), https://doi.org/10.1177/1179573519832014.

31. Silpak Biswas and Jean-Marc Rolain, "Bartonella Infection: Treatment and Drug Resistance," *Future Microbiology* 5, no. 11 (2010): pp. 1719–1731, https://doi.org/10.2217/fmb.10.133.

32. K. Pfister et al., "Diminished Ciprofloxacin-Induced Chondrotoxicity by Supplementation with Magnesium and Vitamin E in Immature Rats," *Antimicrobial Agents and Chemotherapy* 51, no. 3 (August 2007): pp. 1022–1027, https://doi.org/10.1128/aac.01175–06.

33. Tingting Li et al., "Identification of FDA-Approved Drugs with Activity against Stationary Phase Bartonella Henselae," *Antibiotics* 8, no. 2 (2019): p. 50, https://doi.org/10.3390/antibiotics8020050.

34. Venkata Pothineni et al., "Identification of New Drug Candidates Against *Borrelia Burgdorferi* Using High-Throughput Screening," *Drug Design, Development and Therapy* 10 (2016): pp. 1307–1322, https://doi.org/10.2147/dddt.s101486.

35. M. D. Fried et al., "*Bartonella Henselae* Is Associated with Heartburn, Abdominal Pain, Skin Rash, Mesenteric Adenitis, Gastritis and Duodenitis," *Journal of Pediatric Gastroenterology and Nutrition* 35, no. 3 (2002): Abstract 158.

36. Francesco Massei et al., "*Bartonella Henselae* and Inflammatory Bowel Disease," *Lancet* 356, no. 9237 (2000): pp. 1245–1246, https://doi.org/10.1016/s0140-6736(00)02796-3

37. Maile Young Karris et al., "*Bartonella Henselae* Infection of Prosthetic Aortic Valve Associated with Colitis," *Vector-Borne and Zoonotic Diseases* 11, no. 11 (2011): pp. 1503–1505, https://doi.org/10.1089/vbz.2010.0169.

38. Alessandro Ventura et al., "Systemic *Bartonella Henselae* Infection with Hepatosplenic Involvement," *Journal of Pediatric Gastroenterology & Nutrition* 29, no. 1 (1999): pp. 52–56, https://doi.org/10.1097/00005176-199907000-00014.

39. Daniel Kinderlehrer, "Primary Sclerosing Cholangitis Caused by Bartonella: A Case Report," in *Nineteenth Annual ILADS Conference* (Chicago, IL, 2018).

CHAPTER 11

1. Garth Nicolson et al., "Mycoplasmal Infections in Chronic Illnesses: Fibromyalgia and Chronic Fatigue Syndromes, Gulf War Illness, HIV-AIDS and Rheumatoid Arthritis," *Medical Sentinel* 4 (1999): pp. 172–176.

2. Garth Nicolson et al., "Diagnosis and Integrative Treatment of Intracellular Bacterial Infections in Chronic Fatigue and Fibromyalgia Syndromes, Gulf War Illness, Rheumatoid Arthritis and Other Chronic Illnesses," *Clinical Practice of Alternative Medicine* 1 (2000): pp. 92–102.

3. Garth Nicolson, Nancy Nicolson, and Joerg Haier, "Chronic Fatigue Syndrome Patients Subsequently Diagnosed with Lyme Disease *Borrelia Burgdorferi*: Evidence for Mycoplasma Species Coinfections," *Journal of Chronic Fatigue Syndrome* 14, no. 4 (2008): pp. 5–17, https://doi.org/10.1080/10573320802091809.

4. Surender Kashyap and Malay Sarkar, "Mycoplasma Pneumonia: Clinical Features and Management," *Lung India* 27, no. 2 (2010): pp. 75–85, https://doi.org/10.4103/0970–2113.63611.

5. Sándor Hornok et al., "Molecular Investigation of Hard Ticks (Acari: Ixodidae) and Fleas (Siphonaptera: Pulicidae) As Potential Vectors of Rickettsial and Mycoplasmal Agents," *Veterinary Microbiology* 140, no. 1–2 (2009): pp. 98–104, https://doi.org/10.1016/j.vetmic.2009.07.013.

6. Walter Berghoff, "Chronic Lyme Disease and Co-Infections: Differential Diagnosis," *Open Neurology Journal* 6, no. 1 (2012): pp. 158–178, https://doi.org/10.2174/1874205x01206010158.

7. J. Yang et al., "Regulation of Proinflammatory Cytokines in Human Lung Epithelial Cells Infected with Mycoplasma Pneumoniae," *Infection and Immunity* 70, no. 7 (2002): pp. 3649–3655, https://doi.org/10.1128/iai.70.7.3649–3655.2002.

8. F. Blasco Patiño, R. Pérez Maestu, and J. M. López de Letona, "Mechanisms of Disease in Mycoplasma Pneumoniae Infection. Clinical Manifestations and Complications," *Revista Clínica Española* 204, no. 7 (2004): pp. 365–368, https://doi.org/10.1157/13063528.

9. K. B. Waites and D. F. Talkington, "Mycoplasma Pneumoniae and Its Role as a Human Pathogen," *Clinical Microbiology Reviews* 17, no. 4 (2004): pp. 697–728, https://doi.org/10.1128/cmr.17.4.697-728.2004.

10. Jennifer Frankovich et al., "Five Youth with Pediatric Acute-Onset Neuropsychiatric Syndrome of Differing Etiologies," *Journal of Child and Adolescent Psychopharmacology* 25, no. 1 (2015): pp. 31–37, https://doi.org/10.1089/cap.2014.0056.

CHAPTER 12

1. M. B. Allen et al., "First Reported Case of *Ehrlichia Ewingii* Involving Human Bone Marrow," *Journal of Clinical Microbiology* 52, no. 11 (2014): pp. 4102–4104, https://doi.org/10.1128/jcm.01670-14.

2. "Geographic Distribution of Ticks That Bite Humans," Centers for Disease Control and Prevention, January 10, 2019, https://www.cdc.gov/ticks/geographic_distribution.html.

3. Sylvie J. De Martino, Jason A. Carlyon, and Erol Fikrig, "Coinfection with *Borrelia Burgdorferi* and the Agent of Human Granulocytic Ehrlichiosis," *New England Journal of Medicine* 345, no. 2 (2001): pp. 150–151, https://doi.org/10.1056/nejm200107123450218.

4. Khalid Abusaada, Saira Ajmal, and Laura Hughes, "Successful Treatment of Human Monocytic Ehrlichiosis with Rifampin," *Cureus* 8, no. 1 (2016): p. e444, https://doi.org/10.7759/cureus.444.

5. Danilo G. Saraiva et al., "Feeding Period Required by Amblyomma Aureolatum Ticks for Transmission of *Rickettsia Rickettsii* to Vertebrate Hosts," *Emerging Infectious Diseases* 20, no. 9 (2014): pp. 1504–1510, https://doi.org/10.3201/eid2009.140189.

6. V M. F. Vaughn et al., "Seroepidemiologic Study of Human Infections with Spotted Fever Group Rickettsiae in North Carolina," *Journal of Clinical Microbiology* 52, no. 11 (2014): pp. 3960–3966, https://doi.org/10.1128/jcm.01733-14.

7. A. Katz, "NADAL—Neuropsychiatric Autoimmune Disorder Associated with Lyme Disease—A PANDAS/PANS Equivalent: Diagnosis and Treatment," in *19th Annual Conference of the International Lyme and Associated Diseases* (Chicago, IL, 2018).

8. Jennifer Frankovich et al., "Five Youth with Pediatric Acute-Onset Neuropsychiatric Syndrome of Differing Etiologies," *Journal of Child and Adolescent Psychopharmacology* 25, no. 1 (2015): pp. 31–37, https://doi.org/10.1089/cap.2014.0056.

9. Edward B Breitschwerdt et al., "*Bartonella Henselae* Bloodstream Infection in a Boy with Pediatric Acute-Onset Neuropsychiatric Syndrome," *Journal of Central Nervous System Disease* 11 (2019), https://doi.org/10.1177/1179573519832014.

10. Hanna Rhee and Daniel Cameron, "Lyme Disease and Pediatric Autoimmune Neuropsychiatric Disorders Associated with Streptococcal Infections (PANDAS): An Overview," *International Journal of General Medicine* 5 (2012): pp. 163–174, https://doi.org/10.2147/ijgm.s24212.

CHAPTER 13

1. "Symptoms, Diagnosis and Treatment," Centers for Disease Control and Prevention, November 19, 2018, https://www.cdc.gov/stari/symptoms/index.html.

2. Edwin J. Masters, Chelsea N. Grigery, and Reid W. Masters, "STARI, or Masters Disease: Lone Star Tick–Vectored Lyme-Like Illness," *Infectious Disease Clinics of North America* 22, no. 2 (2008): pp. 361–376, https://doi.org/10.1016/j.idc.2007.12.010.

3.   E. J. Masters and H. D. Donnell, "Lyme and/or Lyme-Like Disease in Missouri," *Missouri Medicine* 92, no. 7 (1995): pp. 346–353.
4.   Pamela Weintraub, "Rebel with a Cause: The Incredible Dr. Masters, Part 1," *Psychology Today*, June 25, 2009, https://www.psychologytoday.com/us/blog/emerging -diseases/200906/rebel-cause-the-incredible-dr-masters-part-1.
5.   Kirby C Stafford et al., "Distribution and Establishment of the Lone Star Tick in Connecticut and Implications for Range Expansion and Public Health," *Journal of Medical Entomology* 55, no. 6 (2018): pp. 1561–1568, https://doi.org/10.1093/jme/tjy115.
6.   Chris Crowder et al., "Prevalence of *Borrelia Miyamotoi* in Ixodes Ticks in Europe and the United States," *Emerging Infectious Diseases* 20, no. 10 (2014): pp. 1678–1682, https://doi. org/10.3201/eid2010.131583.
7.   Peter J. Krause et al., "Human Borrelia Miyamotoi Infection in the United States," *New England Journal of Medicine* 368, no. 3 (2013): pp. 291–293, https://doi.org/10.1056 /nejmc1215469.
8.   Sam R. Telford et al., "Borrelia Miyamotoi Disease: Neither Lyme Disease Nor Relapsing Fever," *Clinics in Laboratory Medicine* 35, no. 4 (2015): pp. 867–882, https://doi.org/10.1016/j .cll.2015.08.002.
9.   Lindsay Rollend, Durland Fish, and James E. Childs, "Transovarial Transmission of *Borrelia Spirochetes* by Ixodes Scapularis: A Summary of the Literature and Recent Observations," *Ticks and Tick-Borne Diseases* 4, no. 1–2 (2013): pp. 46–51, https://doi .org/10.1016/j.ttbdis.2012.06.008.

CHAPTER 14

1.   Holly M. Frost et al., "Serologic Evidence of Powassan Virus Infection in Patients with Suspected Lyme Disease," *Emerging Infectious Diseases* 23, no. 8 (2017): pp. 1384–1388, https://doi.org/10.3201/eid2308.161971.
2.   Frost, "Serologic Evidence of Powassan Virus Infection in Patients with Suspected Lyme Disease," 1384–1388.
3.   A. Thomm and K. Knox, "Development of a Serologic Test Panel for Detection of Powassan Virus Infection," *Clinical Virology Symposium* Abstract 249 (2016).
4.   Gregory D. Ebel and Laura D. Kramer, "Short Report: Duration of Tick Attachment Required for Transmission of Powassan Virus by Deer Ticks," *American Journal of Tropical Medicine and Hygiene* 71, no. 3 (2004): pp. 268–271, https://doi.org/10.4269 /ajtmh.2004.71.3.0700268.
5.   Meghan E. Hermance and Saravanan Thangamani, "Powassan Virus: An Emerging Arbovirus of Public Health Concern in North America," *Vector-Borne and Zoonotic Diseases* 17, no. 7 (2017): pp. 453–462, https://doi.org/10.1089/vbz.2017.2110.

CHAPTER 15

1.   Hans Selye, "A Syndrome Produced by Diverse Nocuous Agents," *Nature* 138, no. 3479 (1936): p. 32, https://doi.org/10.1038/138032a0.
2.   W. M. Jefferies, "Cortisol and Immunity," *Medical Hypotheses* 34, no. 3 (1991): pp. 198–208, https://doi.org/10.1016/0306-9877(91)90212-h.
3.   William McK. Jefferies, *Safe Uses of Cortisone* (Springfield, IL: Charles C Thomas Publisher, 1981).
4.   Mitch D. Vanbruggen et al., "The Relationship Between Serum and Salivary Cortisol Levels in Response to Different Intensities of Exercise," *International Journal of Sports Physiology and Performance* 6, no. 3 (2011): pp. 396–407, https://doi.org/10.1123/ijspp.6.3.396.
5.   Jeffries, *Safe Uses of Cortisone.*

6.   Juergen Kratzsch et al., "New Reference Intervals for Thyrotropin and Thyroid Hormones Based on National Academy of Clinical Biochemistry Criteria and Regular Ultrasonography of the Thyroid," *Clinical Chemistry* 51, no. 8 (2005): pp. 1480–1486, https://doi.org/10.1373/clinchem.2004.047399.

7.   Stig Andersen et al., "Narrow Individual Variations in Serum T4 and T3 in Normal Subjects: A Clue to the Understanding of Subclinical Thyroid Disease," *Journal of Clinical Endocrinology & Metabolism* 87, no. 3 (2002): pp. 1068–1072, https://doi.org/10.1210/jcem.87.3.8165.

8.   Nicolas Rodondi et al., "Subclinical Hypothyroidism and the Risk of Coronary Heart Disease and Mortality," *JAMA* 304, no. 12 (2010): pp. 1365–1374, https://doi.org/10.1001/jama.2010.1361.

9.   Christian Meier et al., "Serum Thyroid Stimulating Hormone in Assessment of Severity of Tissue Hypothyroidism in Patients with Overt Primary Thyroid Failure: Cross Sectional Survey," *BMJ* 326, no. 7384 (2003): pp. 311–312, https://doi.org/10.1136/bmj.326.7384.311.

10.   H. F. Escobar-Morreale et al., "Replacement Therapy for Hypothyroidism with Thyroxine Alone Does Not Ensure Euthyroidism in All Tissues, as Studied in Thyroidectomized Rats.," *Journal of Clinical Investigation* 96, no. 6 (January 1995): pp. 2828–2838, https://doi.org/10.1172/jci118353.

11.   H. F. Escobar-Morreale et al., "Only the Combined Treatment with Thyroxine and Triiodothyronine Ensures Euthyroidism in All Tissues of the Thyroidectomized Rat," *Endocrinology* 137, no. 6 (1996): pp. 2490–2502, https://doi.org/10.1210/endo.137.6.8641203.

12.   Robertas Bunevičius et al., "Effects of Thyroxine as Compared with Thyroxine plus Triiodothyronine in Patients with Hypothyroidism," *New England Journal of Medicine* 340, no. 6 (1999): pp. 424–429, https://doi.org/10.1056/nejm199902113400603.

13.   Vijay Panicker et al., "Common Variation in the DIO2 Gene Predicts Baseline Psychological Well-Being and Response to Combination Thyroxine Plus Triiodothyronine Therapy in Hypothyroid Patients," *Journal of Clinical Endocrinology & Metabolism* 94, no. 5 (2009): pp. 1623–1629, https://doi.org/10.1210/jc.2008–1301.

14.   Jacqueline Jonklaas et al., "Single Dose T3 Administration: Kinetics and Effects on Biochemical and Physiologic Parameters," *Therapeutic Drug Monitoring* 37, no. 1 (2015): pp. 110–118, https://doi.org/10.1097/ftd.0000000000000113.

15.   S. Kohler et al., "Timing of Thyroxine Dose Adjustment in Hypothyroid Patients: When Are TSH Levels Stable?," *Journal of Thyroid Disorders & Therapy* 3, no. 3 (2014), https://doi.org/10.4172/2167-7948.1000161.

16.   Forest Tennant and Lisa Lichota, "Testosterone Replacement in Chronic Pain Patients," *Practical Pain Management* 10, no. 6 (2010): pp. 1–8.

17.   Chris J. Malkin et al., "The Effect of Testosterone Replacement on Endogenous Inflammatory Cytokines and Lipid Profiles in Hypogonadal Men," *Journal of Clinical Endocrinology & Metabolism* 89, no. 7 (2004): pp. 3313–3318, https://doi.org/10.1210/jc.2003–031069.

18.   Carlo Pergola et al., "Testosterone Suppresses Phospholipase D, Causing Sex Differences in Leukotriene Biosynthesis in Human Monocytes," *FASEB Journal* 25, no. 10 (2011): pp. 3377–3387, https://doi.org/10.1096/fj.11–182758.

19.   Lindsey E Crosnoe-Shipley et al., "Treatment of Hypogonadotropic Male Hypogonadism: Case-Based Scenarios," *World Journal of Nephrology* 4, no. 2 (2015): pp. 245–253, https://doi.org/10.5527/wjn.v4.i2.245.

20.   Crosnoe-Shipley, "Treatment of Hypogonadotropic Male Hypogonadism: Case-Based Scenarios," 245–253.

21.   Andrea D. Coviello et al., "Low-Dose Human Chorionic Gonadotropin Maintains Intratesticular Testosterone in Normal Men with Testosterone-Induced Gonadotropin Suppression," *Journal of Clinical Endocrinology & Metabolism* 90, no. 5 (2005): pp. 2595–2602, https://doi.org/10.1210/jc.2004–0802.

22. M. Maggio et al., "Circulating Inflammatory Cytokine Expression in Men With Prostate Cancer Undergoing Androgen Deprivation Therapy," *Journal of Andrology* 27, no. 6 (2006): pp. 725–728, https://doi.org/10.2164/jandrol.106.000141.

23. Oliver Seyfried and Joan Hester, "Opioids and Endocrine Dysfunction," *British Journal of Pain* 6, no. 1 (2012): pp. 17–24, https://doi.org/10.1177/2049463712438299.

24. S Telisman et al., "Semen Quality and Reproductive Endocrine Function in Relation to Biomarkers of Lead, Cadmium, Zinc, and Copper in Men," *Environmental Health Perspectives* 108, no. 1 (2000): pp. 45–53, https://doi.org/10.1289/ehp.0010845.

25. Kamila Sitwell, "Sugar Consumption Now vs 100 Years Ago ," Divine Eating Out, accessed February 14, 2018, http://www.divineeatingout.com/food-1/sugar-consumption -now-vs-100-years-ago.

26. Obesity Society, accessed February 14, 2018, http://www.obesity.org/obesity/news/press -releases/us-adult.

27. John Yudkin, "Diet and Coronary Thrombosis Hypothesis and Fact," *Lancet* 273, no. 6987 (1957): pp. 155–162, https://doi.org/10.1016/s0140-6736(57)90614-1.

28. John Yudkin, "Dietary Fat and Dietary Sugar in Relation to Ischæmic Heart-Disease and Diabetes," *Lancet* 284, no. 7349 (1964): pp. 4–5, https://doi.org/10.1016/s0140 -6736(64)90002-9.

29. "Nutrition and Your Health: Dietary Guidelines for Americans, 1990," US Department of Health and Human Services and Department of Agriculture, 1990, https://doi.org/10.1037 /e566932010-001.

30. Cristin E. Kearns, Laura A. Schmidt, and Stanton A. Glantz, "Sugar Industry and Coronary Heart Disease Research. A Historical Analysis of Internal Industry Documents," *JAMA Internal Medicine* 176, no. 11 (January 2016): pp. 1680–1685, https://doi.org/10.1001 /jamainternmed.2016.5394.

31. Victoria Larned, "Obesity Among All US Adults Reaches All-Time High," CNN (Cable News Network, October 13, 2017), https://www.cnn.com/2017/10/13/health/adult-obesity- -increase-study/index.html.

32. David C. Klonoff, "The Increasing Incidence of Diabetes in the 21st Century," *Journal of Diabetes Science and Technology* 3, no. 1 (2009): pp. 1–2, https://doi.org/10.1177/19322968 0900300101).

33. Steven E. Shoelson, Jongsoon B. Lee, and Allison undefined Goldfine, "Inflammation and Insulin Resistance," *Journal of Clinical Investigation* 116, no. 7 (January 2006): pp. 1793– 1801, https://doi.org/10.1172/JCI29069.

CHAPTER 16

1.   Kaitlin Occhipinti and James W. Smith, "Irritable Bowel Syndrome: A Review and Update," *Clinics in Colon and Rectal Surgery* 25, no. 1 (2012): pp. 46–52, https://doi.org /10.1055/s-0032-1301759.

2.   V. Alun-Jones et al., "Food Intolerance: A Major Factor in the Pathogenesis of Irritable Bowel Syndrome," *Lancet* 320, no. 8308 (1982): pp. 1115–1117, https://doi.org/10.1016 /s0140-6736(82)92782-9.

3.   Theron G. Randolph and Ralph W. Moss, *An Alternative Approach to Allergies* (New York: Bantam Books, 1982).

4.   Martin B Van Der Weyden, Ruth M Armstrong, and Ann T Gregory, "The 2005 Nobel Prize in Physiology or Medicine," *Medical Journal of Australia* 183, no. 11–12 (2005): pp. 612–614, https://doi.org/10.5694/j.1326-5377.2005.tb00052.x.

5.   Helge L. Waldum, Per M. Kleveland, and Øystein F. Sørdal, "Helicobacter Pyloriand Gastric Acid: An Intimate and Reciprocal Relationship," *Therapeutic Advances in Gastroenterology* 9, no. 6 (2016): pp. 836–844, https://doi.org/10.1177/1756283x16663395.

6.   A. Sencer Yurtsever et al., "Proton Pump Inhibitors Omeprazole, Lansoprazole and Pantoprazole Induce Relaxation in the Rat Lower Oesophageal Sphincter," *Journal of Pharmacy and Pharmacology* 63, no. 10 (2011): pp. 1295–1300, https://doi.org /10.1111/j.2042–7158.2011.01333.x.

7.   "Testing for Low Stomach Acidity," Well Life Family Medicine, accessed January 29, 2018, http://welllifefm.com/wp-content/uploads/2017/04/Testing-Low-Stomach-Acidity.pdf.

8.   K. S. W. Tan, "New Insights on Classification, Identification, and Clinical Relevance of *Blastocystis Spp.*," *Clinical Microbiology Reviews* 21, no. 4 (2008): pp. 639–665, https://doi .org/10.1128/cmr.00022–08.

9.   Emanuel Lebenthal and R. Guerrant, "Parasitic Causes of Disease," in *Textbook of Secretory Diarrhea* (New York: Raven Press, 1990), pp. 273–280.

10. Fangli Lu and Shiguang Huang, "The Roles of Mast Cells in Parasitic Protozoan Infections," *Frontiers in Immunology* 8 (2017): p. 363, https://doi.org/10.3389/fimmu .2017.00363.

11. Rick M. Maizels and Henry J. McSorley, "Regulation of the Host Immune System by Helminth Parasites," *Journal of Allergy and Clinical Immunology* 138, no. 3 (2016): pp. 666–675, https://doi.org/10.1016/j.jaci.2016.07.007.

12. Mahmoud Abu-Shakra and Yehuda Shoenfeld, "Parasitic Infection and Autoimmunity," *Autoimmunity* 9, no. 4 (1991): pp. 337–344, https://doi.org/10.3109/08916939108997136.

13. I. H. Mchardy et al., "Detection of Intestinal Protozoa in the Clinical Laboratory," *Journal of Clinical Microbiology* 52, no. 3 (June 2013): pp. 712–720, https://doi.org/10.1128/jcm .02877–13.

14. A. C. Dukowicz, B. E. Lacy, and G. M. Levine, "Small Intestinal Bacterial Overgrowth: A Comprehensive Review," *Gastroenterology Hepatology* 3, no. 2 (2007): pp. 112–122.

15. A. R. Khalighi et al., "Evaluating the Efficacy of Probiotic on Treatment in Patients With Small Intestinal Bacterial Overgrowth (SIBO)—a Pilot Study," *Indian Journal of Medical Research* 140, no. 5 (2014): pp. 604–608.

16. Luis O. Soifer et al., "Comparative Effectiveness of a Probiotic vs An Antibiotic in the Treatment of Patients with Intestinal Bacterial Overgrowth (SIBO) and Chronic Abdominal Functional Distension: A Pilot Study," *Acta Gastroenterology Latinoam* 40, no. 4 (2010): pp. 323–327.

17. Kenneth Brown, Brandi Scott-Hoy, and Linda Jennings, "Efficacy of a Quebracho, Conker Tree, and M. Balsamea Willd Blended Extract in a Randomized Study in Patients with Irritable Bowel Syndrome with Constipation," *Journal of Gastroenterology and Hepatology Research* 4, no. 9 (2015): pp. 1762–1767, https://doi.org/10.17554/j.issn.2224–3992.2015.04.560.

18. Victor Chedid et al., "Herbal Therapy Is Equivalent to Rifaximin for the Treatment of Small Intestinal Bacterial Overgrowth," *Global Advances in Health and Medicine* 3, no. 3 (2014): pp. 16–24, https://doi.org/10.7453/gahmj.2014.019.

19. Virginia T. Sherr, "'Bell's Palsy of the Gut' and Other GI Manifestations of Lyme and Associated Diseases," *Practical Gastroenterology*, April 2006, pp. 74–91, http://www .lymepa.org/02 BELLS PALSY of the GUT--Sherr.pdf

20. V. Alun-Jones et al., "Crohn's Disease: Maintenance of Remission by Diet," *Lancet* 826, no. 8448 (1985): pp. 177–180, https://doi.org/10.1016/s0140-6736(85)91497-7.

21. Arezo Judaki et al., "Evaluation of Dairy Allergy Among Ulcerative Colitis Patients," *Bioinformation* 10, no. 11 (2014): pp. 693–696, https://doi.org/10.6026/97320630010693.

22. Martin D. Fried et al., "The Spectrum of Gastrointestinal Manifestations in Children and Adolescents with Lyme Disease," *Journal of Pediatric Gastroenterology & Nutrition* 29, no. 4 (1999): pp. 495–499, https://doi.org/10.1097/00005176-199910000-00050.

23. M. D. Fried et al., "*Borrelia Burgdorferi* Persists in the Gastrointestinal Tract of Children and Adolescents with Lyme Disease," *Journal of Spirochetal and Tick-Borne Diseases* 9 (2002): pp. 11–15.

24.   M. D. Fried et al., "*Bartonella Henselae* Is Associated with Heartburn, Abdominal Pain, Skin Rash, Mesenteric Adenitis, Gastritis and Duodenitis," *Journal of Pediatric Gastroenterology and Nutrition* 35, no. 3 (2002): Abstract 158.

25.   Martin D. Fried, Martin E. Adelson, and Eli Mordechai, "Simultaneous Gastrointestinal Infections in Children and Adolescents," *Practical Gastroenterology*, November 2004, pp. 78–80.

26.   Francesco Massei et al., "*Bartonella Henselae* and Inflammatory Bowel Disease," *Lancet* 356, no. 9237 (2000): pp. 1245–1246, https://doi.org/10.1016/s0140-6736(00)02796-3.

27.   Maile Young Karris et al., "*Bartonella Henselae* Infection of Prosthetic Aortic Valve Associated with Colitis," *Vector-Borne and Zoonotic Diseases* 11, no. 11 (2011): pp. 1503–1505, https://doi.org/10.1089/vbz.2010.0169.

28.   Alessandro Ventura et al., "Systemic *Bartonella Henselae* Infection with Hepatosplenic Involvement," *Journal of Pediatric Gastroenterology & Nutrition* 29, no. 1 (1999): pp. 52–56, https://doi.org/10.1097/00005176-199907000-00014.

CHAPTER 17

1.   Geeta Ramesh et al., "Inflammation in the Pathogenesis of Lyme Neuroborreliosis," *American Journal of Pathology* 185, no. 5 (2015): pp. 1344–1360, https://doi.org/10.1016/j.ajpath.2015.01.024.

2.   Adam Garkowski et al., "Cerebrovascular Manifestations of Lyme Neuroborreliosis—A Systematic Review of Published Cases," *Frontiers in Neurology* 8 (2017): p. 146, https://doi.org/10.3389/fneur.2017.00146.

3.   Brian A. Fallon et al., "Inflammation and Central Nervous System Lyme Disease," *Neurobiology of Disease* 37, no. 3 (2010): pp. 534–541, https://doi.org/10.1016/j.nbd.2009.11.016.

4.   Luciana Besedovsky, Tanja Lange, and Jan Born, "Sleep and Immune Function," *Pflugers Archive* 463, no. 1 (2012): pp. 121–137, https://doi.org/10.1007/s00424-011-1044-0.

5.   Nadia Aalling Jessen et al., "The Glymphatic System: A Beginner's Guide," *Neurochemical Research* 40, no. 12 (2015): pp. 2583–2599, https://doi.org/10.1007/s11064-015-1581-6.

6.   R. J. Wurtman, "Age-Related Decreases in Melatonin Secretion—Clinical Consequences," *Journal of Clinical Endocrinology & Metabolism* 85, no. 6 (2000): pp. 2135–2136, https://doi.org/10.1210/jc.85.6.2135.

7.   Kimberly A. Babson, James Sottile, and Danielle Morabito, "Cannabis, Cannabinoids, and Sleep: a Review of the Literature," *Current Psychiatry Reports* 19, no. 4 (2017): p. 23, https://doi.org/10.1007/s11920-017-0775-9.

8.   M. Andersen et al., "Effects of Progesterone on Sleep: A Possible Pharmacological Treatment for Sleep-Breathing Disorders?," *Current Medicinal Chemistry* 13, no. 29 (2006): pp. 3575–3582, https://doi.org/10.2174/092986706779026200.

9.   M. Oettel and A. K. Mukhopadhyay, "Progesterone: The Forgotten Hormone in Men?," *Aging Male* 7, no. 3 (2004): pp. 236–257, https://doi.org/10.1080/13685530400004199.

10.   Adam Wichniak et al., "Effects of Antidepressants on Sleep," *Current Psychiatry Reports* 19, no. 9 (2017): p. 63, https://doi.org/10.1007/s11920-017-0816-4.

11.   Bruce S. McEwen, "Protective and Damaging Effects of Stress Mediators: Allostasis and Allostatic Load," *New England Journal of Medicine* 338, no. 3 (1998): pp. 171–179, https://doi.org/10.1056/nejm199801153380307.

12.   Douglas Carroll et al., "The Effects of an Oral Multivitamin Combination with Calcium, Magnesium, and Zinc on Psychological Well-Being in Healthy Young Male Volunteers: A Double-Blind Placebo-Controlled Trial," *Psychopharmacology* 150, no. 2 (2000): pp. 220–225, https://doi.org/10.1007/s002130000406.

13.   Carroll, "The Effects of an Oral Multivitamin Combination with Calcium, Magnesium, and Zinc on Psychological Well-Being in Healthy Young Male Volunteers," 220–225.

14. Kennon M. Garrett et al., "Extracts of Kava (*Piper Methysticum*) Induce Acute Anxiolytic-Like Behavioral Changes in Mice," *Psychopharmacology* 170, no. 1 (2003): pp. 33–41, https://doi.org/10.1007/s00213-003-1520-0.

15. Jerome Sarris et al., "L-Theanine in the Adjunctive Treatment of Generalized Anxiety Disorder: A Double-Blind, Randomised, Placebo-Controlled Trial," *Journal of Psychiatric Research* 110 (2019): pp. 31–37, https://doi.org/10.1016/j.jpsychires.2018.12.014.

16. R. Bruce Lydiard, "The Role of GABA in Anxiety Disorders," *Journal of Clinical Psychiatry* 64, no. S3 (2003): pp. 21–27.

17. John E. Lewis et al., "The Effect of Methylated Vitamin B Complex on Depressive and Anxiety Symptoms and Quality of Life in Adults with Depression," *ISRN Psychiatry* 2013 (2013): pp. 1–7, https://doi.org/10.1155/2013/621453.

18. Andrew H. Miller and Charles L. Raison, "The Role of Inflammation in Depression: from Evolutionary Imperative to Modern Treatment Target," *Nature Reviews Immunology* 6, no. 1 (2016): pp. 22–34, https://doi.org/10.1038/nri.2015.5.

19. Michael Irwin, Ute Lacher, and Cindy Caldwell, "Depression and Reduced Natural Killer Cytotoxicity: A Longitudinal Study of Depressed Patients and Control Subjects," *Psychological Medicine* 22, no. 4 (1992): pp. 1045–1050, https://doi.org/10.1017/s0033291700038617.

20. E. Schrader, "Equivalence of St. John's Wort Extract (Ze 117) and Fluoxetine: a Randomized, Controlled Study in Mildmoderate Depression," *International Clinical Psychopharmacology* 15, no. 2 (2000): pp. 61–68, https://doi.org/10.1097/00004850-200015020-00001.

21. Richard C. Shelton, Martin B. Keller, and Alan Gelenberg, "Effectiveness of St John's Wort in Major Depression: A Randomized Controlled Trial," *JAMA* 285, no. 15 (2001): pp. 1978–1986, https://doi.org/10.1001/jama.285.15.1978.

22. Kaustubh G. Joshi and Matthew D. Faubion, "Mania and Psychosis Associated with St. John's Wort and Ginseng," *Psychiatry (Edgmont)* 2, no. 9 (2005): pp. 56–61.

23. Leslie Knowlton, "Investigating SAM-e for Depression," *Psychiatric Times*, May 1, 2001, http://www.psychiatrictimes.com/depression/investigating-sam-e-depression.

24. O. M. Wolkowitz et al., "Dehydroepiandrosterone (DHEA) Treatment of Depression," *Biological Psychiatry* 41, no. 3 (1997): pp. 311–318, https://doi.org/10.1016/s0006-3223(96)00043-1)

25. Anna Serefko et al., "Magnesium in Depression," *Pharmacological Reports* 65, no. 3 (2013): pp. 547–554, https://doi.org/10.1016/s1734-1140(13)71032-6.

26. Alan J. Gelenberg et al., "Tyrosine for the Treatment of Depression," *American Journal of Psychiatry* 137, no. 5 (1980): pp. 622–623, https://doi.org/10.1176/ajp.137.5.622.

27. Helmut Beckmann et al., "DL-Phenylalanine versus Imipramine: A Double-Blind Controlled Study," *Archiv Psychiatrie Und Nervenkrankheiten* 227, no. 1 (1979): pp. 49–58, https://doi.org/10.1007/bf00585677.

28. William F. Byerley et al., "5-Hydroxytryptophan: A Review of Its Antidepressant Efficacy and Adverse Effects," *Journal of Clinical Psychopharmacology* 7, no. 3 (1987): pp. 127–137, https://doi.org/10.1097/00004714-198706000-00002.

29. S. Meyers, "Use of Neurotransmitter Precursors for Treatment of Depression," *Alternative Medicine Review* 5, no. 1 (2000): pp. 64–71.

30. Yanni Papanikolaou et al., "U.S. Adults Are Not Meeting Recommended Levels for Fish and Omega-3 Fatty Acid Intake: Results of an Analysis Using Observational Data from NHANES 2003–2008," *Nutrition Journal* 13, no. 1 (2014): p. 31, https://doi.org/10.1186/1475-2891-13-64.

31. Alan C. Logan, "Neurobehavioral Aspects of Omega-3 Fatty Acids: Possible Mechanisms and Therapeutic Value in Major Depression," *Alternative Medicine Review* 8, no. 4 (2003): pp. 410–425.

32. M. W. P. Carney et al., "Thiamine, Riboflavin and Pyridoxine Deficiency in Psychiatric In-Patients," *British Journal of Psychiatry* 141, no. 3 (1982): pp. 271–272, https://doi.org/10.1192/bjp.141.3.271.

33. Ming Zhang et al., "Methylcobalamin: A Potential Vitamin of Pain Killer," *Neural Plasticity* 2013 (2013): pp. 1–6, https://doi.org/10.1155/2013/424651.
34. physio-pedia.com/Vitamin_B12_Deficiency.com (Accessed November 29, 2020).
35. A. Coppen and J. Bailey, "Enhancement of the Antidepressant Action of Fluoxetine By Folic Acid: A Randomised, Placebo Controlled Trial," *Journal of Affective Disorder* 60, no. 2 (2000): pp. 121–130, https://doi.org/10.1037/e323122004-002.
36. Katie T.B. Touma, Allysa M. Zoucha, and Jonathon R. Scarff, "Liothyronine for Depression: A Review and Guidance for Safety Monitoring," *Innovations in Clinical Neuroscience* 14, no. 3–4 (2017): pp. 24–29.
37. Dale Bredesen, *End of Alzheimer's: The First Program to Prevent and Reverse Cognitive Decline* (New York: Avery Press, 2017).
38. Dana Parish, "'A Slow Slipping Away'—Kris Kristofferson's Long-Undiagnosed Battle with Lyme Disease," *HuffPost*, July 6, 2016, https://www.huffpost.com /entry/a-slow-slipping-away-kris-kristoffersons-long_b_577c047be4b00a3ae4ce6609.
39. Min-Soo Kim et al., "Ginkgo Biloba L. Extract Protects Against Chronic Cerebral Hypoperfusion by Modulating Neuroinflammation and the Cholinergic System," *Phytomedicine* 23, no. 12 (2016): pp. 1356–1364, https://doi.org/10.1016/j.phymed .2016.07.013.
40. Akito Kato-Kataoka et al., "Soybean-Derived Phosphatidylserine Improves Memory Function of the Elderly Japanese Subjects with Memory Complaints," *Journal of Clinical Biochemistry and Nutrition* 47, no. 3 (2010): pp. 246–255, https://doi.org/10.3164/jcbn .10–62.
41. S. Y. Chung et al., "Administration of Phosphatidylcholine Increases Brain Acetylcholine Concentration and Improves Memory in Mice With Dementia," *Journal of Nutrition* 125, no. 6 (1995): pp. 1484–1489, https://doi.org/10.1093/jn/125.6.1484.
42. Satoru Kobayashi et al., "Acetyl-l-Carnitine Improves Aged Brain Function," *Geriatrics & Gerontology International* 10, no. Supp. 1 (February 2010): pp. S99–S106, https://doi .org/10.1111/j.1447–0594.2010.00595.x.
43. Dongsoo Kim, "Practical Use and Risk of Modafinil, a Novel Waking Drug," *Environmental Health and Toxicology* 27 (2012), https://doi.org/10.5620/eht.2012.27.e2012007.
44. Joseph Jankovic and L. G. Aguilar, "Current Approaches to the Treatment of Parkinson's Disease," *Neuropsychiatric Disease and Treatment* 4, no. 4 (2008): pp. 743757, https: //doi.org/10.2147/ndt.s2006.
45. P. Anand and K. Bley, "Topical Capsaicin for Pain Management: Therapeutic Potential and Mechanisms of Action of the New High-Concentration Capsaicin 8% Patch," *British Journal of Anaesthesia* 107, no. 4 (2011): pp. 490–502, https://doi.org/10.1093/bja /aer260.
46. Gerritje S. Mijnhout et al., "Alpha Lipoic Acid for Symptomatic Peripheral Neuropathy in Patients with Diabetes: A Meta-Analysis of Randomized Controlled Trials," *International Journal of Endocrinology* 2012 (2012): pp. 1–8, https://doi.org/10.1155/2012/456279.
47. B. S. Alghamdi, "The Neuroprotective Role of Melatonin in Neurological Disorders," *Journal of Neuroscience Research* 96, no. 7 (2018): pp. 1136–1149, https://doi.org/10.1002 /jnr.24220.
48. Mikael Kowal, Arno Hazekamp, and Franjo Grotenhermen, "Review on Clinical Studies with Cannabis and Cannabinoids 2010–2014," *Cannabinoids* 11, no. Special Issue (2016): pp. 1–18.
49. I Svizenska, P Dubovy, and A Sulcova, "Cannabinoid Receptors 1 and 2 (Cb1 and Cb2), Their Distribution, Ligands and Functional Involvement in Nervous System Structures—A Short Review," *Pharmacology Biochemistry and Behavior* 90, no. 4 (2008): pp. 501–511, https://doi.org/10.1016/j.pbb.2008.05.010.
50. E. S. Onaivi, "Commentary: Functional Neuronal CB2 Cannabinoid Receptors in the CNS," *Current Neuropharmacology* 9, no. 1 (2011): pp. 205–208, https://doi.org /10.2174/157015911795017416.

51. Gemma Navarro et al., "Targeting Cannabinoid CB2 Receptors in the Central Nervous System. Medicinal Chemistry Approaches with Focus on Neurodegenerative Disorders," *Frontiers in Neuroscience* 10, no. 406 (2016): pp. 1–11, https://doi.org/10.3389/fnins.2016.00406.

52. Marcus A. Bachhuber et al., "Medical Cannabis Laws and Opioid Analgesic Overdose Mortality in the United States, 1999–2010," *JAMA Internal Medicine* 174, no. 11 (2014): p. 1875, https://doi.org/10.1001/jamainternmed.2014.4005.

53. David Powell, Rosalie Liccardo Pacula, and Mireille Jacobson, "Do Medical Marijuana Laws Reduce Addictions and Deaths Related to Pain Killers?," *NBER Working Paper No. 2135*, July 2015.

54. Ayikoe G. Mensah-Nyagan et al., "Evidence for a Key Role of Steroids in the Modulation of Pain," *Psychoneuroendocrinology* 34, no. Supp. 1 (2009): pp. s169–s177, https://doi.org/10.1016/j.psyneuen.2009.06.004.

55. Suntanu Dalal and Ronald Melzack, "Potentiation of Opioid Analgesia by Psychostimulant Drugs: A Review," *Journal of Pain and Symptom Management* 16, no. 4 (1998): pp. 245–253, https://doi.org/10.1016/s0885-3924(98)00084-0.

56. Hinton Jonez, "The Allergic Aspects of Multiple Sclerosis," *California Medicine* 79, no. 5 (1953): pp. 376–380.

57. Merit Cudkowicz et al., "Safety and Efficacy of Ceftriaxone for Amyotrophic Lateral Sclerosis: A Multi-Stage, Randomised, Double-Blind, Placebo-Controlled Trial," *Lancet Neurology* 13, no. 11 (2014): pp. 1083–1091, https://doi.org/10.1016/S1474-4422(14)70222-4.

58. Jennifer Frankovich et al., "Five Youth with Pediatric Acute-Onset Neuropsychiatric Syndrome of Differing Etiologies," *Journal of Child and Adolescent Psychopharmacology* 25, no. 1 (2015): pp. 31–37, https://doi.org/10.1089/cap.2014.0056.

59. G. P. Tisi, M. Marzolini, and G. Biffi, "Pediatric Acute Onset Neuropsychiatric Syndrome Associated with Epstein–Barr Infection in Child with Noonan Syndrome," *European Psychiatry* 41, no. Supp. (2017): p. s456, https://doi.org/10.1016/j.eurpsy.2017.01.492.

60. Edward B Breitschwerdt et al., "Bartonella Henselae Bloodstream Infection in a Boy with Pediatric Acute-Onset Neuropsychiatric Syndrome," *Journal of Central Nervous System Disease* 11 (2019), https://doi.org/10.1177/1179573519832014.

61. Hanna Rhee and Daniel Cameron, "Lyme Disease and Pediatric Autoimmune Neuropsychiatric Disorders Associated with Streptococcal Infections (PANDAS): An Overview," *International Journal of General Medicine* 5 (2012): pp. 163–174, https://doi.org/10.2147/ijgm.s24212.

62. Aristo Vojdani, K. Michael Pollard, and Andrew W. Campbell, "Environmental Triggers and Autoimmunity," *Autoimmune Diseases* 2014 (2014): pp. 1–2, https://doi.org/10.1155/2014/798029.

63. Tamara Tuuminen and Kyösti Sakari Rinne, "Severe Sequelae to Mold-Related Illness as Demonstrated in Two Finnish Cohorts," *Frontiers in Immunology* 8 (2017): p. 382, https://doi.org/10.3389/fimmu.2017.00382.

64. Abhishek Chandra et al., "Anti-Neural Antibody Reactivity in Patients with a History of Lyme Borreliosis and Persistent Symptoms," *Brain, Behavior, and Immunity* 24, no. 6 (2010): pp. 1018–1024, https://doi.org/10.1016/j.bbi.2010.03.002.

65. E. S. Raveche et al., "Evidence of Borrelia Autoimmunity-Induced Component of Lyme Carditis and Arthritis," *Journal of Clinical Microbiology* 43, no. 2 (January 2005): pp. 850–856, https://doi.org/10.1128/jcm.43.2.850–856.2005.

66. Carol J. Cox et al., "Antineuronal Antibodies in a Heterogeneous Group of Youth and Young Adults with Tics and Obsessive-Compulsive Disorder," *Journal of Child and Adolescent Psychopharmacology* 25, no. 1 (2015): pp. 76–85, https://doi.org/10.1089/cap.2014.0048.

67. Allen C. Steere, Edward Dwyer, and Robert Winchester, "Association of Chronic Lyme Arthritis with HLA-DR4 and HLA-DR2 Alleles," *New England Journal of Medicine* 323, no. 4 (1990): pp. 219–223, https://doi.org/10.1056/nejm199007263230402.

68. A. Katz, "NADAL—Neuropsychiatric Autoimmune Disorder Associated With Lyme Disease –A PANDAS/PANS Equivalent: Diagnosis and Treatment," in *19th Annual Conference of the International Lyme and Associated Diseases* (Chicago, IL, 2018).

69. Miro Kovacevic, Paul Grant, and Susan E. Swedo, "Use of Intravenous Immunoglobulin in the Treatment of Twelve Youths with Pediatric Autoimmune Neuropsychiatric Disorders Associated with Streptococcal Infections," *Journal of Child and Adolescent Psychopharmacology* 25, no. 1 (2015): pp. 65–69, https://doi.org/10.1089/cap.2014.0067.

70. Denise Calaprice, Janice Tona, and Tanya K. Murphy, "Treatment of Pediatric Acute-Onset Neuropsychiatric Disorder in a Large Survey Population," *Journal of Child and Adolescent Psychopharmacology* 28, no. 2 (2018): pp. 92–103, https://doi.org/10.1089/cap.2017.0101.

71. D. Katz, I. Katz, and Y. Shoenfeld, "Cannabis and Autoimmunity—The Neurologic Perspective: A Brief Review," *Journal of Neurology and Neuromedicine* 1, no. 4 (2016): pp. 11–15.

72. Margaret E. Walker, Julianne K. Hatfield, and Melissa A. Brown, "New Insights Into the Role of Mast Cells in Autoimmunity: Evidence for a Common Mechanism of Action?," *Biochimica Et Biophysica Acta* 1822, no. 1 (2012): pp. 57–65, https://doi.org/10.1016/j.bbadis.2011.02.009.

73. A. Dempsey, "Mast Cell Activation as an Initiator of Autoimmunity," in *Autoimmune Encephalopathy of Infectious Etiology* (Washington, D.C., 2019).

74. Calaprice, "Treatment of Pediatric Acute-Onset Neuropsychiatric Disorder in a Large Survey Population," 92–103.

CHAPTER 18

1. Taha Rashid and Alan Ebringer, "Autoimmunity in Rheumatic Diseases Is Induced by Microbial Infections via Crossreactivity or Molecular Mimicry," *Autoimmune Diseases* 2012 (2012): pp. 1–9, https://doi.org/10.1155/2012/539282.

2. Abhishek Chandra et al., "Anti-*Borrelia Burgdorferi* Antibody Profile in Post-Lyme Disease Syndrome," *Clinical and Vaccine Immunology* 18, no. 5 (2011): pp. 767–771, https://doi.org/10.1128/cvi.00002–11.

3. S. Kuenzle et al., "Pathogen Specificity and Autoimmunity Are Distinct Features of Antigen-Driven Immune Responses in Neuroborreliosis," *Infection and Immunity* 75, no. 8 (2007): pp. 3842–3847, https://doi.org/10.1128/iai.00260–07.

4. J. Chmielewska-Badora, E. Cisak, and J. Dutkiewicz, "Lyme Borreliosis and Multiple Sclerosis: Any Connection? A Seroepidemic Study," *Annals of Agriculture and Environmental Medicine* 7, no. 2 (2000): pp. 141–143.

5. Allen C. Steere, Edward Dwyer, and Robert Winchester, "Association of Chronic Lyme Arthritis with HLA-DR4 and HLA-DR2 Alleles," *New England Journal of Medicine* 323, no. 4 (1990): pp. 219–223, https://doi.org/10.1056/nejm199007263230402.

6. F. Guarneri and C. Guarneri, "Molecular Mimicry in Cutaneous Autoimmune Disease," *World Journal of Dermatology* 2, no. 4 (2013): pp. 36–43, https://doi.org/10.5314/wjd.v2.i4.36

7. Despoina N. Maritsi et al., "*Bartonella Henselae* Infection: An Uncommon Mimicker of Autoimmune Disease," *Case Reports in Pediatrics* 2013 (2013): pp. 1–4, https://doi.org/10.1155/2013/726826.

8. Ricardo G. Maggi et al., "*Bartonella Spp.* Bacteremia and Rheumatic Symptoms in Patients from Lyme Disease–Endemic Region," *Emerging Infectious Diseases* 18, no. 11 (2012): pp. 783–791, https://doi.org/10.3201/eid1811.121226.

9. Francesco Massei et al., "*Bartonella Henselae* and Inflammatory Bowel Disease," *Lancet* 356, no. 9237 (2000): pp. 1245–1246, https://doi.org/10.1016/s0140-6736(00)02796–3.

10. B. Stockmeyer et al., "Chronic Vasculitis and Polyneuropathy Due to Infection with *Bartonella Henselae,*" *Infection* 35, no. 2 (2007): pp. 107–109, https://doi.org/10.1007/s15010-007-6021-3.

11. K. B. Waites and D. F. Talkington, "Mycoplasma Pneumoniae and Its Role as a Human Pathogen," *Clinical Microbiology Reviews* 17, no. 4 (January 2004): pp. 697–728, https://doi.org/10.1128/cmr.17.4.697-728.2004.

12. Daniel A. Kinderlehrer, "Primary Sclerosing Cholangitis and Bartonella: A Case Report" (Chicago, IL, 2018).

13. Jacek Tabarkiewicz et al., "The Role of IL-17 and Th17 Lymphocytes in Autoimmune Diseases," *Archivum Immunologiae Et Therapiae Experimentalis* 63, no. 6 (2015): pp. 435–449, https://doi.org/10.1007/s00005-015-0344-z.

14. Ronald H. Stead et al., "Vagal Influences over Mast Cells," *Autonomic Neuroscience* 125, no. 1–2 (2006): pp. 53–61, https://doi.org/10.1016/j.autneu.2006.01.002.

15. J. Talkington and S. P. Nickell, "*Borrelia Burgdorferi* Spirochetes Induce Mast Cell Activation and Cytokine Release," *Infection and Immunity* 67, no. 3 (1999): pp. 1107–1115.

16. Melody C. Carter, Dean D. Metcalfe, and Hirsch D. Komarow, "Mastocytosis," *Immunology and Allergy Clinics of North American* 34, no. 1 (2014): pp. 186–191, https://doi.org/10.1016/j.iac.2013.09.001.

17. Laura Maintz and Natalija Novak, "Histamine and Histamine Intolerance," *American Journal of Clinical Nutrition* 85, no. 5 (2007): pp. 1185–1196, https://doi.org/10.1093/ajcn/85.5.1185.

18. Yunzhi Xu and Guangjie Chen, "Mast Cell and Autoimmune Diseases," *Mediators of Inflammation* 2015 (2015): pp. 1–8, https://doi.org/10.1155/2015/246126.

19. I Svizenska, P Dubovy, and A Sulcova, "Cannabinoid Receptors 1 and 2 (Cb1 and Cb2), Their Distribution, Ligands and Functional Involvement in Nervous System Structures—A Short Review," *Pharmacology Biochemistry and Behavior* 90, no. 4 (2008): pp. 501–511, https://doi.org/10.1016/j.pbb.2008.05.010.

20. Andrea L. Small-Howard et al., "Anti-Inflammatory Potential of CB1-Mediated CAMP Elevation in Mast Cells," *Biochemical Journal* 388, no. 2 (2005): pp. 465–473, https://doi.org/10.1042/bj20041682.

21. E. S. Onaivi, "Commentary: Functional Neuronal CB2 Cannabinoid Receptors in the CNS," *Current Neuropharmacology* 9, no. 1 (2011): pp. 205–208, https://doi.org/10.2174/157015911795017416.

22. Gemma Navarro et al., "Targeting Cannabinoid CB2 Receptors in the Central Nervous System. Medicinal Chemistry Approaches with Focus on Neurodegenerative Disorders," *Frontiers in Neuroscience* 10, no. 406 (2016): pp. 1–11, https://doi.org/10.3389/fnins.2016.00406.

23. Prakash Nagarkatti et al., "Cannabinoids as Novel Anti-Inflammatory Drugs," *Future Medicinal Chemistry* 1, no. 7 (2009): pp. 1333–1349, https://doi.org/10.4155/fmc.09.93.

24. Bharat B. Aggarwal et al., "Curcumin: The Indian Solid Gold," *Advances In Experimental Medicine and Biology* 595 (2007): pp. 1–75, https://doi.org/10.1007/978-0-387-46401-5_1.

25. Shatadal Ghosh, Sharmistha Banerjee, and Parames C. Sil, "The Beneficial Role of Curcumin on Inflammation, Diabetes and Neurodegenerative Disease: A Recent Update," *Food and Chemical Toxicology* 83 (2015): pp. 111–124, https://doi.org/10.1016/j.fct.2015.05.022.

26. N. Sreejayan and M. N. Rao, "Free Radical Scavenging Activity of Curcuminoids," *Arzneimittelforschung* 46, no. 2 (1996): pp. 169–171.

27. Binu Chandran and Ajay Goel, "A Randomized, Pilot Study to Assess the Efficacy and Safety of Curcumin in Patients with Active Rheumatoid Arthritis," *Phytotherapy Research* 26, no. 11 (2012): pp. 1719–1725, https://doi.org/10.1002/ptr.4639.

28. Hiroyuki Hanai et al., "Curcumin Maintenance Therapy for Ulcerative Colitis: Randomized, Multicenter, Double-Blind, Placebo-Controlled Trial," *Clinical Gastroenterology and Hepatology* 4, no. 12 (2006): pp. 1502–1506, https://doi.org/10.1016/j.cgh.2006.08.008.

29. Philip C. Calder, "Omega-3 Fatty Acids and Inflammatory Processes," *Nutrients* 2, no. 3 (2010): pp. 355–374, https://doi.org/10.3390/nu2030355.

30. Natalie Sinn, Catherine Milte, and Peter R. Howe, "Oiling the Brain: A Review of Randomized Controlled Trials of Omega-3 Fatty Acids in Psychopathology across the Lifespan," *Nutrients* 2, no. 2 (2010): pp. 128–170, https://doi.org/10.3390/nu2020128.

31. Elizabeth A. Miles and Philip C. Calder, "Influence Of Marinen-3 Polyunsaturated Fatty Acids on Immune Function and a Systematic Review of Their Effects on Clinical Outcomes in Rheumatoid Arthritis," *British Journal of Nutrition* 107, no. S2 (2012): pp. S171–S184, https://doi.org/10.1017/s0007114512001560.

32. Joseph Charles Maroon and Jeffrey W. Bost, "Ω-3 Fatty Acids (Fish Oil) as an Anti-Inflammatory: An Alternative to Nonsteroidal Anti-Inflammatory Drugs For Discogenic Pain," *Surgical Neurology* 65, no. 4 (2006): pp. 326–331, https://doi.org/10.1016/j.surneu.2005.10.023.

33. Fereidoon Shahidi and Priyatharini Ambigaipalan, "Omega-3 Polyunsaturated Fatty Acids and Their Health Benefits," *Annual Review of Food Science and Technology* 9, no. 1 (2018): pp. 345–381, https://doi.org/10.1146/annurev-food-111317-095850.

34. K. Bryniarski et al., "Modulation of Macrophage Activity by Proteolytic Enzymes. Differential Regulation of IL-6 and Reactive Oxygen Intermediates (ROIs) Synthesis as a Possible Homeostatic Mechanism in the Control of Inflammation," *Inflammation* 27, no. 6 (2003): pp. 333–340, https://doi.org/10.1023/b:ifla.0000006701.52150.43.

35. Atsushi Kakinuma et al., "Repression of Fibrinolysis in Scalded Rats by Administration of Serratia Protease," *Biochemical Pharmacology* 31, no. 18 (1982): pp. 2861–2866, https://doi.org/10.1016/0006-2952(82)90255-6.

36. M. Z. Siddiqui, "Boswellia Serrata, a Potential Antiinflammatory Agent: An Overview," *Indian Journal of Pharmaceutical Science* 73, no. 3 (2011): pp. 255–261, https://doi.org/10.4103/0250-474X.93507.

37. R. R. Kulkarni et al., "Treatment of Osteoarthritis with a Herbomineral Formulation: a Double-Blind, Placebo-Controlled, Cross-Over Study," *Journal of Ethnopharmacology* 33, no. 1–2 (1991): pp. 91–95, https://doi.org/10.1016/0378-8741(91)90167-c.

38. A. Chopra et al., "Randomized Double Blind Trial of an Ayurvedic Plant Derived Formulation for Treatment of Rheumatoid Arthritis," *Journal of Rheumatology* 27, no. 6 (2000): pp. 1365–1372.

39. Josephc Maroon, Jeffrey Bost, and Adara Maroon, "Natural Anti-Inflammatory Agents For Pain Relief," *Surgical Neurology International* 1, no. 1 (2010): p. 80, https://doi.org/10.4103/2152-7806.73804.

40. W. M. Jefferies, "Cortisol and Immunity," *Medical Hypotheses* 34, no. 3 (1991): pp. 198–208, https://doi.org/10.1016/0306-9877(91)90212-h.

41. T. P. Greco Jr., A. M. Conti-Kelly, and T. P. Greco, "Antiphospholipid Antibodies in Patients with Purported 'Chronic Lyme Disease,'" *Lupus* 20, no. 13 (2011): pp. 1372–1377, https://doi.org/10.1177/0961203311414098.

42. D. Berg et al., "Chronic Fatigue Syndrome and/or Fibromyalgia as a Variation of Antiphospholipid Antibody Syndrome," *Blood Coagulation & Fibrinolysis* 10, no. 7 (1999): pp. 435–438, https://doi.org/10.1097/00001721-199910000-00006.

43. H. A. Ruggiero et al., "Heparin Effect on Blood Viscosity," *Clinical Cardiology* 5, no. 3 (1982): pp. 215–218, https://doi.org/10.1002/clc.4960050303.

44. Sarah Mousavi et al., "Anti-Inflammatory Effects of Heparin and Its Derivatives: A Systematic Review," *Advances in Pharmacological Sciences* 2015 (2015): pp. 1–14, https://doi.org/10.1155/2015/507151.

45. Yunqi Weng et al., "Nattokinase: An Oral Antithrombotic Agent for the Prevention of Cardiovascular Disease," *International Journal of Molecular Sciences* 18, no. 3 (2017): p. 523, https://doi.org/10.3390/ijms18030523.

CHAPTER 19

1. Priya Rajagopalan et al., "Common Folate Gene Variant, Mthfr C677t, Is Associated with Brain Structure in Two Independent Cohorts Of People with Mild Cognitive Impairment," *NeuroImage Clinical* 1, no. 1 (2012): pp. 179–187, https://doi.org/10.1016/j .nicl.2012.09.012.

2. P. Frosst et al., "A Candidate Genetic Risk Factor for Vascular Disease: a Common Mutation in Methylene-Tetrahydrofolate Reductase," *Nature Genetics* 10, no. 1 (1995): pp. 111–113, https://doi.org/10.1038/ng0595-111.

3. S. J. Lewis et al., "The Thermolabile Variant of Mthfr Is Associated with Depression in the British Women's Heart and Health Study and a Meta-Analysis," *Molecular Psychiatry* 11, no. 4 (2006): pp. 352–360, https://doi.org/10.1038/sj.mp.4001790.

4 Xudong Liu et al., "Population- and Family-Based Studies Associate the MTHFR Gene with Idiopathic Autism in Simplex Families," *Journal of Autism and Developmental Disorders* 41, no. 7 (2011): pp. 938–944, https://doi.org/10.1007/s10803-010-1120-x.

5. Amir Karban et al., "The Association of the MTHFR C677T Polymorphism with Inflammatory Bowel Diseases in the Israeli Jewish Population," *Medicine (Baltimore)* 95, no. 51 (2016): p. e5611, https://doi.org/10.1097/md.0000000000005611.

6. S. Y. Chung et al., "Administration of Phosphatidylcholine Increases Brain Acetylcholine Concentration and Improves Memory in Mice with Dementia," *Journal of Nutrition* 125, no. 6 (1995): pp. 1484–1489, https://doi.org/10.1093/jn/125.6.1484.

7. M. J. Glade and K. Smith, "Phosphatidylserine and the Human Brain," *Nutrition* 31, no. 6 (2015): pp. 781–786, https://doi.org/10.1016/j.nut.2014.10.014.

8. Adam M. Zawada et al., "S-Adenosylhomocysteine Is Associated with Subclinical Atherosclerosis and Renal Function in a Cardiovascular Low-Risk Population," *Atherosclerosis* 234, no. 1 (2014): pp. 17–22, https://doi.org/10.1016/j.atherosclerosis.2014.02.002.

9. Joseph Brewer et al., "Detection of Mycotoxins in Patients with Chronic Fatigue Syndrome," *Toxins* 5, no. 4 (2013): pp. 605–617, https://doi.org/10.3390/toxins5040605.

10. Joseph Brewer, Jack Thrasher, and Dennis Hooper, "Chronic Illness Associated with Mold and Mycotoxins: Is Naso-Sinus Fungal Biofilm the Culprit?," *Toxins* 6, no. 1 (2014): pp. 66–80, https://doi.org/10.3390/toxins6010066.

11. Janette Hope, "A Review of the Mechanism of Injury and Treatment Approaches for Illness Resulting from Exposure to Water-Damaged Buildings, Mold, and Mycotoxins," *Scientific World Journal* 6 (2013): pp. 1–20, https://doi.org/10.1155/2013/767482.

12. L. D. Empting, "Neurologic and Neuropsychiatric Syndrome Features of Mold and Mycotoxin Exposure," *Toxicology and Industrial Health* 25, no. 9–10 (2009): pp. 577–581, https://doi.org/10.1177/0748233709348393.

13. J. W. Bennett and M. Kilch, "Mycotoxins," *Clinical Microbiology Reviews* 16, no. 3 (2003): pp. 497–516, https://doi.org/10.1128/cmr.16.3.497-516.2003.

14. Heidi Demaegdt et al., "Endocrine Activity of Mycotoxins and Mycotoxin Mixtures," *Food and Chemical Toxicology* 96 (2016): pp. 107–116, https://doi.org/10.1016/j.fct.2016.07.033.

15. C. Frizzell et al., "Endocrine Disrupting Effects of Zearalenone, Alpha- and Beta-Zearalenol at the Level of Nuclear Receptor Binding and Steroidogenesis," *Toxicology Letters* 206, no. 2 (2011): pp. 210–217, https://doi.org/10.1016/j.toxlet.2011.07.015.

16. Victor Owino, Carolin Cornelius, and Cornelia Loechl, "Elucidating Adverse Nutritional Implications of Exposure to Endocrine-Disrupting Chemicals and Mycotoxins through Stable Isotope Techniques," *Nutrients* 10, no. 4 (2018): p. 401, https://doi.org/10.3390 /nu10040401.

17. Hope, "A Review of the Mechanism of Injury and Treatment for Illness Resulting from Exposure to Water Damaged Buildings, Mold and Mycotoxins," 1–20.

18. Jente Boonen et al., "Human Skin Penetration of Selected Model Mycotoxins," *Toxicology* 301, no. 1–3 (2012): pp. 21–32, https://doi.org/10.1016/j.tox.2012.06.012.

19. L. Nagy, "2012 ILADS Annual Scientific Conference," in *2012 ILADS Annual Scientific Conference* (Boston, MA, 2012).
20. "Surviving Mold," Mold Illness & Surviving Mold, accessed June 8, 2018, http://www.survivingmold.com.
21. Hope, "A Review of the Mechanism of Injury and Treatment for Illness Resulting from Exposure to Water Damaged Buildings, Mold and Mycotoxins," 1–20.
22. Shiro Nakano, Hideo Takekoshi, and Masuo Nakano, "Chlorella (*Chlorella Pyrenoidosa*) Supplementation Decreases Dioxin and Increases Immunoglobulin A Concentrations in Breast Milk," *Journal of Medicinal Food* 10, no. 1 (2007): pp. 134142, https://doi.org/10.1089/jmf.2006.023.
23. G. L. Renju, G. Muraleedhara Kurup, and C. H. Saritha Kumari, "Anti-Inflammatory Activity of Lycopene Isolated from Chlorella Marina on Type II Collagen Induced Arthritis Insprague Dawley Rats," *Immunopharmacology and Immunotoxicology* 35, no. 2 (2013): pp. 282291, https://doi.org/10.3109/08923973.2012.742534.
24. M. T. Simonich et al., "Natural Chlorophyll Inhibits Aflatoxin B1-Induced Multi-Organ Carcinogenesis in the Rat," *Carcinogenesis* 28, no. 6 (2007): pp. 1294–1302, https://doi.org/10.1093/carcin/bgm027.
25. C. Jubert et al., "Effects of Chlorophyll and Chlorophyllin on Low-Dose Aflatoxin B1 Pharmacokinetics in Human Volunteers," *Cancer Prevention Research* 2, no. 12 (2009): pp. 1015–1022, https://doi.org/10.1158/1940–6207.capr-09-0099.
26. J. Brewer, "2014 ILADS Annual Scientific Conference," in *2014 ILADS Annual Scientific Conference* (San Diego, CA, 2014).
27. Bakkiyaraj Dhamodharan et al., "Anti-Biofilm Properties of a Mupirocin Spray Formulation against Escherichia Coli Wound Infections," *Biofouling* 33, no. 7 (2017): pp. 1–10, https://doi.org/10.1080/08927014.2017.1337100.
28. Saranna Fanning and Aaron Mitchell, "Fungal Biofilms," *PLoS Pathogens* 8, no. 4 (2012), https://doi.org/10.1371/journal.ppat.1002585.
29. Montserrat Marí et al., "Mitochondrial Glutathione, a Key Survival Antioxidant," *Antioxidants & Redox Signaling* 11, no. 11 (2009): pp. 2685–2700, https://doi.org/10.1089/ars.2009.2695.
30. S. B. Agawane and P. S. Lonkar, "Effect of Probiotic Containing Saccharomyces Boulardii on Experimental Ochratoxicosis in Broilers: Hematobiochemical Studies," *Journal of Veterinary Science* 5, no. 4 (2004): pp. 359–367, https://doi.org/10.4142/jvs.2004.5.4.359.
31. Samir Abbes et al., "Ability of Lactobacillus Rhamnosus GAF01 to Remove AFM1 in Vitro and to Counteract AFM1 Immunotoxicity in Vivo," *Journal of Immunotoxicology* 10, no. 3 (2012): pp. 279–286, https://doi.org/10.3109/1547691X.2012.718810.
32. William J Rea, Yaqin Pan, and Bertie Griffiths, "The Treatment of Patients with Mycotoxin-Induced Disease," *Toxicology and Industrial Health* 25, no. 9–10 (2009): pp. 711–714, https://doi.org/10.1177/0748233709348281.
33. "FDA Advice about Eating Fish and Shellfish," EPA, March 13, 2020, https://www.epa.gov/fish-tech/2017-epa-fda-advice-about-eating-fish-and-shellfish.
34. "Mercury in Medicine—Are We Taking Unnecessary Risks?," House Hearing, 106 Congress, accessed May 17, 2019, https://www.govinfo.gov/content/pkg/CHRG-106hhrg72722/html/CHRG-106hhrg72722.htm.
35. "Statement on Dental Amalgam," American Dental Association, accessed June 14, 2018, https://www.ada.org/en/about-the-ada/ada-positions-policies-and-statements/statement-on-dental-amalgam.
36. "Symptoms of Elemental Mercury Vapor Exposure and Toxicity," IAOMT, 2016, https://files.iaomt.org/wp-content/uploads/Fact-Sheet-Mercury-Vapor-Toxicity.pdf.
37. Ivo Iavicoli, Luca Fontana, and Antonio Bergamaschi, "The Effects of Metals as Endocrine Disruptors," *Journal of Toxicology and Environmental Health B Critical Reviews* 12, no. 3 (2009): pp. 206–223, https://doi.org/10.1080/10937400902902062.

38. K. P. Mishra, "Lead Exposure and Its Impact on Immune System: A Review," *Toxicology in Vitro* 23, no. 6 (2009): pp. 969–972, https://doi.org/10.1016/j.tiv.2009.06.014.

39. T. W. Clarkson, "Metal Toxicity in the Central Nervous System.," *Environmental Health Perspectives* 75 (1987): pp. 59–64, https://doi.org/10.1289/ehp.877559.

40. K. Michael Pollard, Per Hultman, and Dwight H. Kono, "Toxicology of Autoimmune Diseases," *Chemical Research in Toxicology* 23, no. 3 (2010): pp. 455–466, https://doi.org/10.1021/tx9003787.

41. Sae-Ron Shin and A-Lum Han, "Improved Chronic Fatigue Symptoms after Removal of Mercury in Patient with Increased Mercury Concentration in Hair Toxic Mineral Assay: A Case," *Korean Journal of Family Medicine* 33, no. 5 (2012): pp. 320–325, https://doi.org/10.4082/kjfm.2012.33.5.320.

42. Gervasio A. Lamas et al., "Heavy Metals, Cardiovascular Disease, and the Unexpected Benefits of Chelation Therapy," *Journal of the American College of Cardiology* 67, no. 20 (2016): pp. 2411–2418, https://doi.org/10.1016/j.jacc.2016.02.066.

43. Vera Stejskal, Karin Ockert, and Geir Bjørklund, "Metal-Induced Inflammation Triggers Fibromyalgia in Metal-Allergic Patients," *Neuro Endocrinology Letters* 34, no. 6 (2013): pp. 559–565.

44. L. Nagy, "2012 ILADS Annual Scientific Conference," in *2012 ILADS Annual Scientific Conference* (Boston, MA, 2012).

45. Joy Hussain and Marc Cohen, "Clinical Effects of Regular Dry Sauna Bathing: A Systematic Review," *Evidence-Based Complementary and Alternative Medicine* 2018 (2018): pp. 1–30, https://doi.org/10.1155/2018/1857413.

46. William J Rea, Yaqin Pan, and Bertie Griffiths, "The Treatment of Patients with Mycotoxin Induced Disease," *Toxicology and Industrial Health* 25, no. 9–10 (2009): pp. 711–714, https://doi.org/10.1177/0748233709348281.

47. Walter Crinnion, "Components of Practical Clinical Detox Programs—Sauna as a Therapeutic Tool," *Alternative Therapies in Health and Medicine* 13, no. 2 (2007): pp. S154–S156.

48. K. L. Schmidt, "Generalized Tendomyopathy (Fibromyalgia): Differential Diagnosis, Therapy and Prognosis," *Z Gesamte Inn Med* 46, no. 10–11 (1991): pp. 370–374.

49. Fredrikus G. J. Oosterveld et al., "Infrared Sauna in Patients with Rheumatoid Arthritis and Ankylosing Spondylitis," *Clinical Rheumatology* 28, no. 1 (2008): pp. 29–34, https://doi.org/10.1007/s10067 008-0977-y.

50. Richard Beever, "Far-Infrared Saunas for Treatment of Cardiovascular Risk Factors: Summary of Published Evidence," *Canadian Family Physician* 55, no. 7 (2009): pp. 691–696.

51. Shang-Ru Tsai and Michael R. Hamblin, "Biological Effects and Medical Applications of Infrared Radiation," *Journal of Photochemistry and Photobiology B: Biology* 170 (2017): pp. 197–207, https://doi.org/10.1016/j.jphotobiol.2017.04.014.

52. Sandra L. Ladd et al., "Effect of Phosphatidylcholine on Explicit Memory," *Clinical Neuropharmacology* 16, no. 6 (1993): pp. 540–549, https://doi.org/10.1097/00002826-199312000-00007.

53. Irina Treede et al., "Tnf-α-Induced Up-Regulation of Pro-Inflammatory Cytokines Is Reduced by Phosphatidylcholine in Intestinal Epithelial Cells," *BMC Gastroenterology* 9, no. 1 (2009): p. 53, https://doi.org/10.1186/1471-230x-9-53.

54. Parris Kidd, "Phosphatidylcholine, A Superior Protectant Against Liver Damage," *Alternative Medicine Review* 1, no. 4 (1996): pp. 258–274.

CHAPTER 20

1. Hafeez Ullah et al., "Effects of Sugar, Salt and Distilled Water on White Blood Cells and Platelet Cells," *Journal of Tumor* 4, no. 1 (2015): pp. 354–358, https://doi.org/10.17554/j.issn.1819-6187.2016.04.73.

2. Yinan Hua et al., "Molecular Mechanisms of Chromium in Alleviating Insulin Resistance," *Journal of Nutritional Biochemistry* 23, no. 4 (2012): pp. 313–319, https://doi.org/10.1016/j.jnutbio.2011.11.001.
3. Pranoti Mandrekar et al., "Alcohol Exposure Regulates Heat Shock Transcription Factor Binding and Heat Shock Proteins 70 and 90 in Monocytes and Macrophages: Implication for Tnf-α Regulation," *Journal of Leukocyte Biology* 84, no. 5 (2008): pp. 1335–1345, https://doi.org/10.1189/jlb.0407256.
4. Karin De Punder and Leo Pruimboom, "The Dietary Intake of Wheat and Other Cereal Grains and Their Role in Inflammation," *Nutrients* 5, no. 3 (2013): pp. 771–787, https://doi.org/10.3390/nu5030771.
5. Julia Baudry et al., "Association of Frequency of Organic Food Consumption with Cancer Risk: Findings From the NutriNet-Santé Prospective Cohort Study," *JAMA Internal Medicine* 178, no. 12 (2018): p. 1597, https://doi.org/10.1001/jamainternmed.2018.4357.
6. Keith E. Latham, Carmen Sapienza, and Nora Engel, "The Epigenetic Lorax: Gene–Environment Interactions in Human Health," *Epigenomics* 4, no. 4 (2012): pp. 383–402, https://doi.org/10.2217/epi.12.31.
7. Paul Lips, "Relative Value of 25(OH)D and 1,25(OH)2D Measurements," *Journal of Bone and Mineral Research* 22, no. 11 (2007): pp. 1668–1671, https://doi.org/10.1359/jbmr.070716.
8. Sylvia Christakos et al., "Vitamin D: Beyond Bone," *Annals of the New York Academy of Sciences* 1287, no. 1 (2013): pp. 45–58, https://doi.org/10.1111/nyas.12129.
9. Cynthia Aranow, "Vitamin D and the Immune System," *Journal of Investigative Medicine* 59, no. 6 (2011): pp. 881–886, https://doi.org/10.231/JIM.0b013e31821b8755.

CHAPTER 21

1. Karine Louati and Francis Berenbaum, "Fatigue in Chronic Inflammation: A Link to Pain Pathways," *Arthritis Research & Therapy* 17, no. 1 (2015): p. 254, https://doi.org/10.1186/s13075-015-0784-1.
2. Garth L. Nicolson et al., "Mitochondrial Dysfunction and Chronic Disease: Treatment with Membrane Lipid Replacement and Other Natural Supplements," *Integrative Medicine: A Clinician's Journal* 13, no. 4 (2014): pp. 35–43.
3. Michele Malaguarnera et al., "Acetyl-l-Carnitine Improves Cognitive Functions in Severe Hepatic Encephalopathy: A Randomized and Controlled Clinical Trial," *Metabolic Brain Disease* 26, no. 4 (2011): pp. 281–289, https://doi.org/10.1007/s11011-011-9260-z.
4. Maryam Akbari et al., "The Effects of Alpha-Lipoic Acid Supplementation on Inflammatory Markers Among Patients with Metabolic Syndrome and Related Disorders: a Systematic Review and Meta-Analysis of Randomized Controlled Trials," *Nutrition & Metabolism* 15, no. 1 (2018): p. 39, https://doi.org/10.1186/s12986-018-0274-y.
5. Linda M Forsyth et al., "Therapeutic Effects of Oral Nadh on the Symptoms of Patients with Chronic Fatigue Syndrome," *Annals of Allergy, Asthma & Immunology* 82, no. 2 (1999): pp. 185–191, https://doi.org/10.1016/s1081-1206(10)62595-1.
6. Nicolson, "Mitochondrial Dysfunction and Chronic Disease: Treatment With Natural Supplements," 35–43.
7. S. Kalghatgi et al., "Bactericidal Antibiotics Induce Mitochondrial Dysfunction and Oxidative Damage in Mammalian Cells," *Science Translational Medicine* 5, no. 192 (March 2013), https://doi.org/10.1126/scitranslmed.3006055.
8. Bobak Robert Mozayeni et al., "Rheumatological Presentation of Bartonella Koehlerae and Bartonella Henselae Bacteremias: A Case Report," *Medicine (Baltimore)* 97, no. 17 (2018): p. e0465, https://doi.org/10.1097/md.0000000000010465.
9. "When Else to Suspect Ehlers-Danlos Syndrome," Oh TWIST, May 24, 2015, http://ohtwist.com/when-else-to-suspect-ehlers-danlos-syndrome.

10.   Tessa Watt et al., "Response to Valganciclovir in Chronic Fatigue Syndrome Patients with Human Herpesvirus 6 and Epstein-Barr Virus Igg Antibody Titers," *Journal of Medical Virology* 84, no. 12 (2012): pp. 1967–1974, https://doi.org/10.1002/jmv.23411.

CHAPTER 22

1.   Scott Forsgren and Dietrich Klinghardt, "Kryptopyrroluria (AKA Hemopyrrollactamuria): A Major Piece of the Puzzle in Overcoming Chronic Lyme Disease," *Townsend Letter*, July 2017.

2.   David T. Robles et al., "Morgellons Disease and Delusions of Parasitosis," *American Journal of Clinical Dermatology* 12, no. 1 (2011): pp. 1–6, https://doi.org/10.2165/11533150 -000000000-00000.

3.   Raphael Stricker and Marianne Middelveen, "Filament Formation Associated with Spirochetal Infection: A Comparative Approach to Morgellons Disease," *Clinical, Cosmetic and Investigational Dermatology* 4 (2011): pp. 167–177, https://doi.org/10.2147 /ccid.s26183.

4.   Virginia R Savely, Mary M Leitao, and Raphael B Stricker, "The Mystery of Morgellons Disease: Infection or Delusion?," *American Journal of Clinical Dermatology* 7, no. 1 (2006): pp. 1–5, https://doi.org/10.2165/00128071-200607010-00001.

5.   Virginia R. Savely and Raphael B. Stricker, "Morgellons Disease: Analysis of a Population with Clinically Confirmed Microscopic Subcutaneous Fibers of Unknown Etiology," *Clinical, Cosmetic and Investigational Dermatology* 3 (2010): pp. 67–78, https://doi.org /10.2147/ccid.s9520.

6.   Marianne J Middelveen et al., "Exploring the Association Between Morgellons Disease and Lyme Disease: Identification of *Borrelia Burgdorferi* in Morgellons Disease Patients," *BMC Dermatology* 15, no. 1 (2015): p. 1, https://doi.org/10.1186/s12895-015-0023-0.

7.   William T. Harvey, "Morgellons Disease," *Journal of the American Academy of Dermatology* 56, no. 4 (2007): pp. 705–706, https://doi.org/10.1016/j.jaad.2007.01.012.

8.   Peter Mayne et al., "Morgellons: A Novel Dermatological Perspective as the Multisystem Infective Disease Borreliosis," *F1000Research* 2 (2013): p. 118, https://doi.org/10.12688 /f1000research.2-118.v1.

9.   "What Are Electromagnetic Fields?," World Health Organization, August 4, 2016, https: //www.who.int/peh-emf/about/WhatisEMF/en/index1.html.

10.   "Electromagnetic Fields and Public Health the Present Evidence," World Health Organization, accessed May 28, 2019, https://www.who.int/peh-emf/publications/en /EMF_Risk_Chpt1.pdf.

11.   Elfidegizem Kivrak et al., "Effects of Electromagnetic Fields Exposure on the Antioxidant Defense System," *Journal of Microscopy and Ultrastructure* 5, no. 4 (2017): pp. 167–176, https://doi.org/10.1016/j.jmau.2017.07.003.

12.   National Research Council (US) Committee on Assessment of the Possible Health Effects of Ground Wave Emergency Network (GWEN), "Effects of Electromagnetic Fields on Organs and Tissues," Assessment of the Possible Health Effects of Ground Wave Emergency Network. (U.S. National Library of Medicine, January 1, 1993), https://www.ncbi.nlm.nih .gov/books/NBK208983.

13.   L Kheifets et al., "Pooled Analysis of Recent Studies of Magnetic Fields and Childhood Leukaemia," *British Journal of Cancer* 103, no. 7 (2010): pp. 1128–1135, https://doi.org /10.1038/sj.bjc.6605838.

14.   "Electromagnetic Fields and Cancer," National Cancer Institute, accessed October 23, 2018, https://www.cancer.gov/about-cancer/causes-prevention/risk/radiation/electro magnetic-fields-fact-sheet#q4.

15.   National Research Council (US) Committee on Assessment of the Possible Health Effects of Ground Wave Emergency Network (GWEN), "Effects of Electromagnetic Fields on Organs and Tissues," Assessment of the Possible Health Effects of Ground Wave Emergency

Network (U.S. National Library of Medicine, January 1, 1993), https://www.ncbi.nlm.nih .gov/books/NBK208983.

16. "Electromagnetic Fields and Cancer," National Cancer Institute, accessed October 23, 2018.

17. "Effects of Electromagnetic Fields on Organs and Tissues," January 1, 1993.

18. G. Abdel-Rassoul et al., "Neurobehavioral Effects Among Inhabitants Around Mobile Phone Base Stations," *Neurotoxicology* 28, no. 2 (2007): pp. 434–440, https://doi.org/10.1016/j .neuro.2006.07.012.

19. Michael J. Abramson et al., "Mobile Telephone Use Is Associated with Changes in Cognitive Function in Young Adolescents," *Bioelectromagnetics* 30, no. 8 (2009): pp. 678–686, https: //doi.org/10.1002/bem.20534.

20. S. E. Chia, H. P. Chia, and J. S. Tan, "Prevalence of Headache Among Handheld Cellular Telephone Users in Singapore: A Community Study.," *Environmental Health Perspectives* 108, no. 11 (2000): pp. 1059–1062, https://doi.org/10.1289/ehp.001081059.

21. N. Hakansson, "Occupational Exposure to Extremely Low Frequency Magnetic Fields and Mortality from Cardiovascular Disease," *American Journal of Epidemiology* 158, no. 6 (2003): pp. 534–542, https://doi.org/10.1093/aje/kwg197.

22. Myung Chan Gye and Chan Jin Park, "Effect of Electromagnetic Field Exposure on the Reproductive System," *Clinical and Experimental Reproductive Medicine* 39, no. 1 (2012): pp. 1–9, https://doi.org/10.5653/cerm.2012.39.1.1.

23. Antonio Sastre, Charles Graham, and Mary R Cook, "Brain Frequency Magnetic Fields Alter Cardiac Autonomic Control Mechanisms," *Clinical Neurophysiology* 111, no. 11 (2000): pp. 1942–1948, https://doi.org/10.1016/s1388-2457(00)00438-7.

24. Martin L. Pall, "Microwave Frequency Electromagnetic Fields (EMFs) Produce Widespread Neuropsychiatric Effects Including Depression," *Journal of Chemical Neuroanatomy* 75, no. Part B (2016): pp. 43–51, https://doi.org/10.1016/j.jchemneu .2015.08.001.

25. Bryan Black et al., "Anthropogenic Radio-Frequency Electromagnetic Fields Elicit Neuropathic Pain in an Amputation Model," *PLoS One* 11, no. 1 (2016), https://doi.org /10.1371/journal.pone.0144268.

CHAPTER 23

1. A. M. Elvis and J. S. Ekta, "Ozone Therapy: A Clinical Review," *Journal of Natural Science, Biology and Medicine* 2, no. 1 (2011): pp. 66–70, https://doi.org/10.4103/0976–9668.82319.

2. Sami Aydogan et al., "Impaired Erythrocytes Deformability in H2o2-Induced Oxidative Stress: Protective Effect of L-Carnosine," *Clinical Hemorheology and Microcirculation* 39, no. 1–4 (2008): pp. 93–98, https://doi.org/10.3233/ch-2008-1072.

3. Caroline Fife, "Explaining the Math for Hyperbaric Oxygen," February 6, 2018, https: //carolinefifemd.com/2018/02/06/explaining-the-math-for-hyperbaric-oxygen.

4. K. Saito et al., "Suppressive Effect of Hyperbaric Oxygenation on Immune Responses of Normal and Autoimmune Mice," *Clinical & Experimental Immunology* 86, no. 2 (1991): pp. 322–327, https://doi.org/10.1111/j.1365–2249.1991.tb05817.x.

5. Mitchell L. Hoggard and L. James Johnson, "An Overview of Lyme Disease and Hyperbaric Oxygen (HBO) Therapy," Richard A. Neubauer Research Institute, accessed November 25, 2018, https://www.ranri.org/Articles/overviewLyme.pdf.

6. Elvis, "Ozone Therapy: A Clinical Review," 66–70.

7. Elvis, "Ozone Therapy: A Clinical Review," 66–70.

8. Nathaniel Altman, *The New Oxygen Prescription: The Miracle of Oxidative Therapies* (Rochester, VT: Healing Arts Press, 2017).

9. Altman, *The New Oxygen Prescription: The Miracle of Oxidative Therapies*.

10. "Ozone: A Wide Spectrum Healer," Ozone Therapy Heals, accessed November 25, 2018, http://www.oxygenhealingtherapies.com/Ozone_Wide_Spectrum_Healer.html.

11. E. K. Knott, "Development of Ultraviolet Blood Irradiation," *American Journal of Surgery* 76, no. 2 (1948): pp. 165–171, https://doi.org/10.1016/0002-9610(48)90068-3.

12. Ximing Wu, Xiaoqing Hu, and Michael R. Hamblin, "Ultraviolet Blood Irradiation: Is It Time to Remember 'The Cure That Time Forgot'?," *Journal of Photochemistry and Photobiology B.* 157 (2016): pp. 89–96, https://doi.org/10.1016/j.jphotobiol.2016.02.007.

13. R. Rowan, "The Cure That Time Forgot," *International Journal of Biomedical Research* 14, no. 2 (1996): pp. 115–132.

14. Altman, *The New Oxygen Prescription: The Miracle of Oxidative Therapies.*

15. P. M. Lantos et al., "Unorthodox Alternative Therapies Marketed to Treat Lyme Disease," *Clinical Infectious Diseases* 60, no. 12 (2015): pp. 1776–1782, https://doi.org/10.1093/cid/civ186.

16. Barry Lynes, *The Cancer Cure That Worked!: Fifty Years of Suppression* (South Lake Tahoe, CA: BioMed Publishers, 2011).

17. Rob Harrill, "Magnetic Fields May Hold Key to Malaria Treatment," *UW News*, March 30, 2000, http://www.washington.edu/news/2000/03/30/magnetic-fields-may-hold-key-to-malaria-treatment-uw-researchers-find.

18. Rajiv Chopra et al., "Employing High-Frequency Alternating Magnetic Fields for the Non-Invasive Treatment of Prosthetic Joint Infections," *Scientific Reports* 7, no. 1 (2017): p. 7520, https://doi.org/10.1038/s41598-017-07321-6.

19. "FDA Seeks Permanent Injunctions Against Two Stem Cell Clinics," U.S. Food and Drug Administration, accessed November 12, 2018, https://www.fda.gov/newsevents/newsroom/pressannouncements/ucm607257.htm,

20. J. L. Clement and P. S. Jarrett, "Antibacterial Silver," *Metal-Based Drugs* 1, no 5 6 (1994): pp. 467–482, https://doi.org/10.1155/MBD.1994.467.

21. M. A. Radzig et al., "Antibacterial Effects of Silver Nanoparticles on Gram-Negative Bacteria: Influence on the Growth and Biofilms Formation, Mechanisms of Action," *Colloids and Surfaces B: Biointerfaces* 102 (2013): pp. 300–306, https://doi.org/10.1016/j.colsurfb.2012.07.039.

22. Jose Ruben Morones et al., "The Bactericidal Effect of Silver Nanoparticles," *Nanotechnology* 16, no. 10 (2005): pp. 2346–2353, https://doi.org/10.1088/0957-4484/16/10/059.

23. Niels Hadrup and Henrik R. Lam, "Oral Toxicity of Silver Ions, Silver Nanoparticles and Colloidal Silver—A Review," *Regulatory Toxicology and Pharmacology* 68, no. 1 (2014): pp. 1–7, https://doi.org/10.1016/j.yrtph.2013.11.002.

24. Filipa Sobral et al., "Chemical Characterization, Antioxidant, Anti-Inflammatory and Cytotoxic Properties of Bee Venom Collected in Northeast Portugal," *Food and Chemical Toxicology* 94 (2016): pp. 172–177, https://doi.org/10.1016/j.fct.2016.06.008.

25. Jae Dong Lee et al., "Anti-Inflammatory Effect of Bee Venom on Type II Collagen-Induced Arthritis," *American Journal of Chinese Medicine* 32, no. 3 (2004): pp. 361–367, https://doi.org/10.1142/s0192415x04002016.

26. T. Wesselius et al., "A Randomized Crossover Study of Bee Sting Therapy for Multiple Sclerosis," *Neurology* 65, no. 11 (2005): pp. 1764–1768, https://doi.org/10.1212/01.wnl.0000184442.02551.4b.

27. Kayla M. Socarras et al., "Antimicrobial Activity of Bee Venom and Melittin Against *Borrelia Burgdorferi*," *Antibiotics (Basel)* 6, no. 4 (2017): p. 31, https://doi.org/10.3390/antibiotics6040031)

28. W. A. Schrader, "Low Dose Allergen Immunotherapy (LDA): The Allergy Treatment of the Future—Here Now," *Townsend Newsletter*, April 2012.

29. Norman Brown and Jaak Panksepp, "Low-Dose Naltrexone for Disease Prevention and Quality of Life," *Medical Hypotheses* 72, no. 3 (2009): pp. 333–337, https://doi.org/10.1016/j.mehy.2008.06.048.

30. Jarred Younger, Luke Parkitny, and David McLain, "The Use of Low-Dose Naltrexone (LDN) as a Novel Anti-Inflammatory Treatment for Chronic Pain," *Clinical Rheumatology* 33, no. 4 (2014): pp. 451–459, https://doi.org/10.1007/s10067-014-2517-2.

31. Daniel Roberto Coradi Freitas, João Barberino Santos, and Cleudson Nery Castro, "Healing with Malaria: A Brief Historical Review Ff Malariotherapy for Neurosyphilis, Mental Disorders and Other Infectious Diseases," *Revista Da Sociedade Brasileira De Medicina Tropical* 47, no. 2 (2014): pp. 260–261, https://doi.org/10.1590/0037-8682-0209-2013.

32. "Hyperthermia:—A–Z on Lyme Disease," A-Zlyme, accessed November 24, 2018, https://a-zlyme.com/treatment/alternative-medicine.

33. "Hyperthermia: A–Z on Lyme Disease," A-Zlyme, accessed November 24, 2018

34. Michelle McKeon, "Hyperthermia Treatment," *Townsend Letter*, July 2017.

35. A. V. Suvernev, G. V. Ivanov, and A. V. Efremov, "Whole Body Hyperthermia at 43.5–44°C: Dreams or Reality?," *Landes BioScience*, 2013.

36. S. Hajdu et al., "Increased Temperature Enhances the Antimicrobial Effects of Daptomycin, Vancomycin, Tigecycline, Fosfomycin, and Cefamandole on Staphylococcal Biofilms," *Antimicrobial Agents and Chemotherapy* 54, no. 10 (2010): pp. 4078–4084, https://doi.org/10.1128/aac.00275-10.

37. Thomas A. Mace et al., "Differentiation of CD8 T Cells into Effector Cells Is Enhanced by Physiological Range Hyperthermia," *Journal of Leukocyte Biology* 90, no. 5 (2011): pp. 951–962, https://doi.org/10.1189/jlb.0511229.

38. Lee AC, Harris JL, Khanna KK, Hong JH. A Comprehensive Review on Current Advances in Peptide Drug Development and Design. *Int J Mol Sci.* 2019;20(10):2383. doi:10.3390/ijms20102383

39. Natural Health Well, accessed November 24, 2018, http://www.natural-health-well.com/ondamed-treatment.

40. "Frequently Asked Questions," EEG Education and Research, accessed November 24, 2018, http://www.eegspectrum.com/faq.

41. Xiaopeng Deng et al., "Randomized Controlled Trial of Adjunctive EEG-Biofeedback Treatment of Obsessive-Compulsive Disorder," *Shanghai Archives of Psychiatry* 26, no. 5 (2014): pp. 272–279, https://doi.org/10.11919/j.issn.1002-0829.214067.

42. "Treating POTS Using Biofeedback, Heart Rate Training, Exercise, Diet," POTS Treatment Center, accessed March 17, 2019, http://www.potstreatmentcenter.com/services/

CHAPTER 24

1.   S. D. Wright and S. W. Nielsen, "Experimental Infection of the White-Footed Mouse with *Borrelia Burgdorferi*," *American Journal of Veterinary Research* 51, no. 12 (1990): pp. 1980–1987.

2.   Elizabeth C. Burgess et al., "Experimental Inoculation of *Peromyscus Spp.* with *Borrelia Burgdorferi*: Evidence of Contact Transmission," *American Journal of Tropical Medicine and Hygiene* 35, no. 2 (January 1986): pp. 355–359, https://doi.org/10.4269/ajtmh.1986.35.355.

3.   Kathleen D. Moody and Stephen W. Barthold, "Relative Infectivity of *Borrelia Burgdorferi* in Lewis Rats by Various Routes of Inoculation," *American Journal of Tropical Medicine and Hygiene* 44, no. 2 (1991): pp. 135–139, https://doi.org/10.4269/ajtmh.1991.44.135.

4.   W. T. Harvey and P. Salvato, "'Lyme Disease': Ancient Engine of an Unrecognized Borreliosis Pandemic?," *Medical Hypotheses* 60, no. 5 (2003): pp. 742–759, https://doi.org/10.1016/s0306-9877(03)00060-4.

5.   Marianne J. Middelveen et al., "Culture and Identification of Borrelia Spirochetes in Human Vaginal and Seminal Secretions," *F1000Research* 3 (2015): p. 309, https://doi.org/10.12688/f1000research.5778.1.

6. Jad A Dandashi and Damir Nizamutdinov, "Texas Occurrence of Lyme Disease and Its Neurological Manifestations," *Journal of Neuroinfectious Diseases* 7, no. 2 (2016): p. 217, https://doi.org/10.4172/2314-7326.1000217.

7. T. Gardner, "Lyme Disease," in *Infectious Diseases of the Fetus and Newborn Infant*, ed. J. S. Remington and J. O. Klein (Philadelphia, PA, 2001), pp. 519–642.

8. Peter J. Krause and Edouard Vannier, "Transplacental Transmission of Human Babesiosis," *Infectious Diseases in Clinical Practice* 20, no. 6 (2012): pp. 365–367, https://doi.org/10.1097/ipc.0b013e3182769089.

9. E. B. Breitschwerdt et al., "Molecular Evidence of Perinatal Transmission of Bartonella *Vinsonii Subsp. Berkhoffii* and *Bartonella Henselae* to a Child," *Journal of Clinical Microbiology* 48, no. 6 (2010): pp. 2289–2293, https://doi.org/10.1128/jcm.00326-10.

10. A. Dhand et al., "Human Granulocytic Anaplasmosis During Pregnancy: Case Series and Literature Review," *Clinical Infectious Diseases* 45, no. 5 (January 2007): pp. 589–593, https://doi.org/10.1086/520659.

11. Joanna Regan et al., "A Confirmed *Ehrlichia Ewingii* Infection Likely Acquired Through Platelet Transfusion," *Clinical Infectious Diseases* 56, no. 12 (2013): pp. e105–e107, https://doi.org/10.1093/cid/cit177.

12. D. A. Steiner, E. W. Uhl, and M. B. Brown, "In Utero Transmission of Mycoplasma Pulmonis in Experimentally Infected Sprague-Dawley Rats.," *Infection and Immunity* 61, no. 7 (1993): pp. 2985–2990, https://doi.org/10.1128/iai.61.7.2985-2990.1993.

13. Gardner, "Lyme Disease," in *Infectious Diseases of the Fetus and Newborn Infant*, 519–642.

14. Robert C. Bransfield et al., "The Association Between Tick Borne Infections, Lyme Borreliosis and Autism Spectrum Disorders," *Medical Hypotheses* 70, no. 5 (2008): pp. 967–974, https://doi.org/10.1016/j.mehy.2007.09.006.

15. Raphael B Stricker and Lorraine Johnson, "Lyme Disease Vaccination: Safety First," *Lancet Infectious Diseases* 14, no. 1 (2014): p. 12, https://doi.org/10.1016/s1473-3099(13)70319-0.

16. Donald H. Marks, "Neurological Complications of Vaccination with Outer Surface Protein A (OspA)," *International Journal of Risk & Safety in Medicine* 23, no. 2 (2011): pp. 89–96, https://doi.org/10.3233/jrs-2011-0527.

17. Holcomb B. Noble, "Three Suits Say Lyme Vaccine Caused Severe Arthritis," *New York Times*, June 13, 2000, https://www.nytimes.com/2000/06/13/science/3-suits-say-lyme-vaccine-caused-severe-arthritis.html.

18. Stricker, "Lyme Disease Vaccination: Safety First," 12.

19. P. J. Molloy et al., "Detection of Multiple Reactive Protein Species by Immunoblotting after Recombinant Outer Surface Protein A Lyme Disease Vaccination," *Clinical Infectious Diseases* 31, no. 1 (2000): pp. 42–47, https://doi.org/10.1086/313920.

20. C Ewing et al., "Isolation of *Borrelia Burgdorferi* from Saliva of the Tick Vector, Ixodes Scapularis," *Journal of Clinical Microbiology* 32, no. 3 (1994): pp. 755–758, https://doi.org/10.1128/jcm.32.3.755-758.1994

21. Nikolai Petrovsky, "Comparative Safety of Vaccine Adjuvants: A Summary of Current Evidence and Future Needs," *Drug Safety* 38, no. 11 (2015): pp. 1059–1074, https://doi.org/10.1007/s40264-015-0350-4.

22. R. C. Johnson et al., "Comparative in Vitro and in Vivo Susceptibilities of the Lyme Disease Spirochete *Borrelia Burgdorferi* to Cefuroxime and Other Antimicrobial Agents," *Antimicrobial Agents and Chemotherapy* 34, no. 11 (1990): pp. 2133–2136, https://doi.org/10.1128/aac.34.11.2133.

23. D. Terekhova et al., "Erythromycin Resistance in *Borrelia Burgdorferi*," *Antimicrobial Agents and Chemotherapy* 46, no. 11 (2002): pp. 3637–3640, https://doi.org/10.1128/aac.46.11.3637-3640.2002.

24. Natacha Sertour et al., "Infection Kinetics and Tropism of Borrelia Burgdorferi Sensu Lato in Mouse After Natural (via Ticks) or Artificial (Needle) Infection Depends on the Bacterial Strain," *Frontiers in Microbiology* 9 (2018): p. 1722, https://doi.org/10.3389/fmicb.2018.01722.

25. Lars Eisen, "Pathogen Transmission in Relation to Duration of Attachment by Ixodes Scapularis Ticks," *Ticks and Tick-Borne Diseases* 9, no. 3 (2018): pp. 535–542, https://doi.org/10.1016/j.ttbdis.2018.01.002.

26. R. B. Nadleman, J. Nowakowski, and D. Fish, "Single-Dose Doxycycline for the Prevention of Lyme Disease After an Ixodes Scapularis Tick Bite," *New England Journal of Medicine* 345 (2001): pp. 79–84, https://doi.org/10.1056/nejm200111013451815.

27. P. A. S. Theophilus et al., "Effectiveness of Stevia Rebaudiana Whole Leaf Extract Against the Various Morphological Forms of Borrelia Burgdorferi in Vitro," *European Journal of Microbiology and Immunology* 5, no. 4 (2015): pp. 268–280, https://doi.org/10.1556/1886.2015.00031.

28. D. Terekhova et al., "Erythromycin Resistance in Borrelia Burgdorferi," *Antimicrobial Agents and Chemotherapy* 46, no. 11 (2002): pp. 3637–3640, https://doi.org/10.1128/aac.46.11.3637-3640.2002.

29. "Effects of Exercise on Immune Function," Gatorade Sports Science Institute, accessed June 22, 2019, https://www.gssiweb.org/sports-science-exchange/article/sse-151-effects-of-exercise-on-immune-function.

CHAPTER 25

1. Vincent J Felitti et al., "Relationship of Childhood Abuse and Household Dysfunction to Many of the Leading Causes of Death in Adults," *American Journal of Preventive Medicine* 14, no. 4 (1998): pp. 245–258, https://doi.org/10.1016/s0749-3797(98)00017-8.

2. Shanta R. Dube et al., "Cumulative Childhood Stress and Autoimmune Diseases in Adults," *Psychosomatic Medicine* 71, no. 2 (2009): pp. 243–250, https://doi.org/10.1097/psy.0b013e3181907888.

3. Huan Song et al., "Association of Stress-Related Disorders With Subsequent Autoimmune Disease," *JAMA* 319, no. 23 (2018): pp. 2388–2400, https://doi.org/10.1001/jama.2018.7028.

4. Jennifer C. Chan, Bridget M. Nugent, and Tracy L. Bale, "Parental Advisory: Maternal and Paternal Stress Can Impact Offspring Neurodevelopment," *Biological Psychiatry* 83, no. 10 (2018): pp. 886–894, https://doi.org/10.1016/j.biopsych.2017.10.005.

5. Rachel Yehuda and Amy Lehrner, "Intergenerational Transmission of Trauma Effects: Putative Role of Epigenetic Mechanisms," *World Psychiatry* 17, no. 3 (2018): pp. 243–257, https://doi.org/10.1002/wps.20568.

6. Alexander C. McFarlane, "The Long-Term Costs of Traumatic Stress: Intertwined Physical and Psychological Consequences," *World Psychiatry* 9, no. 1 (2010): pp. 3–10, https://doi.org/10.1002/j.2051-5545.2010.tb00254.x.

7. Lea Winerman, "By the Numbers: Antidepressant Use on the Rise," *Monitor on Psychology* (American Psychological Association, November 2017), https://www.apa.org/monitor/2017/11/numbers.

8. Sandra Lopez-Leon et al., "Psychotropic Medication in Children and Adolescents in the United States in the Year 2004 vs 2014," *DARU Journal of Pharmaceutical Sciences* 26, no. 1 (2018): p. 204, https://doi.org/10.1007/s40199-018-0204-6.

9. Winderman, "By the Numbers."

10. "Health, United States, 2017," Health, United States, 2017 (U.S. Department of Health and Human Services, 2017), https://www.cdc.gov/nchs/data/hus/hus17.pdf.

Index